AF840749

Holistic Approach to Assisted Reproductive Technology

Kenan Demir and Rümeysa Yılmaz Göç

Holistic Approach to Assisted Reproductive Technology

nova
science publishers
New York

Copyright © 2023 by Nova Science Publishers, Inc.

All rights reserved. No part of this book may be reproduced, stored in a retrieval system or transmitted in any form or by any means: electronic, electrostatic, magnetic, tape, mechanical photocopying, recording or otherwise without the written permission of the Publisher.

We have partnered with Copyright Clearance Center to make it easy for you to obtain permissions to reuse content from this publication. You can visit copyright.com and search by Title, ISBN, or ISSN.

For further questions about using the service on copyright.com, please contact:
Copyright Clearance Center
Phone: +1-(978) 750-8400 Fax: +1-(978) 750-4470 E-mail: info@copyright.com

NOTICE TO THE READER

The Publisher has taken reasonable care in the preparation of this book, but makes no expressed or implied warranty of any kind and assumes no responsibility for any errors or omissions. No liability is assumed for incidental or consequential damages in connection with or arising out of information contained in this book. The Publisher shall not be liable for any special, consequential, or exemplary damages resulting, in whole or in part, from the readers' use of, or reliance upon, this material. Any parts of this book based on government reports are so indicated and copyright is claimed for those parts to the extent applicable to compilations of such works.

Independent verification should be sought for any data, advice, or recommendations contained in this book. In addition, no responsibility is assumed by the Publisher for any injury and/or damage to persons or property arising from any methods, products, instructions, ideas or otherwise contained in this publication.

This publication is designed to provide accurate and authoritative information with regards to the subject matter covered herein. It is sold with the clear understanding that the Publisher is not engaged in rendering legal or any other professional services. If legal or any other expert assistance is required, the services of a competent person should be sought. FROM A DECLARATION OF PARTICIPANTS JOINTLY ADOPTED BY A COMMITTEE OF THE AMERICAN BAR ASSOCIATION AND A COMMITTEE OF PUBLISHERS.

Library of Congress Cataloging-in-Publication Data

Print ISBN: 979-8-89113-017-3
PDF ISBN: 979-8-89113-064-7
ePUB ISBN: 979-8-89113-158-3

Published by Nova Science Publishers, Inc. † New York

We hope that book will serve as a valuable resource for researchers, practitioners, and patients, providing a comprehensive understanding of the science, techniques, and emotional aspects of in vitro fertilization. May this book contribute to the advancement of reproductive medicine and bring joy and hope to countless individuals and families.

I present this book as a souvenir to my dear brother Mehmet Yılmaz, who left an indelible void in our lives with his untimely departure.

Rümeysa Yılmaz Göç

Contents

Preface

It is with great pleasure and gratitude that we present this book, "Holistic Approach to Assisted Reproductive Technology", to our esteemed colleagues in the fields of Histology and Embryology, as well as Obstetrics and Gynecology. This collaborative effort represents our collective dedication to advancing the knowledge and understanding of in vitro fertilization (IVF).

Furthermore, we would like to express our heartfelt appreciation to our families for their unwavering support and understanding during the arduous process of researching and writing this book. Their love, patience, and encouragement have been our driving force, reminding us of the importance of our work and motivating us to go beyond our limits.

Editors

Chapter 1

The Anatomy and Physiology of Reproduction

Deniz Kalemci[1], MD*, and Ayşe Nur Damar[2], MD
[1,2]Department of Medicine, Pamukkale Universty, Denizli, Turkiye

Abstract

Organs and glands of the reproductive system are necessary for the creation of new life (Lyons, 2021). The components of the female reproductive system are the uterus, fallopian tubes, ovary, vagina, and vulva (Standring, 2020). The components of the male reproductive system are the testes, scrotum, epididymis, ejaculatory duct, penis, and accessory sex glands (Standring, 2020). Ovarian and testicular cells are gonads with endocrine gland characteristics that support the development and maturation of the reproductive system. Furthermore, the ovaries are responsible for the synthesis and secretion of the sex steroid hormones estrogen and progesterone, and the testes are responsible for the synthesis and secretion of testosterone (Costanzo, 2022). In this chapter, the objective is to explain the anatomy and functions of the male and female reproductive systems.

Key Words: Reproductive system, Ovaries, Testes, Estrogen, Testosterone

Introduction

The male reproductive system includes internal structures: testes, epididymis, vas deferens, funiculus spermaticus, in addition to accessory glands such as the prostate, glandula seminalis and glandula bulbourethralis,

---

* Corresponding Author's E-mail: kalemcideniz@gmail.com

In: Holistic Approach to Assisted Reproductive Technology
Editor: Kenan Demir and Rümeysa Yılmaz Göç
ISBN: 979-8-89113-017-3
© 2023 Nova Science Publishers, Inc.

and external structures: scrotum, penis and urethra masculina (Jens Waschke, 2016).The main roles of the testes, the male gonads, are spermatogenesis and steroidogenesis, thus responsible for reproductive function as well as normal physical and sexual development and behavior. The secretions of the prostate and seminal glands form the main part of the seminal fluid, which contains nutrients, growth factors, and enzymes necessary for the function of sperm. The external genitalia optimize the environment of the testes and allow the seminal fluid to pass through the female reproductive system (Standring, 2020).

The components of the female reproductive system are the uterus, fallopian tubes, ovary, vagina, and vulva. The external genital system is called Vulva and consists of mons pubis, labium major, labium minor, clitoris, vaginal vestibule, and bartholin glands (Standring, 2020). As a result of the lack of fusion of the urogenital folds, the female genital organs do not have an external urethra, unlike men (Puppo, 2011). Fertilization occurs in the fallopian tubes after oogenesis, which is essential for the female reproductive system and takes place in the ovaries (Lyons, 2021; Standring, 2020). One of the functions of the uterus is to preserve the fertilized egg until birth (Lyons, 2021). Males and females have similar reproductive hormones. All hormones must interact and work together to provide the monthly cycle of women, release the egg, and prepare the uterus for implantation (Hall & Hall, 2016).

Male Reproductive System

The Testes and Scrotum

The testes, a pair of oval-shaped reproductive organs, are suspended in the scrotum by spermatic cords, and the left testicle is located lower than the right testicle (Moore et al., 2018). At approximately 26 weeks of gestation, the testes descend from the abdominal cavity into the scrotum through the inguinal canal as a result of testosterone-induced shortening of the gubernaculum (a fetal connective tissue that connects the caudal part of the epididymis, testis, and lower part of the scrotum) (Ross & Pawlina, 2011). As it descends, it is accompanied by blood vessels, autonomic nerves, lymphatic vessels, and layers of fascia and muscle derived from the layers of the abdominal wall through which it passes (external spermatic, cremasteric, and internal spermatic fascia) (Lyons, 2021; Ross & Pawlina, 2011) .

Each testes is surrounded from the inside out by a three-layered tough capsule consisting of a vascular layer, tunica albuginea, and tunica vaginalis derived from the peritoneum. On the posterior surface of the testis, which is the attachment site of the epididymis, the tunica albuginea protrudes inward to form the mediastinum of the testis, and the tunica vaginalis protrudes outward to cover the epididymis. The septations arising from the mediastinum divide the testes into lobules containing 1-4 convoluted seminiferous tubules and interstitial tissue (Standring, 2020). In the mediastinum, the tubules straighten and anastomose to form the rete testis and drain into the caput epididymis through efferent ducts (Smith & Turek, 2017).

The testicular arteries originate from the anterolateral part of the abdominal aorta and inferior to the renal arteries and follow an oblique course in the retroperitoneal region, crossing the ureters and external iliac arteries, into the deep inguinal rings and from there to the superficial inguinal rings and enter the spermatic cords. The testicular and epididymis veins form the pampiniform venous plexus, which surrounds the testicular artery (Moore et al., 2018). The testes, their position in the scrotum, the cremaster reflex, and the current heat exchange mechanism of the pampiniform plexus keep the testes 3-4 degrees below body temperature (Standring, 2020). The

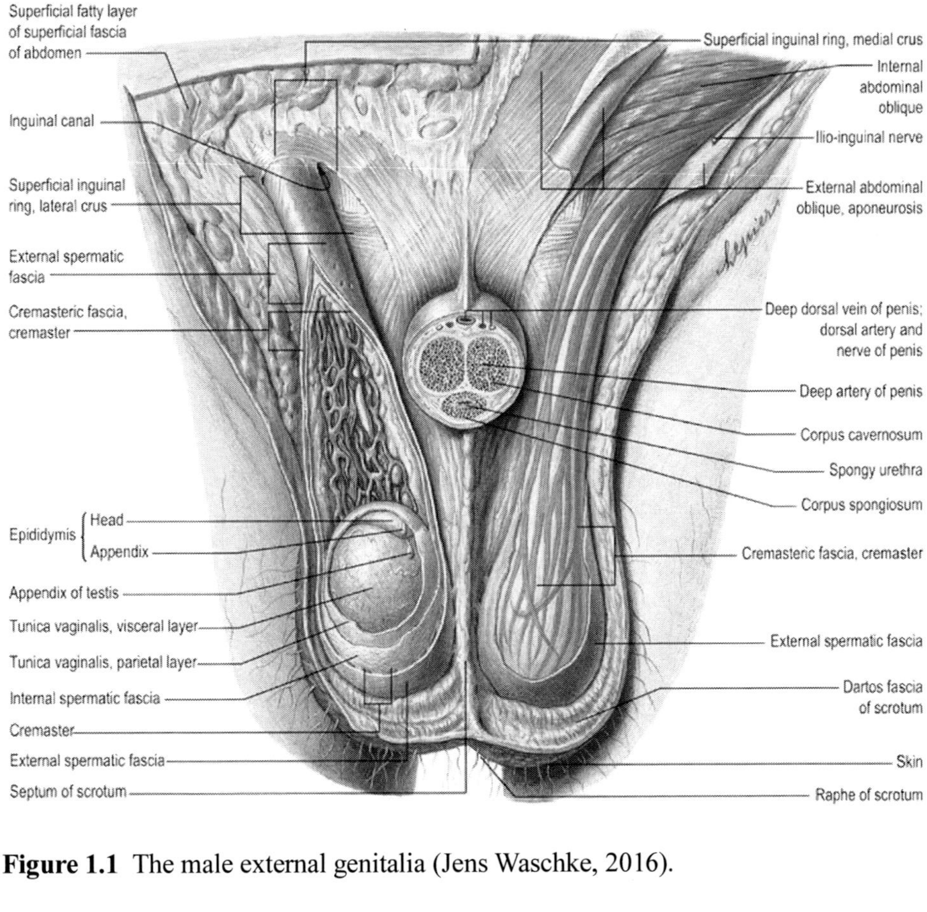

Figure 1.1 The male external genitalia (Jens Waschke, 2016).

plexus veins merge superiorly and enter the vena cava inferior on the right side and the renal vein on the left (Moore et al., 2018).

Epididymis

The epididymis, located posterior to the testis, is separated from the testis by the epididymal sinus (a deep groove located laterally) (Standring, 2020). Sperm undergo a number of changes here and gradually become more functional and mobile as they pass through (Smith & Turek, 2017). Anatomically, it is divided into three parts: The head, where the 8-12 ductus efferents empty, the body, and the tail, which is continued by the tortuous part of the ductus deferens (Standring, 2020).

Ductus Deferens- Ejaculatory Duct

The ductus deferens, a thick, muscular tubular structure derived from the mesonephric duct, carries sperm from the epididymis to the urethra and also has absorbent and secretory functions. It passes through the spermatic cord and enters the inguinal canal (Standring, 2020). When it reaches the posterior part of the bladder, it becomes curved and dilated and here it merges with the seminal vesicle duct and forms the ejaculatory duct (Lyons, 2021).

The double ejaculatory ducts pass through the prostate gland and merge with the prostatic urethra (Lyons, 2021). Unlike the ductus deferens, it has a thin wall structure (Standring, 2020).

Penis

The penis consists of erectile tissues called the double corpora cavernosa and corpus cavernosum, the penile urethra in the corpus spongiosum and vessels, the fascia and nerves associated with these structures (Standring, 2020). The corpus spongiosum expands in the proximal part and becomes the penile bulbus, which is attached to the perineal membrane. The corpora cavernosa separate from each other proximally to form the crura and attach to the ischiopubic ramus. The two crura and bulbus form the root of the penis, while the remaining unfixed part is called the trunk (Lyons, 2021).

At the distal end of the penis, the corpus spongiosum expands and forms the glans penis. The double layer membrane attached to the ventral surface of the glans and surrounding it in various ways is called the prepuceum. The superficial penile fascia is a loose connective tissue without fat, whereas the deep fascia is a dense and tight fascial sheath, and distally it merges with the tunica albuginea, which envelopes all three corporal bodies (Standring, 2020).

Seminal Glands

Seminal vesicles are a pair of spiral tubes with irregular diverticula, partly covered by the peritoneum, in a fibromuscular sheath at the base of the prostate, between the urinary bladder and the rectum (Standring, 2020). Seminal vesicles produce the main components of the seminal fluid, including fructose, which is a source of energy (Lyons, 2021). In most men, the right seminal vesicle is larger than the left and both glands shrink with age (Standring, 2020).

Prostate

The prostate is a round fibromuscular gland located in the lower part of the bladder and surrounding the prostatic urethra (Lyons, 2021; Standring, 2020). Synthesizes alkaline secretions that protect sperm from the acidic environment in the female reproductive system and opens to the prostatic urethra (Lyons, 2021). Secretions of glands constitute 90% of the volume of semen, while the remaining volume is composed of sperm (Costanzo, 2022).

Bulbo-Urethral Glands (Cowper's Glands)

The bulbourethral gland is a small, round, yellow, lobed, bilateral gland located within the muscles of the perineum (Standring, 2020). It produces a mucus-rich secretion that lubricates the urethra and neutralizes residual urine, and opens proximal to the pars spongiaosa of the urethra (Lyons, 2021).

Male Reproduction Physiology

Most control of sexual functions begins when gonadotropin-releasing hormone (GnRH) passes to the anterior pituitary gland through the hypothalamic-pituitary portal vascular system by neurons in the arcuate nucleus of the hypothalamus and stimulates the release of gonadotropic hormones, luteinizing hormone (LH) and follicle stimulating hormone (FSH). GnRH is a peptide secreted every 1-3 hours at intervals of a few minutes, and the intensity of the hormone's stimulation depends on the amount of GnRH released together with the frequency of the secretion cycles. LH secretion, like GnRH, is cyclical and depends on the pulsatile release of GnRH. Unlike LH, FSH secretion is more influenced by long-term changes in GnRH than by the pulsatile release of GnRH. Therefore, GnRH is also known as LH releasing hormone.

Testosterone is secreted by Leydig cells only when stimulated by LH, and the proportion of testosterone secreted is almost directly proportional to the amount of LH. Leydig cells are present for a few weeks after birth, but then absent until approximately 10 years of age. However, injection of purified LH into a child of any age or secretion of LH during puberty converts testicular interstitial cells to Leydig cells (Hall & Hall, 2020).

FSH binds to Sertoli cell FSH receptors in seminiferous tubules and stimulates Sertoli cell growth and secretion of spermatogenic substances. Both FSH and testosterone are necessary for spermatogenesis. FSH increases when sperm cannot be produced, while FSH secretion decreases when spermatogenesis proceeds very rapidly. The reason for this negative feedback mechanism is believed to be the inhibin produced by Sertoli cells, which has a direct suppressive effect on the anterior pituitary gland.

During pregnancy, the hormone human chorionic gonadotropin (hCG) is secreted by the placenta and has similar effects on the sexual organs as LH. hCG causes testosterone secretion to begin at 7 weeks intrauterine from the testes if the fetus is male. Testosterone promotes the formation of the internal male genital tract and suppresses the formation of the female genital tract (Hall & Hall, 2020).

Some tissues are affected by testosterone and other tissues by dihydrotestosterone, which is formed by activating testosterone with the enzyme 5α-reductase. Testosterone is responsible for increased muscle mass, growth spurt, enlargement of the penis and seminal vesicles, deepening of the voice, spermatogenesis, and libido during puberty. Dihydrotestosterone is responsible for external genitalia differentiation, hair distribution, sebaceous gland activity, and prostate enlargement (Costanzo, 2022).

Female Reproductive System

Vestibule

This area is between the urethra, vagina, Bartholin glands, and labium minor where the small vestibular glands open and has an erectile characteristic (Lyons, 2021; Standring, 2020).

Mons Pubis

This is the area of adipose tissue and hairy skin in pubic symphysis. Hairs here are formed after puberty (Standring, 2020).

Labium Major

This structure is the skin folds containing hairy, pigmented fat follicles that extend bilaterally between the mons pubis-perineum and form the lateral borders of the vulva. Labium majors converge under the mons pubis and form the anterior commissure, but do not converge posteriorly. In the posterior, they merge with the adjacent skin and end close to the parallel form. The posterior commissure forms the skin between the labium majors and draws the posterior border to the vulva (Standring, 2020).

Labium Minor

Labium minors are 3-4 cm long, fat-free, and hairless skin folds containing erectile tissue that is located inside the labium majors and surrounding the vaginal orifice (Puppo, 2011; Standring, 2020). Occasionally, an extra labial fold (labium tertium) may be found on one or both sides between the labia minor and major (Standring, 2020).

Clitoris

It is homologous to the male glans penis and corpora cavernosa and is innervated by the pudendal nerve (Eickmeyer, 2017; Puppo, 2013). This is an erectile structure consisting of crus, root, cylindrical body, and glans structures (Lyons, 2021; Standring, 2020).

Bartholin Glands

The bartholin glands are large vestibular glands composed of tubuloacinar tissue and homologous to male bulbourethral glands (Lyons, 2021; Standring, 2020). The bartholin glands, which contain cells that produce serotonin, bombesin, calcitonin, and α-hCG, surround the vaginal opening (Puppo, 2011; Standring, 2020). It secretes mucus through the bulbospongiosus muscle to lubricate the vestibule and vagina during sexual arousal (Eickmeyer, 2017; Lyons, 2021).

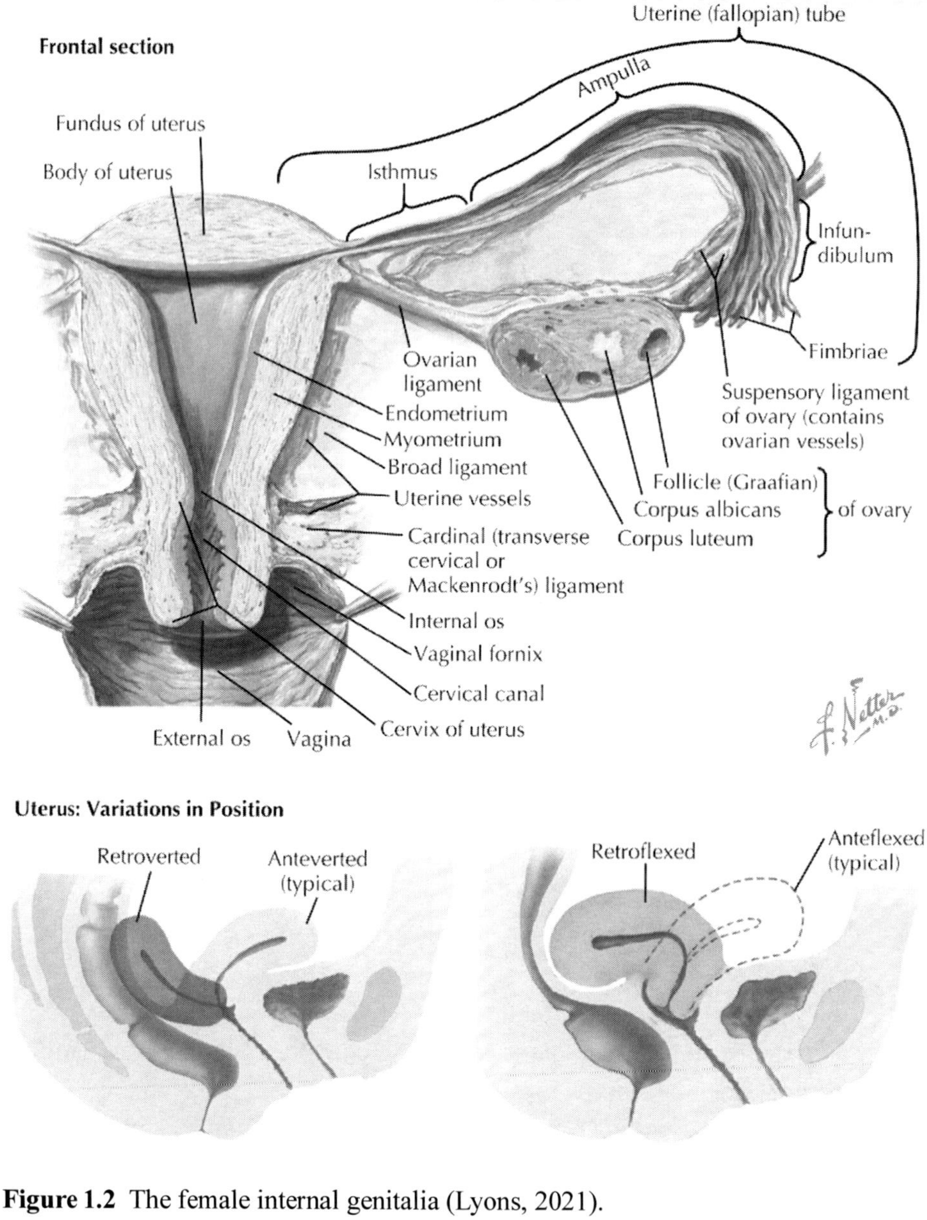

Figure 1.2 The female internal genitalia (Lyons, 2021).

Vagina

The vagina is a distensible fibromuscular tube without glands that surrounds the cervix with its parts called the fornix and opens into the vestibule of the vulva (Lyons, 2021; Puppo, 2011). The anterior wall (approx. 7,5 cm) is shorter than the posterior wall (approx. 9 cm) because the vaginal mucosa attaches to a higher point in the posterior wall. The vagina supports the fundus and urethra of the urinary bladder anteriorly and the rectum posteriorly (Standring,

2020). The proximal vagina is supported laterally by the levator ani muscle together with the cardinal and uterosacral ligaments, while the distal vagina is surrounded by the bulbospongiosus, which plays a role in the inferior vaginusmus. The pubovaginal muscle responsible for superior vaginusmus hangs around the vagina (Puppo & Puppo, 2015; Standring, 2020). Below the external urethral orifice, there is a thin mucosal fold just inside the vaginal orifice that opens into the vestibule and is called the hymen (Standring, 2020).

Uterus

The uterus is a muscular and luminous organ located in the pelvis between the posterior of the bladder and the anterior of the rectum (Lyons, 2021; Standring, 2020). The uterus is anatomically divided into corpus (upper 2/3) and cervix (lower 1/3) (Ross & Pawlina, 2011; Standring, 2020). The part above the corpus where the fallopian tubes enter is called the fundus, and the part that connects the corpus to the cervix is called the isthmus (approximately 1 cm) (Lyons, 2021; Standring, 2020).

The cervix is approximately 2.5 cm long (Standring, 2020). The proximal of the lumen of the cervix opens to the uterus with the internal os, and the distal of the lumen of the cervix opens to the vagina by the external os (Eroschenko, 2017; Lyons, 2021). The cervix is usually tilted forward (anteversion) relative to the vagina. The body of the uterus is bent toward the cervix, so it is in a slightly anteflexed position (Lyons, 2021). In a minority of women, they may be in retroflexion and retroversion positions (Standring, 2020). The cervix undergoes changes such as dilation caused by uterine contractions during pregnancy (Ludmir & Sehdev, 2000). The cervix expands due to the elastin in its stroma, allowing the baby to pass at birth (Lyons, 2021; Standring, 2020).

The uterus consists of three layers called endometrium, myometrium, and perimetrium from the inside out (Eroschenko, 2017).

The endometrium has 2 layers, these are the functional stratum, which is close to the lumen, which is shed during menstruation, which contains the bodies of the uterine glands and blood vessels, and the basalis stratum, which regenerates the functional layer (Eroschenko, 2017; Ross & Pawlina, 2011).

The uterine arteries form arcuate arteries, and the arcuate arteries form straight and spiral arteries that supply the endometrium. Straight arteries supply the stratum basalis layer, while spiral arteries supply the stratum functionalis layer. Since spiral arteries are long, curved, and more sensitive to hormonal changes than straight arteries, they cause shedding of the stratum functionalis during menstruation. The myometrium consists of interstitial connective tissue, blood vessels, and a thick layer of smooth muscle. The perimetrium is covered with serosa (Eroschenko, 2017).

The uterus is supplied by the uterine artery, which is a branch of the internal iliac artery. One branch of the uterine artery, which has many branches, anastomoses with the branches of the ovarian artery and another branch anastomoses with the branches of the vaginal artery to form the vaginal azygos arteries. The uterine veins drain into the internal iliac veins. It anastomoses with vaginal and ovarian venous plexuses as in the arteries (Standring, 2020).

Fallopian Tubes

They are a pair of tubes approximately 12 cm long, consisting of 4 successive parts from the ovary to the uterus, respectively, infindibulum, ampulla, isthmus, and intramural (Eroschenko, 2017). The intramural part is within the uterine wall (Standring, 2020). The ampulla forms the widest part of the tube and is also where fertilization takes place (Lyons, 2021; Standring, 2020). Finger-shaped extensions of the infundibulum, covered with ciliated epithelium, that capture the oocyte that is thrown into the peritoneal cavity and direct it to the fallopian tubes are called fimbriae (Eroschenko, 2017; Lyons, 2021; Standring, 2020).

Ovaries

The ovaries are where oogenesis takes place (Lyons, 2021). Ovaries are connected to the uterus by the ovarian ligament and are suspended by the peritoneal fold called the mesoovarium (Lyons, 2021; Standring, 2020). Although their size increases gradually with body growth, they decrease greatly after menopause (Standring, 2020). The ovaries, surrounded by the germinal epithelium and the underlying tunica albuginea, have a cortex and medulla (Eroschenko, 2017; Standring, 2020). The ovaries, which are surrounded by the germinal epithelium and the tunica albuginea below it, have a cortex and medulla (Eroschenko, 2017; Standring, 2020). While there are follicles in the cortex, there are plenty of vessels and nerves in the medulla (Eroschenko, 2017; Standring, 2020). Unlike other structures in the pelvic cavity (which are fed by branches of the internal iliac artery), the ovaries are fed by the branch of the ovarian artery of the abdominal aorta (Lyons, 2021; Standring, 2020). The ovarian artery is within the ovarian suspension ligament (Lyons, 2021). The ovarian veins drain into the inferior vena cava on the right and the renal vein on the left (Standring, 2020).

Female Reproduction Physiology

The beginning of adult sexual life in which estrogen increases rapidly in women is called puberty, the first menstruation is called menarche, while the end of sexual cycles is called menopause. Gonadotropin-releasing hormone (GnRH), which is secreted from the hypothalamus and inhibited by estrogen progesterone, triggers the anterior pituitary gland for the secretions of luteinizing hormone (LH), which provides the development of the corpus luteum, and follicle stimulating hormone (FSH), which ensures the development of follicles in the ovary.

At the beginning of the average 28-day monthly cycle of women, since there are no mature follicles and corpus luteum, GnRH secretion cannot be inhibited due to the low amount of estrogen and progesterone released from them, and FSH-LH is released and starts follicle development. Thanks to the positive feedback in only the dominant follicle, a single follicle matures while the others undergo atresia (Hall & Hall, 2016). Estrogen secreted from the mature follicle has been recognized as the main neural trigger for the preovulatory surge of ovulation-promoting gonadotropins (Mahesh & Brann, 1998; Mahesh & Muldoon, 1987). Ovulation occurs on the 14th day due to the LH surge, and the high amount of LH enables the formation of lutein cells and corpus luteum from granulosa and theca cells. As the levels of estrogen and progesterone secreted by the corpus luteum increase, both GnRH and direct FSH-LH release are inhibited, their amounts decrease, and the corpus luteum degenerates. Therefore, menstrual bleeding begins (Hall & Hall, 2016).

Estrogen, progesterone, inhibin (mainly inhibits FSH, to a lesser extent LH), and androgens are produced in the ovaries. Estrogen stimulates bone development, stromal-ductal development of female genitalia and breasts, and slightly accelerates metabolism. Progesterone prepares the endometrium for implantation and stimulates the lobular-alveolar development of the breasts (Hall & Hall, 2016).

During pregnancy, many changes such as lengthening of abdominal muscles, increased pelvic width, and increased lumbar lordosis ensure adaptation to the fetus and prepare the woman for childbirth (Eickmeyer, 2017).

Conclusion

To understand clinical andrology, gynecology, and the underlying causes of female and male infertility, it is necessary to know the anatomy and basic physiology of the reproductive system (Jequier, 2011).

References

Costanzo, L. S. (2022). *Costanzo Physiology E-Book*. Elsevier - OHCE.

Eickmeyer, S. M. (2017). Anatomy and Physiology of the Pelvic Floor. *Phys Med Rehabil Clin N Am*, *28*(3), 455-460. https://doi.org/10.1016/j.pmr.2017.03.003

Eroschenko, V. P. (2017). Female Reproductive System. In W. Kluwer, C. Taylor, & A. Vosburgh (Eds.), *Atlas Of Histology With Functional Correlations* (Thirteenth Edition ed., pp. 520-569). Wolters Kluwer.

Hall, J. E., & Hall, M. E. (2020). *Guyton and Hall Textbook of Medical Physiology E-Book* (14 ed.). Elsevier - OHCE.

Hall, J. E., & Hall, M. E. (2016). Female Physiology Before Pregnancy and Female Hormones. In *Pocket Companion to Guyton and Hall Textbook of Medical Physiology* (Fourteenth ed., pp. 606-613). Elsevier-Elyse O'Grady.

Jens Waschke, T. M. B. (2016). *Sobotta, Anatomie Das Lehrbuch*. Elsevier Limited (Turkey).

Jequier, A. M. (2011). Anatomy and physiology of the male reproductive tract. In *Male Infertility: A Clinical Guide* (2 ed., pp. 7-28). Cambridge University Press. https://doi.org/10.1017/CBO9780511997402.003

Ludmir, J., & Sehdev, H. M. (2000). Anatomy and physiology of the uterine cervix. *Clin Obstet Gynecol*, *43*(3), 433-439. https://doi.org/10.1097/00003081-200009000-00003

Lyons, V. T. (2021). *Netter's Essential Systems-Based Anatomy*. Elsevier-OHCE.

Mahesh, V. B., & Brann, D. W. (1998). Regulation of the preovulatory gonadotropin surge by endogenous steroids. *Steroids*, *63*(12), 616-629. https://doi.org/10.1016/s0039-128x(98)00075-0

Mahesh, V. B., & Muldoon, T. G. (1987). Integration of the effects of estradiol and progesterone in the modulation of gonadotropin secretion. *J Steroid Biochem*, *27*(4-6), 665-675. https://doi.org/10.1016/0022-4731(87)90135-x

Moore, K. L., Dalley, A. F., Agur A. (2018). *Clinically oriented anatomy* (8 ed.). Lippincott Williams and Wilkins.

Puppo, V. (2011). Embryology and anatomy of the vulva: the female orgasm and women's sexual health. *Eur J Obstet Gynecol Reprod Biol*, *154*(1), 3-8. https://doi.org/10.1016/j.ejogrb.2010.08.009

Puppo, V. (2013). Anatomy and physiology of the clitoris, vestibular bulbs, and labia minora with a review of the female orgasm and the prevention of female sexual dysfunction. *Clin Anat*, *26*(1), 134-152. https://doi.org/10.1002/ca.22177

Puppo, V., & Puppo, G. (2015). Anatomy of sex: Revision of the new anatomical terms used for the clitoris and the female orgasm by sexologists. *Clin Anat*, *28*(3), 293-304. https://doi.org/10.1002/ca.22471

Ross, M. H., & Pawlina, W. (2011). *Histology A Text And Atlas With Correlated Cell And Moleculer Biology*.

Smith, R. P., & Turek, P. (2017). *Netter Collection of Medical Illustrations: Reproductive System* (2nd ed.). Elsevier - OHCE.

Standring, S. (2020). *Gray's Anatomy E-Book* (42nd ed.). Elsevier Limited-OHCE.

Chapter 2

Oogenesis

Sena Özcan Yıldırım, MD*

IVF Centre of Elazig Fethi Sekin City Hospital, Elazig, Turkiye

Abstract

Oogenesis is the process of formation of the mature follicle that can ovulate from the primordial follicle and takes place in the ovarian cortex. It is also called folliculogenesis, as it describes the development of an ovarian follicle that contains an immature oocyte. Folliculogenesis begins before birth, becomes active at puberty, and ends with menopause. The follicle passes through stages called primordial, primary, secondary, and Graafian, until mature follicles are formed in the ovaries. Primordial follicles consist of the primary oocyte along with a single layer of flat follicle cells surrounding it and are separated from the ovarian stroma by a basement membrane. Primary follicles are formed when the follicle cells surrounding the primary oocyte are transformed into a cubical form. Depending on the number of layers of follicular cells, there are two types of primary follicles, unilaminar and multilaminar. When the antral space begins to appear between the granulosa cells of the secondary follicle, the follicle is called a secondary oocyte. Graafian follicles, also known as mature follicles, form at the end of follicular development; these are the follicles that enter ovulation.

Key Words: Oogenesis, Folliculogenesis, Ovarian embryonic development

* Corresponding Author's E-mail: senaozcan23@hotmail.com

In: Holistic Approach to Assisted Reproductive Technology
Editor: Kenan Demir and Rümeysa Yılmaz Göç
ISBN: 979-8-89113-017-3
© 2023 Nova Science Publishers, Inc.

Introduction

The formation of healthy and functional gametes is the most fundamental step in the reproductive system.

Oogenesis is a lengthy and meticulously controlled developmental process that results in the formation of a female gamete (sometimes referred to as an ovum or oocyte) from a primordial germ cell. It includes the transformation of a diploid germ cell into a haploid oocyte, which is followed by the maturity of an oocyte capable of fertilization (Zhai et al., 2018).

During oogenesis, the oocyte passes through three basic stages, namely proliferation, growth, and maturation (Zhai et al., 2018). Primordial follicles are considered growing follicles (primary and secondary) and Graafian follicles (Figure 2.1, Figure 2.2). The process of folliculogenesis, which starts before birth and becomes active at puberty, the reproductive period of the woman ends with menopause (Ross & Pawlina, 2018).

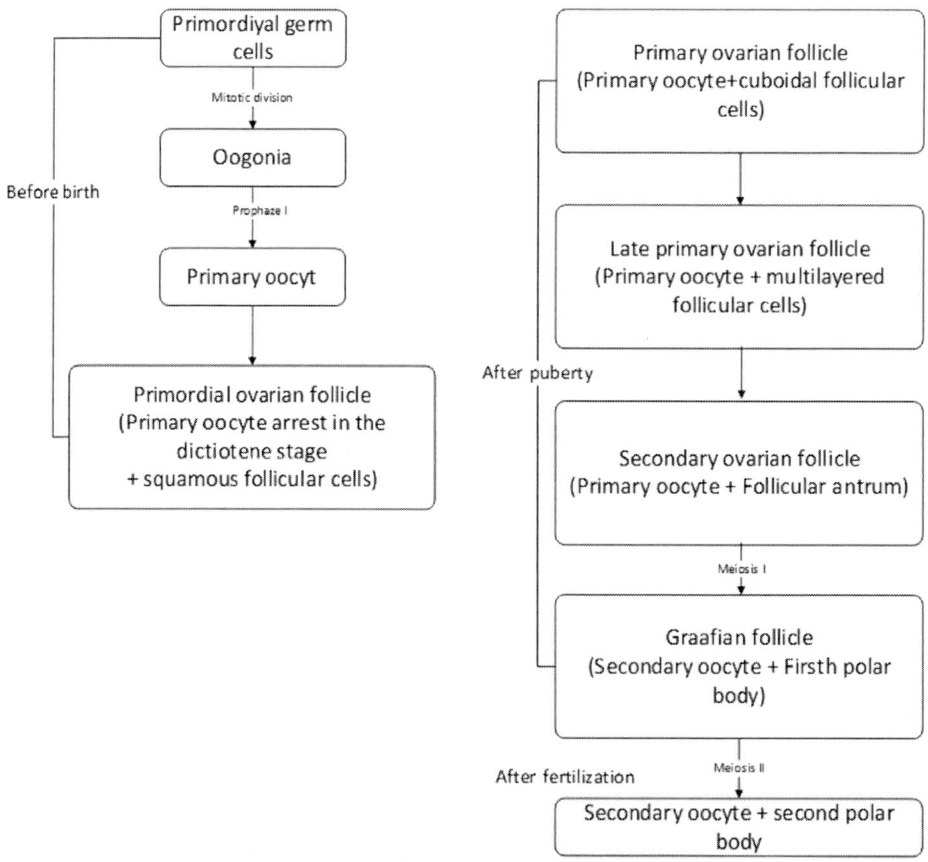

Figure 2.1 Stages in oogenesis (Created by the author).

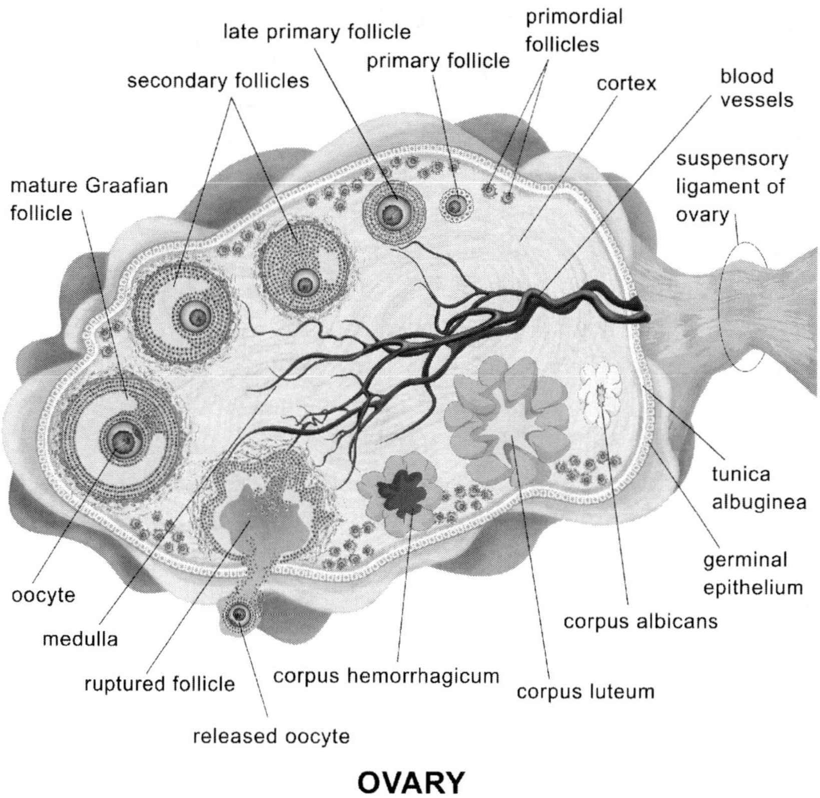

Figure 2.2 An ovarian slice is schematically shown. The early primary follicle and mature follicle (Graafian) represent different stages of follicular development (Created by the author).

Follicle Development Before Birth

Sperm, which is the male germ cell, fertilizes the egg, which is the female germ cell, and forms the zygote, and thus the development process begins. After the blastocyst implants in the uterus and starts to develop into the three main germ layers, a group of unique cells called primordial germ cells develops. Primordial germ cells arise just behind the primitive streak in the extraembryonic mesoderm of the yolk sac (Moore et al., 2016). These cells will form the gametes in a developing individual. Proper development of these unique cell populations will define an individual's fertility in the future. Primordial germ cells are located transiently in the mesoderm and endoderm of the primitive streak. In humans, primordial germ cells can be identified at approximately 3 weeks of gestation, near the yolk sac endoderm at the root of the allantois (Elder & Dale, 2019). From the fourth to the end of the fifth week, they migrate from the yolk sac wall to the gonads. In an embryo that has two X chromosomes, primordial germ cells reaching the gonads are called oogonia. Primordial germ cells increase in number by undergoing several mitotic divisions during migration and after reaching the gonads. This stage is called the *proliferation phase* and begins and ends in the embryonic period (Zhai et al., 2018).

Migration and proliferation of primordial germ cells are regulated by activin, BMPs (bone morphogenetic proteins), which are part of the transforming growth factor beta (TGFβ) family, and several germ cell-derived transcription factors. BMP2 and BMP4 increase the amount of primordial germ cells in the mouse ovaries, while BMP7 decreases it. Activin boosts the number of primordial germ cells in humans. Factors vital for the survival, migration and proliferation of primordial germ cells include SOX17 (Irie et al., 2015), BLIMP1, PRDM14, among others (Bowles & Koopman, 2010).

At the end of the third month of development, primordial germ cells that reach the gonads become clusters of cells surrounded by a flat epithelial cell epithelium originating from the surface epithelium. While most oogonia originating from the same cell in the group continue to divide by mitosis, some enter meiosis to produce primary oocytes. When the embryo is between 11 and 20 weeks old, the first meiotic division starts (Sadler, 2019). Signaling through STRA8 (stimulated by the retinoic acid gene 8), retinoic acid-dependent factor, is required for the initiation of meiosis. RNA-binding proteins such as DAZL and BOLL are also involved in several meiotic division phases in humans (He et al., 2013).

The growth phase of oogenesis begins when the oogonia complete mitosis, expand to produce primary oocytes, and begin meiosis, which continues after birth. After the oogonia transform into a primary oocyte, each primary oocyte in the cluster becomes surrounded by flat epithelial cells that are now called follicular cells. The primary oocyte and surrounding follicular cells are collectively called the primordial follicle (Sadler, 2019) (Figure 2.3).

In the fifth month before birth, the number of oogonia reaches its maximum. At this time, the process of cell death begins and many oogonia and primary oocytes degenerate. In the primordial follicle formation process, pro-apoptotic proteins such as BAX and caspases, and antiapoptotic proteins such as members of the B-cell lymphoma-leukemia (BCL) family, BCL2 and BCLX, are known to play a role. The lack of BCL2 or BCLX has been shown to lead to a decrease in the number of primordial follicles, while the deletion of the BAX or Caspase 2 function can lead to a rise in the number of primordial follicles (Sánchez & Smitz, 2012).

The early growth of primordial follicles is independent of the hormone gonadotropin. Primordial follicles are found in the cortex below the tunica albuginea in the ovary. The outer surface of the follicle cells, which consists of a single row of flat cells, is surrounded by a basal lamina. At this stage, the

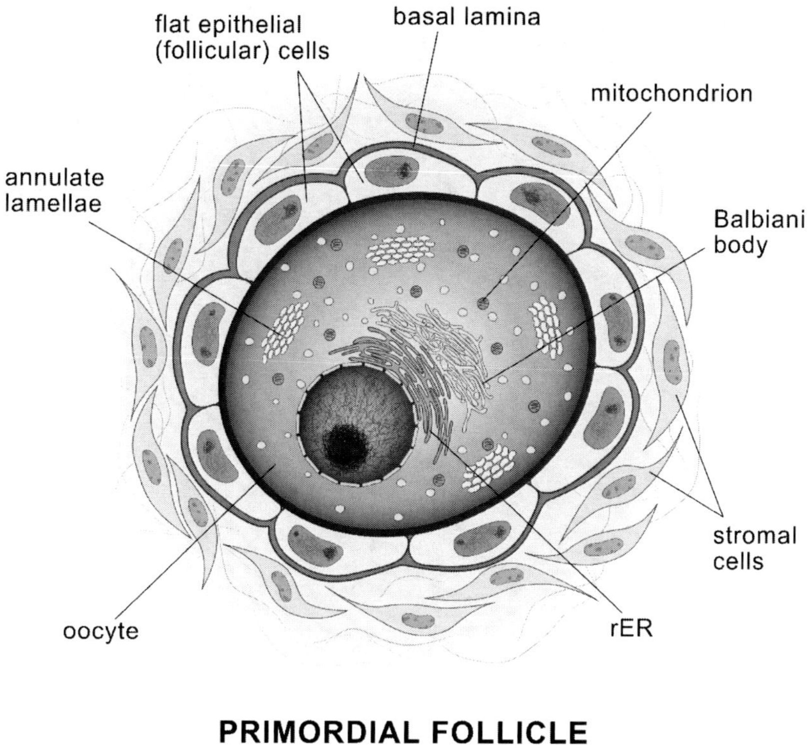

Figure 2.3 Schematic drawing of a primordial follicle (Created by the author).

oocyte inside the follicle is approximately 20-30 μm in diameter and has an eccentric nucleus containing finely dispersed chromatin and one or more large nucleoli. In the cytoplasm of the oocyte, called the ooplasm, granular endoplasmic reticulum sacs, membranes, and vesicles of the Golgi complex, mitochondria, centrioles, and lysosomes exist as cytoplasmic condensations called Balbiani bodies that can be detected with light microscopy. Furthermore, the ooplasm contains annular lamellae, numerous mitochondria, and vesicles (Ross & Pawlina, 2018).

Follicle Development After Puberty

Near birth, all primary oocytes enter meiosis. However, rather than completing meiosis I, these cells are paused in the diplotene phase of the prophase and enter a prolonged dormant phase known as the dictyate (germinal vesicle) that lasts to puberty. Meiosis is interrupted by the oocyte maturation inhibitor (OMI), a small peptide secreted by follicular cells. Although there are between 600,000 and 800,000 primary oocytes at birth, most of them undergo atresia in

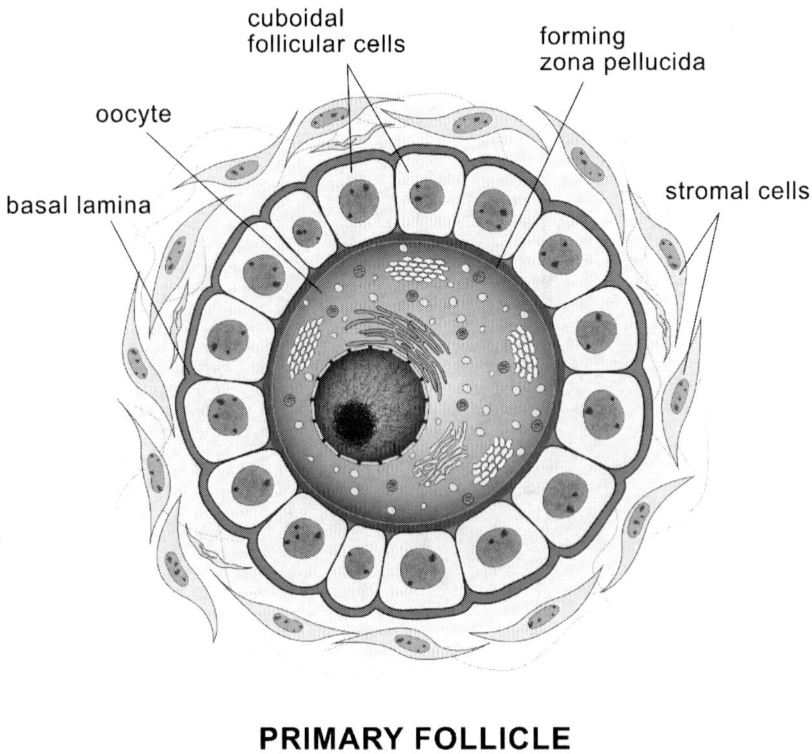

Figure 2.4 Schematic drawing of a primary follicle (Created by the author).

childhood and approximately 40,000 primary oocytes remain at the beginning of puberty, of which less than 500 ovulate (Sadler, 2019).

During the transformation of the primordial follicles into the primary (pre-antral) follicle (Figure 2.4) several changes are known to occur in the oocyte, follicle cells, and adjacent stroma. First, the oocyte enlarges in diameter and grows to 60-120 μm in diameter. Parallel with the growth of the oocyte, the diameter of the follicle grows to 200-400 μm in diameter. Dictyate chromosomes consist of large amounts of condensed DNA; nonetheless, during this period, active synthesis of ribosomal and messenger RNA continues to be carried out, as these preparations are important for the formation of organelles and protein stores in the cell. As the oocyte grows, secreted glycoproteins form the zona pellucida (ZP), a translucent layer without cells between the oocyte and follicular cells (Johnson, 2018). The ZP is important for events that occur during oocyte formation, fertilization, and early embryo development. Therefore, ZP plays a role in folliculogenesis, organization, and differentiation of granulosa cells, recognition and attachment of sperm, induction of the acrosome reaction, prevention of polyspermia, and preservation of the preimplanted embryo (Moros-nicol et al., 2021). The human ZP glycoproteins are named as ZP-1, ZP-2, ZP-3, and ZP-4. The proteins ZP-1, ZP-3,, and ZP-4 act as receptors for sperm attachment and induce acrosome reaction, while ZP-2 participates in the binding of secondary sperm (Gupta, 2018). As the diameter of the oocyte and follicle increases, the flat follicular cells surrounding the oocyte transform into cuboids. Follicular cells are separated from stromal cells around the ovary by a basement membrane.

Primordial follicle stimulation is an ongoing system. Signaling via PTEN/PI3K was shown to be important for the transition from primordial to primary follicles. PI3K (phosphatidylinositol 3 kinase) is a serine/threonine protein kinase that promotes cell growth while inhibiting the expression of FOXO3 (Forkhead Box O3) expression, which promotes apoptosis. PTEN (Phosphatase and tensin homolog) is a protein that inactivates PI3K. Studies in mouse and human ovaries have shown that inhibition of PTEN inhibition and activation of PI3K can induce primordial follicle activation (Dale, 2018). TSC / mTORC1 is another pathway that has been shown to regulate the development of primordial follicles. The Kit ligand and its receptor, neurotrophins, transcription factors such as Sohln1 and Nobox, TGF family proteins such as BMP4 and BMP7, and AMH (anti Mullerian hormone) are other crucial components of the process (Zhai et al., 2018).

As the follicles continue to grow and mature, the follicular cells undergo mitotic proliferation that then stratifies to form the granulosa layer of the follicle. The follicle cells are called granulosa cells after this stage. Although there are extensive corrugated junctions between granulosa cells, the basal layer of granulosa cells lacks tight junctions of type occludens, and there is no blood follicle barrier. Thus, nutrients and other molecules necessary for the normal development of the follicle can easily pass from the blood to the follicle fluid (Gartner, 2017).

During the growth phase of the follicle, various changes occur in the connective tissue around it. When the follicle contains three to six layers of granulosa cells, stromal cells form the theca follicle adjacent to the basal lamina (Figure 2.5) (Elder & Dale, 2019). Theca cells increase vascularity by secreting angiogenic factors, increasing nutrient availability to the follicle and supporting its growth. The theca layer then differentiates into two layers called theca interna and theca externa. The theca interna is the inner layer of secreting cubical cells and is rich in blood vessels. The theca externa is the outer layer consisting of smooth muscle cells and collagen fibers. Cells in the theca interna layer express luteinizing hormone (LH) receptors and synthesize androgens that can be converted to estrogens upon stimulation with LH. The synthesis of estrogens from androgens is catalyzed by the enzyme aromatase, which is expressed in granulosa cells. These synthesized estrogens both increase the number of LH receptors in granulosa cells and spread

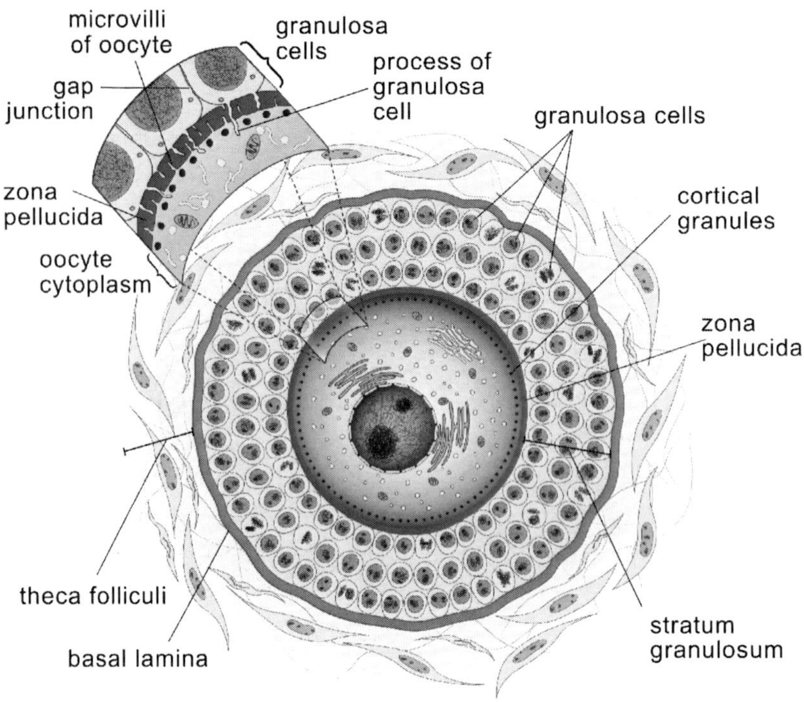

Figure 2.5 Schematic drawing of a late primary follicle (Created by the author).

throughout the body by returning to the theca layer. Although there is no clear boundary between the theca externa and the surrounding connective tissue, there is a basement membrane called the glasy membrane between the theca interna and the layers of the granulosa (Schoenwolf et al., 2021).

During the ongoing follicular maturation in primary follicles, the distribution of organelles in the oocyte changes. The Balbiani body disintegrates and the Golgi body diffuses into the cytoplasm. The rough endoplasmic reticulum, mitochondria, tiny vesicles, and free ribosomes expand in number. Secretory vesicles called cortical granules are formed just below the plasma membrane of the oocyte. Upon activation of proteases in these vesicles by the sperm, they move to the perivitelline space located between the oocyte and the granulosa cells surrounding the oocyte via exocytosis and carry out the cortical reaction.

Numerous microvilli extend from the oocyte to the perivitelline space. Additionally, along the zona pellucida, follicular cells also expand in the form of tiny, fingerlike extensions that entangle with the plasma membrane microvilli of the oocyte. These procedures are crucial for the passage of elements needed by the oocyte from the follicular cells (Ross & Pawlina, 2018; Sadler,

2019). After the antrum appears between the granulosa cells, the follicle is now called the *secondary/antral follicle.*

While development continues, oocyte growth stops when the stratum granulosum reaches 6-12 layers, and a viscous fluid begins to appear between the granulosa cells. This follicular fluid is made in part of granulosa cell secretions and partly of serum transudate. Drops of secreted fluid combine to form a single follicular antrum. The appearance of the follicular antrum indicates the beginning of the antral phase of development (Figure 2.6). The antrum, which is initially crescent-shaped, enlarges over time. When the eccentrically located oocyte increases in size to approximately 125 μm, the growth of the oocyte is suppressed by OMI secreted from the granulosa cells into the antral fluid. The increase in follicular size after this stage is mainly due to an increase in the size of the follicular antrum and the volume of the follicular fluid, although granulosa cells continue to proliferate (Johnson, 2018; Ross & Pawlina, 2018).

During the development of secondary follicles from primary follicles, proteins such as TBP2 (TATA box binding protein 2) and TAF4B (TATA box

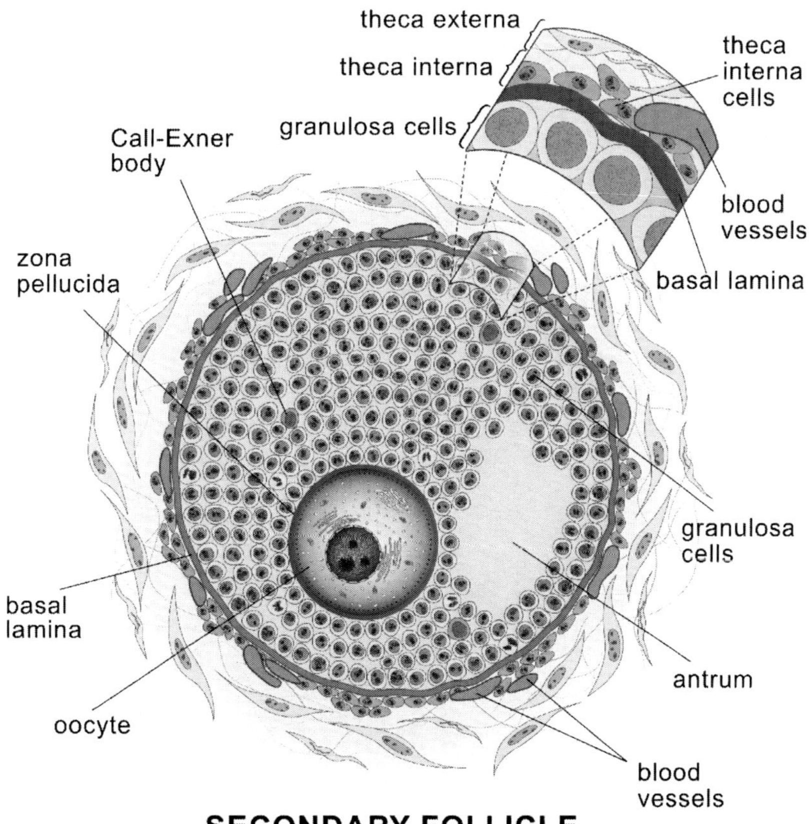

Figure 2.6 Schematic drawing of a secondary follicle (Created by the author).

binding protein related factor) that are secreted by oocytes, surrounding granulosa and theca cells play an important role. Furthermore, in the early stages, ovarian follicles develop the help of locally released factors independently of FSH and only become dependent on FSH when they enter the antral stage (Gazdag et al., 2009).

As the secondary follicle increases in size, the antrum also expands, and where the stratum granulosum is associated with the oocyte, the granulosa cells form a mound called the cumulus oophorus. The cumulus oophorus cells are located immediately around the oocyte and are excreted together with the oocyte at ovulation; this is called the corona radiata. These cells send microvilli to the zona pellucida, which connect with the microvilli of the oocyte. As follicular maturation progresses, the number of microvilli and LH receptors of corona radiata cells increases. During this period, Call-Exner bodies are seen between granulosa cells. These bodies are released from granulosa cells and contain hyaluronan and proteoglycans (Gartner, 2017). The follicle in this period is called a *mature/Graafian follicle* (Figure 2.7). During this period, the oocyte goes through a *maturation phase,* and the primary oocyte completes

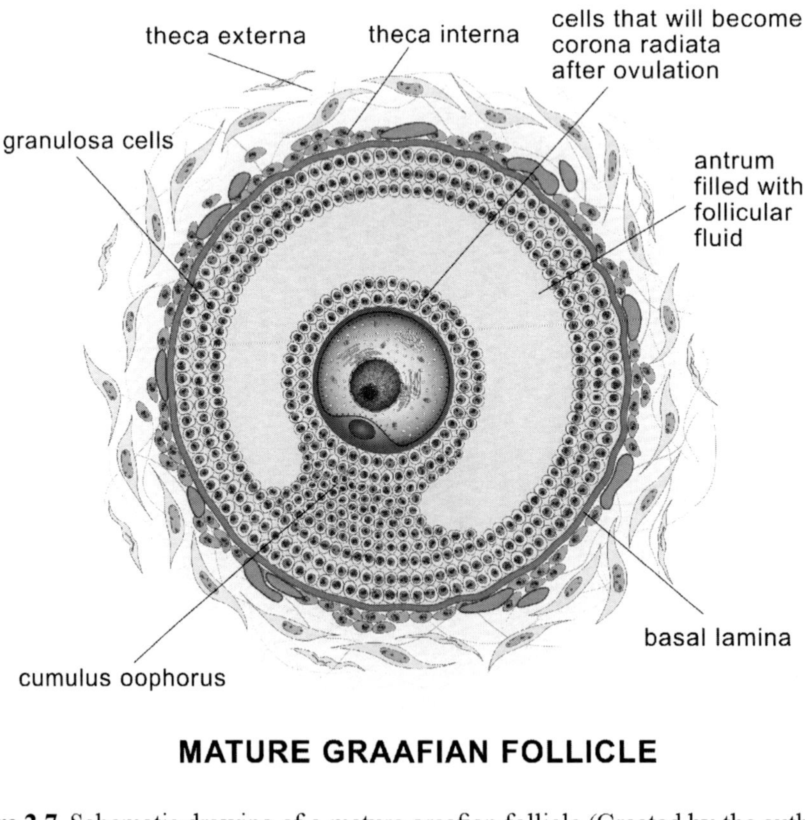

Figure 2.7 Schematic drawing of a mature graafian follicle (Created by the author).

meiosis I and is converted to a secondary oocyte. The Graafian follicle therefore contains mature secondary oocytes (Sontakke, 2018).

The diameter of the Graafian follicle can be up to 25 mm. Due to its large size, it protrudes from the surface of the ovary. As the diameter of the follicle increases, the mitotic activity of the granulosa cells decreases and the space between the granulosa cells increases. An opening appears between the oocyte and cumulus cells and other granulosa cells and preparations for ovulation are initiated. The theca interna, which is made up of cells rich in blood vessels and can secrete steroid hormones, is surrounded by the theca externa, which is associated with the connective tissue of the the ovary. In humans, LH stimulates theca interna cells to secrete androgens. Since the aromatase enzyme is not expressed in theca interna cells, estrogen is not produced there. Rather, androgens are converted to estrogens by FSH action in the smooth endoplasmic reticulum of granulosa cells (Sadler, 2019).

Stimulation of NOTCH signaling in gonadal somatic cells by ligands from nearby germ cells is one of the processes that controls oocyte maturation. In addition, oocyte-derived factors GDF9 and BMP15, which are participants in the TGF-β superfamily, have been shown to be crucial in oocyte maturation (Su et al., 2008).

Estrogen, which is secreted both from the follicle and systemically, increases the sensitivity of gonadotropes to the gonadotropin-releasing hormone. Approximately 24 hours before ovulation, there is an increase in FSH or LH secretion in the adenohypophysis. In response to the LH surge, LH receptors in granulosa cells are desensitized and stop producing estrogen in response to LH. As a result, primary meiosis (meiosis I) is completed, generating a large secondary oocyte and a much smaller polar body, each with 23 chromosomes. The first polar body is located in the perivitelline space, which is between the zona pellucida and the secondary oocyte's cell membrane. Both granulosa and theca cells then undergo luteinization and produce progesterone. Approximately three hours before ovulation, the cell initiates meiosis II but stops at metaphase. Meiosis II is only completed if the oocyte is fertilized; In the absence of fertilization, the cell degenerates roughly 24 hours after ovulation (Ross & Pawlina, 2018; Sadler, 2019).

Conclusion

Oogenesis is a process that begins in the embryonic period, becomes periodic after puberty, and ends with menopause. In this process, the oocytes, follicular cells around the oocyte, and the somatic cells surrounding the follicles undergo numerous changes. Primordial germ cells first transform into oogania, then primary oocytes, and before ovulation, into secondary oocytes. Primordial follicles formed by the primary oocyte and its surrounding flat epithelial cells transform into primary follicles containing cubical follicular cells. The follicle is transformed into secondary follicles when the fluid-filled antrum becomes visible in the primary follicles. Secondary follicles finally transform into Graafian follicles with the formation of the cumulus oophorus, together with the oocyte that completes meiosis I to form a secondary oocyte. In order for this whole process to be completed, the complex interactions between the oocyte, follicular cells, and surrounding somatic cells, as well as systemic hormonal and molecular mechanisms, must proceed in a highly regulated and temporal manner. The completion of this process is vital for female fertility, since deregulation in any of these mechanisms can lead to incomplete oogenesis and thereby infertility.

References

Bowles, J., & Koopman, P. (2010). Sex determination in mammalian germ cells: extrinsic versus intrinsic factors. *Reproduction, 139*(6), 943–957. https://doi.org/10.1530/REP-10-0075

Dale, B. (2018). *Fertilization The Beginning of Life* (pp. 4–23). https://doi.org/10.1017/9781316650318.003

Elder, K., & Dale, B. (2019). Gametes and Gametogenesis. In *In-Vitro Fertilization* (pp. 53–76). Cambridge University Press. https://doi.org/10.1017/9781108611633.004

Gartner, L. (2017). *Textbook of Histology* (4th ed.). Elsevier.

Gazdag, E., Santenard, A., Ziegler-Birling, C., Altobelli, G., Poch, O., Tora, L., & Torres-Padilla, M.-E. (2009). TBP2 is essential for germ cell development by regulating transcription and chromatin condensation in the oocyte. *Genes Dev, 15;23*(18), 2210–2223. https://doi.org/10.1101/gad.535209

Gupta, S. K. (2018). The Human Egg ' s Zona Pellucida. In *Extracellular Matrix and Egg Coats* (1st Edition, Vol. 130). Elsevier Inc. https://doi.org/10.1016/bs.ctdb.2018.01.001

He, J., Stewart, K., Kinnell, H. L., Anderson, R. A., & Childs, A. J. (2013). A Developmental Stage-Specific Switch from DAZL to BOLL Occurs during Fetal Oogenesis in Humans, but Not Mice. *Plos One, 25;8(9):e7.* https://doi.org/10.1371/journal.pone.0073996

Irie, N., Leehee, W., Tang, W. C. W., Kobayashi, T., Viukov, S., Manor, Y. S., Dietmann, S., Hanna, J. H., & Surani, M. A. (2015). SOX17 Is a Critical Specifier of Human Primordial Germ Cell Fate. *CELL, 160*(1–2), 253–265. https://doi.org/10.1016/j.cell.2014.12.013

Johnson, M. H. (2018). *Essential Reproduction* (8th Edition). Wiley Blackwell.

Moore, K., Persaud, T. V., & Torchia, M. (2016). *The Developing Human* (10th Edition). Elsevier.

Moros-nicol, C., Chevret, P., Algarra, B., Cots-rodr, P., Gonz, L., Avil, M., & Izquierdo-rico, M. J. (2021). *New Insights into the Mammalian Egg Zona Pellucida*. https://doi.org/https://doi.org/10.3390/ijms22063276

Ross, M. H., & Pawlina, W. (2018). *Histology a Text and Atlas* (8th ed.). Wolters Kluwer.

Sadler, T. (2019). Langman's Medical Embryology. In T. Sadler (Ed.), *Sadler* (14th Edition). Wolters Kluwer.

Sánchez, F., & Smitz, J. (2012). Molecular control of oogenesis. *Biochim Biophys Acta*, *1822*(12), 1896–1912. https://doi.org/10.1016/j.bbadis.2012.05.013

Schoenwolf, G. C., Steven, B. B., Philip, R. B., & Francis-West, P. H. (2021). *Larsen' Human Embryology* (6th Edition). Elsevier.

Sontakke, Y. (2018). *Textbook of Human Embryology* (Firsth). CBC.

Su, Y.-Q., Sugiura, K., Wigglesworth, K., O'Brien, M. J., Affourtit, J. P., Pangas, S. A., Matzuk, M. M., & Eppig, J. J. (2008). Oocyte regulation of metabolic cooperativity between mouse cumulus cells and oocytes: BMP15 and GDF9 control cholesterol biosynthesis in cumulus cells. *Development*, *135*(1), 111–121. https://doi.org/10.1242/dev.009068

Zhai, F., Ma, X., Yan, L., & Qiao, J. (2018). The molecular genetics of oogenesis. In *Human Reproductive and Prenatal Genetics*. Elsevier Inc. https://doi.org/10.1016/B978-0-12-813570-9.00007-3

Chapter 3

Development and Structural Features of Sperm

Derya Özdemir Taş, MD*
Center for Assisted Reproduction, Obstetrics and Gynecology Clinics, Ankara City Hospital, Ankara, Turkiye

Abstract

Testicle differentiation begins with the development of testicular cords, including gonocytes and Sertoli cells, at the 6th week of gestation. Testicles have exocrine secretory and endocrinological functions, as a part of the hypothalamic-pituitary-gonadal (HPG) axis, in sperm and androgen production, respectively. The testicular compartments contain tightly packed seminiferous tubules and loose interstitial connective tissue. The seminiferous tubules are lined with a stratified germinal epithelium composed of Sertoli cells and spermatogenic. Spermatogenic cells develop from type A spermatogonial stem cells. Type A spermatogonia produces type A dark and type A pale spermatogonia, respectively. Then, type a pale spermatagonias differentiate into type b spermatagonias. Type B spermatogonia form primary spermatocytes and then enter secondary spermatocytes, Sa, Sb, Sc, Sd1 and Sd2 spermatids. Spermatids mature to mature, motile spermatozoa at spermiogenesis. After meiosis, round haploid spermatids enter spermiogenesis as small, nonpolarized cells with cytoskeletal network and form a mature sperm structure. Mature sperm consists of two parts, the head and the flagellum. The flagellum consists of the nucleus and an oval acrosome that covers 40-70% of the nucleus. Flagellum has a special ciliary shape with a complex structure and involves more than 1000 proteins. The basic structure that provides the movement in the Flagellum is the axoneme. The axoneme contains

* Corresponding Author's E-mail: derya-ozdemir61@hotmail.com

In: Holistic Approach to Assisted Reproductive Technology
Editor: Kenan Demir and Rümeysa Yılmaz Göç
ISBN: 979-8-89113-017-3
© 2023 Nova Science Publishers, Inc.

microtubular pairs. Flagellum has an axoneme along its entire length. The axoneme is surrounded by a plasma membrane at the end.

Key Words: Testicle, Spermatogenesis, Sertoli cell, Acrosome

Introduction

Testicle differentiation begins with the development of testicular cords, including gonocytes and Sertoli cells, at the 6th week of gestation. Sertoli cells begin to secrete anti-Mullerian hormone (AMH) just after differentiation and lead to Mullerian canal regression, which is completed mid-pregnancy. Leydig cells begin to appear in the interstitium of the fetal testes at week 8, but at 6-7 weeks the testicles will have in vitro steroidogenic activity. Testosterone can be detected in the fetal circulation at the 8th week and reach its peak values between the 11th and 13th weeks. This time frame, which encompasses the end of the first trimester and the first half of the second, is crucial for the good reproductive development of the male fetus. The probable masculinization programming window (MPW) occurs in humans at this time and testosterone must be present for normal masculinization to occur. Due to the androgen effect, MPW occurs when the anogenital distance (AGD), penis, urethra, and testicles descend, as well as adult fertility (O'Shaughnessy & Fowler, 2014).

During the first 6 months after birth, serum concentrations of testosterone, FSH, and LH increase transiently. In addition, the number of testicular germ cells also increases in parallel with changes in androgen levels and serum gonadotropin. Subsequently, the number of testicular germ cells decreases and reaches the lowest number per tubule at 2 years of age. It is then followed by a gradual increase up to puberty. With the onset of active spermatogenesis from the onset of puberty, serum gonadotropin, and androgen concentrations, the number of spermatogonia per tubule and tubular diameter increases rapidly (Dunkel et al., 1997).

Spermatogenesis

Spermatogenesis is a complex and sequential process responsible for the production of the male gamete cell, namely sperm. The seminiferous tubules, which are tiny tubular structures that are thought of as functional units of the testicles, are where this process occurs. The human testes can produce approximately 275 million sperm each day and has 600–1200 seminiferous tubules (Neto et al., 2021).

Testicles

Male gonads, the other name testicles, are the sex glands that have both an exocrine secretory function in sperm production and an endocrinological function as part of the HPG axis in men through androgen production. The testes are between 2-3 cm in width and 3-5 cm in length and are divided into compartments by the scrotal septum. They have an oval shape and lie in the scrotum (Titi-Lartey & Khan, 2022). The testicular compartments contain loose interstitial connective tissue and tightly packed seminiferous tubules. The seminiferous tubules are lined with a stratified germinal epithelium composed of spermatogenic germ cells and Sertoli cells (supporting sustentacular) (Figures 3.1, 3.2). Each tubule is surrounded by loose connective tissues, capillaries, lymphatic vessels, nerves, macrophages, as well as neurovascular bundles, groups of testosterone-secreting interstitial cells (Leydig) among those structures (Olaniyan et al., 2020).

The testicles are in a capsule consisting of 3 layers. These; tunica vaginalis (outermost), Tunica albuginea (middle), and Tunica vasculosa (innermost). The tunica vaginalis is an extension of the peritoneal structure, the processus vaginalis. When the processus vaginalis is not destroyed, a direct connection occurs between the scrotum and the peritoneal cavity. Tunica albuginea consists of dense collagen fibers. Posteriorly, it inserts inward to

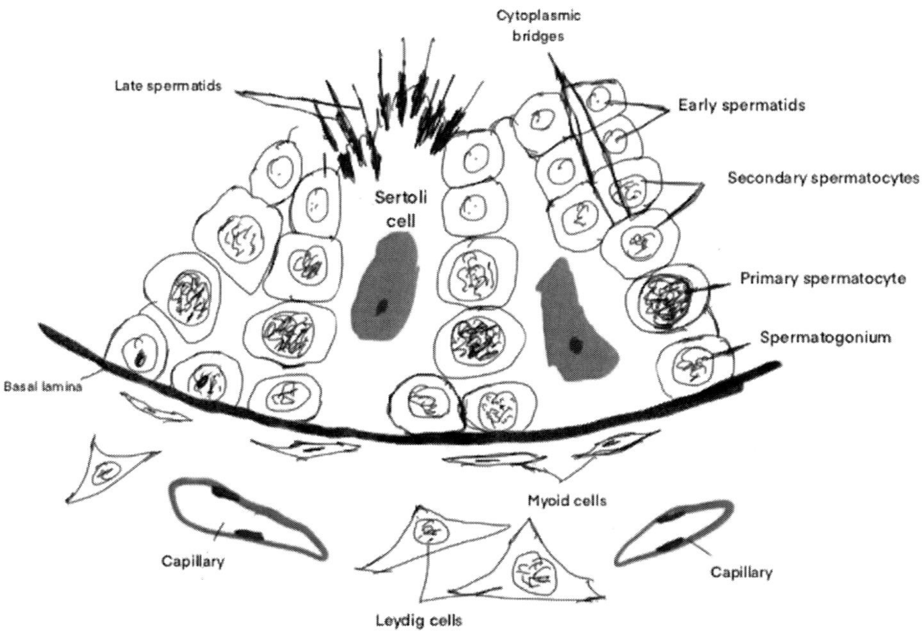

Figure 3.1 Cellular organization of seminiferous tubules (Created by the author).

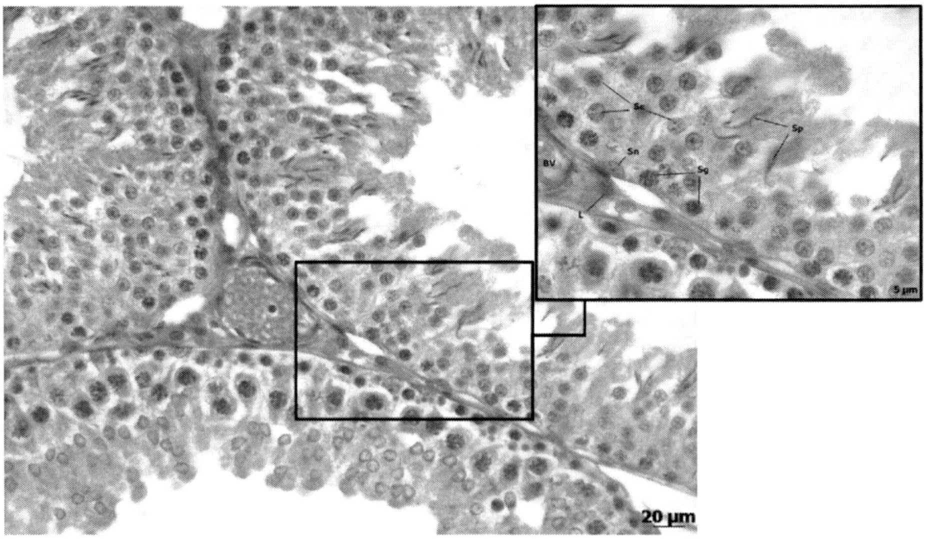

Figure 3.2 Histological sections stained with hematoxylin and eosin of testis ×400; inset ×1000. Sg, spermatogonia; Sn, Sertoli nuclei; Sc, spermatocytes; Sp, spermatids; L,Leydig cell; BV, blood vessel (Author's own archive).

create an incomplete fibrous septum within the testes. The tunica vasculosa is the vascular layer of the testes that is held together by the delicate areolar tissue composed of a plexus of blood vessels (Tullington & Blecker, 2022).

Seminiferous tubules

Seminiferous tubules are composed of germ cells in the stages of progressive differentiation to form mature sperm and the epithelium containing Sertoli cells that surround and support them. The seminiferous tubules, which can be up to 70 cm long and tightly coiled within the testicular lobules, transport the sperm released into the lumen to the rete testis. After that, it enters the epididymis and the efferent ducts. It is then sent to the vas deferens where the ejaculation will take place. The basal lamina encircles the tubules. The extracellular matrix is made up of the basal lamina, which provides structural integrity and controls the function of the cells in contact with it. It divides the tubules from the interstitial compartment. Leydig cells can be seen in the interstitial section between each tubule and numerous different seminiferous tubules are surrounded by basal lamina in a testicular biopsy specimen that underwent cross sectional histological analysis (Matsumoto & Bremner, 2016). There is a layer outside the basal lamina, called the tunica propria, which consists of 3-5 layers of myoid cells and collagen fibrils. Myoid cells are believed to play a role in the production of extracellular matrix proteins and in the regulation of the functions of Sertoli cells. At the same time, they are known to have the ability to contract (Davidoff et al., 1990).

Two types of cells, *Sertoli and spermatogenic cells*, are present in a stratified layer from the basal lamina towards the lumen.

Sertoli cells have columnar shapes, thin and long mitochondria, and usually contain lipid droplets and lipofuscin at the base of their cytoplasm. Sertoli cell nuclei have different shapes and are usually pear-shaped or oval with folds in their nuclear membranes. This folding in the nucleolemma and large evident euchromatic nucleoplasm nucleolus are the characteristics of cells with high metabolic activity (Johnson et al., 2008). Microtubules, intermediate filaments, and actin filaments, which are cytoskeletal structures, are abundant in Sertoli cells. These structures are concentrated in certain regions and are dynamic. Interestingly, all three elements of the cytoskeleton are associated with intercellular binding sites and play important roles in the displacement, positioning, and fixation of spermatogenic cells in the seminiferous tubules (Vogl et al., 2008).

The Sertoli-Sertoli tight junction (ScTj), which aids in the formation of the blood-testis barrier, is where the intricate physical interaction between Sertoli and germ cells begins for the first time. The barrier may be thought to be tight; however, it was discovered that the contribution of germ cells and peritubular myoid to the increase in transepithelial resistance varies depending on whether it is studied in vivo or in vitro. The intricate transition of preleptotene and leptotene spermatocytes from the basal to the adluminal compartment through the ScTj is one of the epithelium's most spectacular morphological activities. Similarly to opening and closing canal locks surrounding a ship, the movement of hundreds of syncytial germ cells occurs without disrupting this crucial barrier and calls for extremely precise synchronization. By crossing cytoplasmic bridges made of three nearby Sertoli cells, or tricellular junctions, germ cells remain connected (França et al., 2016).

Sertoli cells have a wide variety of essential functions. These include; providing nutrition and structural support to developing germ cells, degenerating germ cells and phagocytosis of residual bodies, relaxation of spermatids in spermiation, and the formation of the blood testicular barrier by the production of a number of proteins that affect the mitotic activity of spermatogonia that regulate and/or respond to hormone release from the pituitary gland (Jégou, 1992).

Another type of cell in the seminiferous tubule is the spermatogenic cell. Spermatogenic cells contain a family of cells that transmit genetic and epigenetic information through generations and whose sole purpose is to form sperm cells. 13 types of human spermatogenic germ cells have been identified so far. These spermatogenic cells begin to develop from type A spermatogonial stem cells. Type A spermatogonia produces type A dark and type A pale spermatogonia, respectively. Then, type a pale spermatagonias differentiate into type b spermatagonias. Type B spermatogonia form primary spermatocytes and then into secondary spermatocytes, Sa, Sb, Sc, Sd1 and Sd2 spermatids (Neto et al., 2016). It is explained in detail at the spermatogenesis part.

Spermatogenesis: The extraembryonic ectoderm and visceral endoderm stimulate bone morphogenetic protein to cause the blastocyst epiblast in the yolk sac to grow into progenitors of primordial germ cells (PGCs) in the mammalian testis. The origin of gamete cells in adults is the primordial germ cell, which develops in the epiblast during the second week of embryonic development and subsequently migrates to the yolk sac during the fourth week. Mitotic divisions of PGC continue for some time during its migration from the yolk sac to the developing gonadal ridges and once it reaches the gonadal ridges. PGC differentiate into gonocytes (prospermatogonia) after reaching the gonadal ridge. Gonocytes gain a distinctive characteristic with a large nucleus and a prominent nucleolus while surrounded by seminiferous cords. Silent prospermatogonia, in a mitotic manner, are connected by intercellular bridges. The presence of intercellular bridges is accepted as a sign of differentiation from PGC to gonocytes. After the proliferation period, gonocytes migrate to the basal membrane of the tubule and form type A spermatogonia (de Kretser et al., 1998; Ibtisham et al., 2017).

Spermatogenesis takes around 74 days. It includes three distinct functional phases that typically occur in the seminiferous tubules: mitosis, meiosis, and spermiogenesis (Cannarella et al., 2020).

Mitosis: Spermatogonial stem cells are undifferentiated spermatogonia that retain their regeneration potential and differentiate into type A_{paired} and type A_{lined} spermatogonia that have lost their regeneration capacity. When this happens, they separate into differentiated spermatogonia that contain type A1-4 and type B spermatogonia. This procedure requires 16 days. Within another 16 days, type B spermatogonia split into primary spermatocytes, marking the end of the mitotic division phase. It is known that numerous markers are expressed in these cells throughout this process and play a role in controlling their differentiation and proliferation. In particular, mouse SSCs express ID4 and PAX7, while human SSCs also show PAX7 expression. Furthermore, human spermatogonia includes the transcription factors PLZF and SALL4, which are necessary for SSCs to regenerate on their own (Cannarella et al., 2019).

Meiosis: During the meiosis phase, two cellular divisions and a single DNA replication result in the ploidy being reduced by half. Homologous chromosomes split during the first meiosis (meiosis I). Although primary spermatocytes (4C, 2n) have secondary chromosomes with haploid DNA, they include 2C DNA (1n). Separation of the sister chromatid and meiosis II division continue in secondary spermatocytes. Round spermatids (1C, 1n) are generated at the end of meiosis II, initiating the spermiogenesis process. In instance, ploidy reduction is necessary for gametogenesis in sexually reproducing organisms. Because the fusion of male and female gametes during fertilization ensures that the number of chromosomes of the species is restored. The exchange of genetic material between homologous chromosomes during prophase I, which also contributes to the reductive nature of meiosis, is crucial. During this phase, a unique proteinaceous structure, called the synaptonemal complex (SC), is created, providing the necessary affinity for homologous recombination. This is the most researched meiotic stage because of the significance of the distinctive activities that take place during meiotic prophase I (SC creation, alignment, pairing, and recombination). Leptotene, zygotene, pachytene, diplotene, and diakinesia are the different substages that are separated from this lengthy stage to aid in study. Leptotene is where SC assembly begins, zygotene is where homologous mating occurs, and pachytene is characterized by recombination (crossing-over). Throughout the diplotene, the SC divides. Any interruption during these processes frequently results in infertility and spermatogenic halt (Rodríguez-Casuriaga & Geisinger, 2021).

Spermiogenesis: It is the last phase of spermatogenesis and a process that sperm have retained throughout evolution. According to microscopic investigations, the four phases of mammalian spermiogenesis are the golgi, cap, acrosome, and maturation stage (Toshimori, 2009) (Figure 3.3). Proacrosomal vesicles of the endocytic pathway and the trans-Golgi network combine to

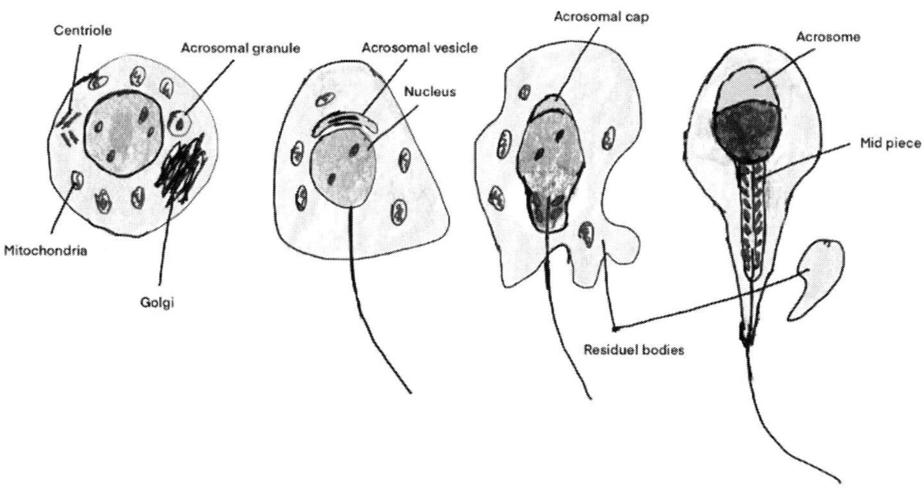

Figure 3.3 Phases of spermiogenesis (Created by the author).

create acrosomal vesicles, which contain acrosomal granules, during the Golgi phase. A cytoskeletal plate known as the acroplasome helps the acrosomal vesicle attach to the nuclear envelope. The acrosomal vesicle flattens and extends over the anterior pole of the spermatid nucleus to form a cap during the cap phase. The adaptable F-actin of the acroplasm mediates this remodeling of the acrosome and spermatid elongation. During the acrosomal phase, actin filaments, which consist of a perinuclear ring and extend into the elongated sperm tail, and another temporary structure, namely the manchette, which contain microtubules, are formed. The manchette contributes to the formation of the head and tail of the sperm by providing protein transport across the cytoskeleton. Finally, in the maturation stage, the elongation of the spermatids is completed. Spermatid cytoplasm and organelles are also excreted by Sertoli cells as residual bodies that are phagocytosed (Zakrzewski et al., 2021). Simultaneously, spermiogenesis involves a distinctive chromatin remodeling process that frequently replaces more than 90% of core histones with testis-specific histone variants, followed by transitional proteins (TPs) and finally protamines (PRMs). Protamines are different from core histones because they are loaded with lysine and cysteine residues. After this histone-protamine exchange, the chromatin structure is six times more compact than that of somatic cells, protecting genetic material from X-rays, germs, oxidation, and harmful molecules found in the female reproductive system (Hao et al., 2019).

Acquisition of Sperm Motility: Testicular sperm are immature and are known to acquire motility and fertilization abilities as they pass through the epididymis (Baldi et al., 2002). The epididymis has anatomical regions such as the first segment, caput, corpus, and cauda. It is a ductlike organ that connects the testicle to the vas deferens (Sullivan et al., 2019). Sperm maturation occurs during the epididymal transition. Before ejaculation, functionally mature sperm are kept in the cauda epididymis. Depending on the species, 50 to 80% of the spermatozoa are in the epididymal lumen in the cauda epididymis at any given time. In the caudate lumen, epithelial cells release substances that support the preservation of the luminal environment that are intended to keep spermatozoa immobile during storage. Although these factors are still unknown, the presence of enzymes and specific proteins is believed to play a role in the regulation of luminal pH (Devi et al., 2021). Although testicular sperm can twitch, it cannot complete a progressive movement. When the sperm reached the caudal part of the epididymis, many cells gained the ability of progressive motility. Sperm cell specific motility is believed to be increased artificially. However, the lumen of the epididymis provides the ideal environment for this motility to occur. From a structural and morphological point of view, many changes occur in spermatozoa that help serve motility. Sperm acrosome narrows as a result of a change in the structure of the plasma membrane of sperm after transit through the epididymis. The tubular lumen is hypothesized to include certain chemicals and enzymes that regulate changes in membrane structure. The genetic material and the sperm head are compressed as a result of the increased disulfide bridge of the sperm nucleus (James et al., 2020).

Hormonal Regulation of Spermatogenesis

Gonadotropins play a role in the differentiation and spermatogenesis of spermatogonia. Hypothalamic gonadotropin-releasing hormone (GnRH) regulates the release of gonadotropins from the pituitary gland, such as follicle stimulating hormone (FSH) and luteinizing hormone (LH) . Gonadotropins act on Sertoli and Leydig cells that express the follicle stimulating hormone receptor (FSHR) and the luteinizing hormone receptor (LHR) to regulate spermatogenesis. Only Sertoli cells and undifferentiated germ cells are present in the seminiferous tubules of the testes in the absence of LH and FSH. In the juvenile or prepubertal stage of testicular development, the epithelium of seminiferous tubules is made entirely of undifferentiated germ cells and Sertoli cells, indicating a prolonged hypogonadotropic state. Undifferentiated spermatogonia, which may multiply largely independently of gonadotropins, make up all testicular germ cells in the early or juvenile phase (Khanehzad et al., 2021).

Leydig Cells: Leydig cells located in the region between the seminiferous tubules are the primary source of androgens. Androgens diffuse into the seminiferous tubules and interstitial blood arteries. By attaching to androgen receptors (AR) in Sertoli cells and peritubular myoid cells under hypothalamic-pituitary-gonadal control, it regulates male germ cell signaling pathways. Leydig cells also play a significant role in controlling steroidogenesis and growth factors, such as Inhibin, insulin peptide 3 (INSL-3), thyroid hormones, estrogens, and others, by influencing spermatogenesis, according to a number of studies. (Zhou et al., 2019).

Testosterone is the main androgen that regulates spermatogenesis in the testes. LH activation causes the Leydig cell to generate testosterone, which diffuses into seminiferous tubules and functions as a paracrine factor there. It does so by acting through the 110 kD protein known as the androgen receptor (AR, also known as NR3C4), which is found in the cytoplasm and nucleus. In germ cells, there is no active androgen receptor. Instead, dispersed testosterone binds to AR in the nucleus and cytoplasm of Sertoli cells, where it causes the functional reactions necessary to maintain spermatogenesis. Additionally, AR expressed in PTM cells, Leydig, vascular endothelial cells, and arteriolar smooth muscle interacts with testosterone. The concentrated synthesis of testosterone in Leydig cells accounts for 25 to 125 times greater testosterone levels in males and rodents than in serum. Uncertainty exists over the physiological implications of large amounts of testosterone in the testicles. Despite this, it has been discovered that when testosterone levels in the testes fall below 70mM, sperm production rapidly decreases (Smith & Walker, 2014; Zirkin et al., 1989).

FSH activates the genes required for the control of spermatogenesis by binding to the Sertoli cell-produced FSHR protein. In the early stages of mammalian spermatogenesis, a number of growth factors also govern the onset of meiosis and the differentiation of spermatogonia (de Rooij, 2009). Numerous growth factors, such as glial cell-derived neurotrophic factor (GDNF), activin A, bone morphogenetic protein 4 (BMP4), kit ligand (KL), and neuregulins (NRGs), are produced by sertoli cells and encourage the self-regeneration and differentiation of spermatogonial tissue (Khanehzad et al., 2021).

Structure of Mature Sperm

Sperm cell has a specific structure and consists of two main parts, the head and tail (flagellum) (Figure 3.4). The sperm cell has a smooth oval-shaped head that is 2.5-3.5 micrometers wide (smaller than the size of a pinhead) and 5-6 micrometers long (Bellastella et al., 2010). The nucleus of the sperm head carries the male haploid genetic material. The acrosome, a unique membrane organelle that houses several hydrolases that aid sperm entry into the zona pellucida of the oocyte, is located at the front of the sperm nucleus. The acrosome is a secretory granule generated in the Golgi during the early stages of spermatogenesis. In three ways, it resembles the cellular lysosome, which

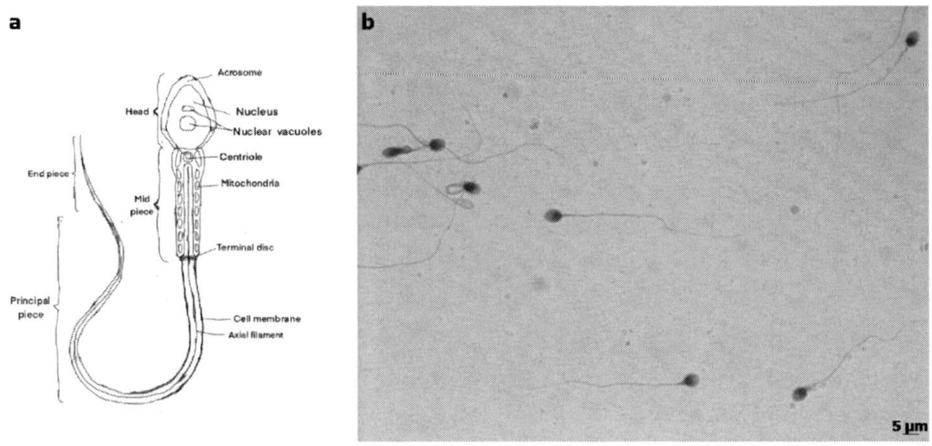

Figure 3.4 Sperm structure (a), Papanicolaou stained semen smear × 1000 (b) (Author's own archive).

ordinarily performs intracellular defense and digesting activities. First, the Golgi apparatus is the source of both organelles. Second, acridine orange and vivid orange-red stain both organelles. This suggests that the internal pH of the organelles is acidic. The two organelles also have a number of similar enzymes in common, including proteases, acidic glycohydrolases, esterases, arylsulfatases, and acidic phosphatases. The acrosome has some different characteristics despite these similarities. In sperm, for instance, the acrosome structure resembles a sac and is encircled by inner and outer acrosome membranes. The outer acrosome membrane immediately merges with the surrounding plasma membrane during sperm-zona binding, releasing acrosomal contents (proteases, glycohydrolases, etc.) to the sperm-oocyte binding point (acrosomal exocytosis). Acrogranin, acrosin, and the sperm protein AM67 are only a few examples of antigens that the acrosome possesses in contrast to the cellular lysosome (Abou-Haila & Tulsiani, 2000; Wu et al., 2020).

Sperm motility is provided by the tail. Generally speaking, as the length of the flagellum increases, so does the velocity of the sperm. The "9 + 2" microtubule-containing axoneme sits in the middle of the sperm tail. The head-tail coupling apparatus (HTCA) joins the sperm head and tail (also called sperm neck or the connecting piece). To bring the head and tail of the sperm together during high velocity, a strong HTCA sperm is required due to its long and fine structure (Wu et al., 2020).

It is a special ciliary structure with a complex design that involves more than 1000 proteins that are involved in the sperm tail. It is divided into three parts; mid-piece, principal-piece, and the end-piece (Figure 3.4). With the exception of the small end portion, which lacks periaxonemal structures, the sperm tail is entirely covered in axonemes and various surrounding structures. Only the axoneme and the plasma membrane are present in the final fragment. The microtubule-based axoneme is made up of nine outer pairs and one core pair of microtubules (9 + 2), which are joined by radial railings and dynein arms. The dynein arms are located in the axoneme and are responsible for the movement of the sperm tail. The periaxonemal structures in the midpiece consist of a spirally arranged mitochondrial sheath, the number of which varies depending on the species. Humans have about 10-12 cycles. The outer dense fibers are another periaxonemal component in the midpiece (ODFs). Nine columns that extend from the connecting component and terminate at various locations along the tail make up the outer fibers. Each fiber is thickest at the beginning and gets thinner as it gets closer to the conclusion. The primary purpose of ODFs is to protect the sperm tail from harm as it travels through the epididymis and during ejaculation. Additionally, these fibers are crucial for sperm capacitation and motility (Kumar & Singh, 2021; Lehti & Sironen, 2017; Tottle, 1974).

Conclusion

In seminiferous tubules, the dynamic spermatogenesis process results in the transformation of diploid spermatogonia into haploid sperm. In addition to providing these cells with paracrine support, sertoli cells also promote the development of germ cells. FSH and LH stimulate Sertoli and Leydig cells, which are a crucial part of spermatogenesis. Special cells known as mature sperm contain the genetic components required to fertilize the egg. Sperm cells have an oval, smooth head, a united body, and a spiral tail. Male infertility, however, can also be caused by aberrant sperm structure, low sperm count and motile sperm ratio, hormonal issues (such as issues with hormones secreted by the pituitary and testicular glands), and genetic disorders.

References

Abou-Haila, A., & Tulsiani, D. R. (2000). Mammalian sperm acrosome: formation, contents, and function. *Arch Biochem Biophys*, *379*(2), 173-182. https://doi.org/10.1006/abbi.2000.1880

Baldi, E., Luconi, M., Bonaccorsi, L., & Forti, G. (2002). Signal transduction pathways in human spermatozoa. *J Reprod Immunol*, *53*(1-2), 121-131. https://doi.org/10.1016/s0165-0378(01)00089-4

Bellastella, G., Cooper, T. G., Battaglia, M., Ströse, A., Torres, I., Hellenkemper, B., Soler, C., & Sinisi, A. A. (2010). Dimensions of human ejaculated spermatozoa in Papanicolaou-stained seminal and swim-up smears obtained from the Integrated Semen Analysis System (ISAS(®)). *Asian J Androl*, *12*(6), 871-879. https://doi.org/10.1038/aja.2010.90

Cannarella, R., Condorelli, R. A., Duca, Y., La Vignera, S., & Calogero, A. E. (2019). New insights into the genetics of spermatogenic failure: a review of the literature. *Hum Genet*, *138*(2), 125-140. https://doi.org/10.1007/s00439-019-01974-1

Cannarella, R., Condorelli, R. A., Mongioì, L. M., La Vignera, S., & Calogero, A. E. (2020). Molecular Biology of Spermatogenesis: Novel Targets of Apparently Idiopathic Male Infertility. *Int J Mol Sci*, *21*(5). https://doi.org/10.3390/ijms21051728

Davidoff, M. S., Breucker, H., Holstein, A. F., & Seidl, K. (1990). Cellular architecture of the lamina propria of human seminiferous tubules. *Cell Tissue Res*, *262*(2), 253-261. https://doi.org/10.1007/bf00309880

de Kretser, D. M., Loveland, K. L., Meinhardt, A., Simorangkir, D., & Wreford, N. (1998). Spermatogenesis. *Hum Reprod*, *13 Suppl 1*, 1-8. https://doi.org/10.1093/humrep/13.suppl_1.1

de Rooij, D. G. (2009). The spermatogonial stem cell niche. *Microsc Res Tech*, *72*(8), 580-585. https://doi.org/10.1002/jemt.20699

Devi, A., Kushwaha, B., Maikhuri, J. P., Singh, R., & Gupta, G. (2021). Cell signaling in sperm midpiece ensures quiescence and survival in cauda epididymis. *Reproduction*, *162*(5), 339-351. https://doi.org/10.1530/rep-21-0202

Dunkel, L., Hirvonen, V., & Erkkilä, K. (1997). Clinical aspects of male germ cell apoptosis during testis development and spermatogenesis. *Cell Death & Differentiation*, *4*(3), 171-179. https://doi.org/10.1038/sj.cdd.4400234

França, L. R., Hess, R. A., Dufour, J. M., Hofmann, M. C., & Griswold, M. D. (2016). The Sertoli cell: one hundred fifty years of beauty and plasticity. *Andrology*, *4*(2), 189-212. https://doi.org/10.1111/andr.12165

Hao, S. L., Ni, F. D., & Yang, W. X. (2019). The dynamics and regulation of chromatin remodeling during spermiogenesis. *Gene*, *706*, 201-210. https://doi.org/10.1016/j.gene.2019.05.027

Ibtisham, F., Wu, J., Xiao, M., An, L., Banker, Z., Nawab, A., Zhao, Y., & Li, G. (2017). Progress and future prospect of in vitro spermatogenesis. *Oncotarget*, *8*(39), 66709-66727. https://doi.org/10.18632/oncotarget.19640

James, E. R., Carrell, D. T., Aston, K. I., Jenkins, T. G., Yeste, M., & Salas-Huetos, A. (2020). The Role of the Epididymis and the Contribution of Epididymosomes to Mammalian Reproduction. *Int J Mol Sci*, *21*(15). https://doi.org/10.3390/ijms21155377

Jégou, B. (1992). The Sertoli cell in vivo and in vitro. *Cell Biol Toxicol*, *8*(3), 49-54. https://doi.org/10.1007/bf00130510

Johnson, L., Thompson, D. L., Jr., & Varner, D. D. (2008). Role of Sertoli cell number and function on regulation of spermatogenesis. *Anim Reprod Sci*, *105*(1-2), 23-51. https://doi.org/10.1016/j.anireprosci.2007.11.029

Khanehzad, M., Abbaszadeh, R., Holakuyee, M., Modarressi, M. H., & Nourashrafeddin, S. M. (2021). FSH regulates RA signaling to commit spermatogonia into differentiation pathway and meiosis. *Reprod Biol Endocrinol*, *19*(1), 4. https://doi.org/10.1186/s12958-020-00686-w

Kumar, N., & Singh, A. K. (2021). The anatomy, movement, and functions of human sperm tail: an evolving mystery. *Biol Reprod*, *104*(3), 508-520. https://doi.org/10.1093/biolre/ioaa213

Lehti, M. S., & Sironen, A. (2017). Formation and function of sperm tail structures in association with sperm motility defects. *Biol Reprod*, *97*(4), 522-536. https://doi.org/10.1093/biolre/iox096

Matsumoto, A., & Bremner, W. (2016). Testicular Disorders. In (pp. 694-784). https://doi.org/10.1016/B978-0-323-29738-7.00019-8

Neto, F. T., Bach, P. V., Najari, B. B., Li, P. S., & Goldstein, M. (2016). Spermatogenesis in humans and its affecting factors. *Semin Cell Dev Biol*, *59*, 10-26. https://doi.org/10.1016/j.semcdb.2016.04.009

Neto, F. T. L., Flannigan, R., & Goldstein, M. (2021). Regulation of Human Spermatogenesis. *Adv Exp Med Biol*, *1288*, 255-286. https://doi.org/10.1007/978-3-030-77779-1_13

O'Shaughnessy, P. J., & Fowler, P. A. (2014). Development of the human fetal testis. *Annales d'Endocrinologie*, *75*(2), 48-53. https://doi.org/https://doi.org/10.1016/j.ando.2014.03.009

Olaniyan, O. T., Dare, A., Okotie, G. E., Adetunji, C. O., Ibitoye, B. O., Bamidele, O. J., & Eweoya, O. O. (2020). Testis and blood-testis barrier in Covid-19 infestation: role of angiotensin-converting enzyme 2 in male infertility. *J Basic Clin Physiol Pharmacol*, *31*(6). https://doi.org/10.1515/jbcpp-2020-0156

Rodríguez-Casuriaga, R., & Geisinger, A. (2021). Contributions of Flow Cytometry to the Molecular Study of Spermatogenesis in Mammals. *Int J Mol Sci*, *22*(3). https://doi.org/10.3390/ijms22031151

Smith, L. B., & Walker, W. H. (2014). The regulation of spermatogenesis by androgens. *Semin Cell Dev Biol*, *30*, 2-13. https://doi.org/10.1016/j.semcdb.2014.02.012

Sullivan, R., Légaré, C., Lamontagne-Proulx, J., Breton, S., & Soulet, D. (2019). Revisiting structure/functions of the human epididymis. *Andrology*, *7*(5), 748-757. https://doi.org/10.1111/andr.12633

Titi-Lartey, O. A., & Khan, Y. S. (2022). Embryology, Testicle. In *StatPearls*. StatPearls Publishing Copyright © 2022, StatPearls Publishing LLC.

Toshimori, K. (2009). Dynamics of the mammalian sperm head: modifications and maturation events from spermatogenesis to egg activation. *Adv Anat Embryol Cell Biol*, *204*, 5-94.

Tottle, C. (1974). Homoepathy. *Self & Society*, *2*(7), 11-12. https://doi.org/10.1080/03060497.1974.11086482

Tullington, J. E., & Blecker, N. (2022). Lower Genitourinary Trauma. In *StatPearls*. StatPearls Publishing Copyright © 2022, StatPearls Publishing LLC.

Vogl, A. W., Vaid, K. S., & Guttman, J. A. (2008). The Sertoli cell cytoskeleton. *Adv Exp Med Biol*, *636*, 186-211. https://doi.org/10.1007/978-0-387-09597-4_11

Wu, B., Gao, H., Liu, C., & Li, W. (2020). The coupling apparatus of the sperm head and tail†. *Biol Reprod*, *102*(5), 988-998. https://doi.org/10.1093/biolre/ioaa016

Zakrzewski, P., Lenartowska, M., & Buss, F. (2021). Diverse functions of myosin VI in spermiogenesis. *Histochem Cell Biol*, *155*(3), 323-340. https://doi.org/10.1007/s00418-020-01954-x

Zhou, R., Wu, J., Liu, B., Jiang, Y., Chen, W., Li, J., He, Q., & He, Z. (2019). The roles and mechanisms of Leydig cells and myoid cells in regulating spermatogenesis. *Cell Mol Life Sci*, *76*(14), 2681-2695. https://doi.org/10.1007/s00018-019-03101-9

Zirkin, B. R., Santulli, R., Awoniyi, C. A., & Ewing, L. L. (1989). Maintenance of advanced spermatogenic cells in the adult rat testis: quantitative relationship to testosterone concentration within the testis. *Endocrinology*, *124*(6), 3043-3049. https://doi.org/10.1210/endo-124-6-3043

Chapter 4

First Stages of Development

Merve Kavak Balgetir, MD*

IVF Center, Elazıg Fethi Sekin City Hospital, Elazig, Turkiye

Abstract

The preimplantation period of human embryo development is highly significant, during which the human embryo undergoes genetic, physiological, and morphological changes. This first stage of embryo development is characterized by the preimplantation stage of development. During this stage, female and male gametes develop and then undergo cytoplasmic and nuclear differentiation, resulting in the production of mature spermatozoa and oocytes. The maturation stages of sperm and oocytes are of prime importance for successful fertilization and its continuation. Fertilization, also known as the union of the spermatozoa and oocyte, occurs in the oviduct. The paternal and maternal chromosomes combine to create a zygote with a single diploid nucleus once oocyte meiosis is complete. At this stage, embryonic development is considered to have begun. The freshly formed embryo goes through numerous rounds of cell division known as cleavage as it travels from the oviduct to the uterus, and each cell produced by cleavage is a blastomere. From the 8 to 16 cell stage, the embryo or morula differentiates into two cell groups: (i) a peripheral outer cell layer and (ii) a central inner cell mass. The cleaving embryo, or morula, develops into two sets of cells: a peripheral outer cell layer and a core inner cell mass, starting at the 8 to 16cell stage. The embryo begins to develop a central chamber filled with fluid during the 30 cell stage known as the blastocyst. The embryo on days 5 to 6 of development is called a blastocyst. The blastocyst grows as the cells divide and the cavity expands. In the final stage, the blastocyst hatches

---

* Corresponding Author's Email: mervekavak89@hotmail.com

In: Holistic Approach to Assisted Reproductive Technology
Editor: Kenan Demir and Rümeysa Yılmaz Göç
ISBN: 979-8-89113-017-3
© 2023 Nova Science Publishers, Inc.

from the zona pellucida to implant in the endometrium. This whole process is a summary of the prenatal period of human beings.

Key Words: Sperm, Oocyte, Fertilization, Zygote, Morula, Blastocyst, Embryo

Introduction

Reproduction requires successful fertilization. In this chapter, we initially elaborate on the dangerous journey of spermatozoa from their production sites to their fertilization sites in the oviduct, and then we move on to the preparation stages of the oogonia that will host the sperm and their preparation for fertilization. To reach the oviduct, human spermatozoa, which are just a few micrometers long, must travel more than 100,000 times their own length, or 30 to 40 cm, through the male and female reproductive tract. Less than one millionth of the sperm produced complete the journey. The voyage alone is challenging, but before spermatozoa can fully develop their ability to fertilize, they must successfully navigate a number of modifications in both the male and female genital tracts. These changes include events such as sperm maturation, capacitation, and activation and acrosome reaction. The spermatozoon performs all these complex changes without expressing any of its own genes, which are transcriptionally inactive and heterochromatic. During fertilization, when a sperm enters an oocyte to create a zygote, development starts. Biochemical mechanisms in all stages of maturation, activation, and fertilization are highly important for healthy zygote/embryo development.

A zygote is a highly specialized totipotent cell that can develop into any form of cell. It has chromosomes and genes inherited from both parents. The zygote divides numerous times and gradually develops into a multicellular human through cell division, migration, growth, and differentiation (Johnson, 2018; Barroso et al., 2009).

Preparation of Gametes for Fertilization

Spermatozoa and oocytes are inactive through various mechanisms, and their transition to competent cells is called gamete activation. The steps in which they gain activity are as important as all maturation steps. The steps in gamete activation are governed by interconnected pathways. Calcium is a key molecule in this process. The success of fertilization depends on the gametes reaching full maturity. (Yanagimachi, 1981).

Oocyte Preparation

Oocyte maturation is a crucial step for successful fertilization. The initial activation event of the oocytes occurs with an increase in the ionic permeability of the plasma membrane. Nuclear and cytoplasmic activation of the oocyte is a key step for the transition to the zygote stage, where intracellular Ca^{2+} release plays a crucial role in the oocyte, following gamete fusion. In humans, sperm causes an outward current in the plasma membrane of the oocyte by activating calcium-gated potassium channels. (Dozortsev et al., 1994). In the endoplasmic reticulum, there are inositol 1,4,5-trisphosphate ($InsP_3$) receptors responsible for calcium release (Wakai et al., 2012). Numerous studies on the physiology of fertilization in mammals have revealed that sperm factor initiates the activation of oocytes. Electrical, mechanical, or pharmacological stimulation that elevates intracellular Ca2+ ion concentrations can induce this activation. Furthermore, oocyte activation ensures that sperm-triggered oocytes that are arrested in metaphase II continue to meiosis (Dozortsev et al., 1994). Cortical granules merge with the plasma membrane of the egg immediately after sperm penetration and by exocytosing their contents in the perivitelline region (Holubcová et al., 2013). The cortical reaction alters the properties of the zona pellucida (ZP), leading to the shingles reaction (hardening of ZP) (Figure 4.1) (Elder & Dale, 2020).

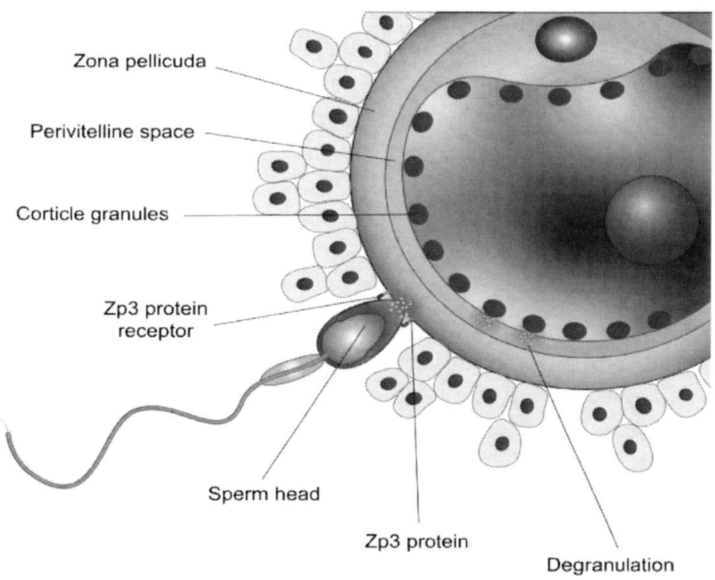

Figure 4.1 Role of Zp3 proteins. Zp3 proteins of the zona pellucida, binding of sperm to Zp3 receptors, and cortical degranulation (Created by the author).

Zona Reaction

Zona pellucida is a glycoprotein layer that acts as a protective cover for the developing oocyte and is secreted by the growing oocyte. ZP2 and ZP3 are the two main subunits of ZP (Wassarman et al., 1996). Sperm ZP2 receptors are found on the inner acrosomal membrane and are exposed once an acrosome reaction (AR) occurs. ZP2 after AR allows the sperm to bind to ZP. Sperm penetrate the ZP and fuse with the oocyte plasma membrane. Sperm penetrates the strong ZP that surrounds the oocyte. SED1, a sperm surface protein, mediates binding to ZP3. Additionally, binding of human sperm to eggs is achieved via a sequence of sugar molecules, called sialyl-LewisX, at the ends of the oligosaccharides of the ZP proteins. The acrosome is induced to release degradative enzymes as a result of this interaction, allowing the sperm to enter ZP. The cell membranes of the two cells merge when a spermatozoon successfully penetrates the zona pellucida and reaches the oocyte. AR occurs when the sperm binds to ZP3. After sperm penetration, shingles take on a protective role and undergo permanent changes, thus blocking new sperm penetration (polyspermy) after fertilization (Figure 4.1) (Schoenwolf et al., 2020).

Sperm Preparation

For successful fertilization, the spermatozoon must be activated after undergoing numerous behavioral, physiological, and structural changes. Some of these modifications are caused by environmental cues, while others are caused by the interaction of the spermatozoon with the oocyte and extracellular structures. If we evaluate, in general, all of these preparations; oolemma binding, capacitation, hyperactivity, crossing of ZP, acrosome reaction, and changes in membrane fusion (Elder & Dale, 2020).

Capacitation

During capacitation, spermatozoa undergo a sequence of modifications that give them the "capacity" to adhere to and penetrate the egg. These alterations include enhanced membrane fluidity, cholesterol efflux, ion fluxes that alter the potential of the sperm membrane, increased protein tyrosine phosphorylation, hypermotility induction, and AR (Forman & Fissore, 2015). During capacitation: Spermatozoa are cleared of covering seminal and epididymal plasma proteins, changes occur in sperm plasma membrane glycoproteins (Gur & Breitbart 2006). In man, in vivo capacitation begins during the passage of sperm into the cervix. Many enzymes and factors in the female canal such as arylsulfatase, fucosidase, and taurine are involved in capacitation.

In the event of capacitation, glycoproteins on the surface of the sperm cell are removed or rearranged. Receptor sites that can respond to oocyte signals are exposed and the acrosome reaction takes place. At this stage, hyperactivation occurs and the sperm penetrates the ZP more easily (Elder & Dale, 2020).

Acrosome reaction

The acrosome is a membrane-bound cap that covers the anterior part of the sperm head, containing a wide variety of hydrolytic enzymes, including hyaluronidase, phospholipase C, collagenase, acrosin, phosphatase, proacrosin, β-galactosidase and arylsulfatase. AR occurs only in the presence of Ca^{2+}. Calcium influx causes fusion of the acrosomal membrane and exocytosis of the acrosomal contents. The permeability of the plasma membrane of sperm changes when a capacitated sperm binds to ZP, temporarily changing the concentration of several intracellular ions. This, in turn, triggers AR, which is the final step in activation of the spermatozoon before gamete fusion. The outer acrosomal membrane fuses with the plasma membrane of the sperm head, allowing the release of the contents. The acrosomal granule breaks down to release lysins, and these enzymes create a pathway along ZP so that the plasma membrane of the sperm head enters contact with the plasma membrane of the oocyte and the two membranes fuse (Figure 4.1) (Elder & Dale, 2020).

Sperm-Oocyte Interaction

Only capacitated sperms are able to respond to the ovulated follicle's unidentified sperm chemotropic component by swimming directly toward the egg, according to in vitro findings.

Several lipids appear to play a role in the membrane fusion process, such as chromosome reaction during fertilization, gamete fusion, cortical exocytosis, receptor regulation, and intracellular oscillations. Lipases such as sphingomyelinase, phospholipase C, D, and A2, autotaxin, and lipin 1 are involved in the production of second messenger lipids in fertilization. In the human oocyte, the microdomains of the lipid raft are rich in the ganglioside GM1 and the tetraspanin protein CD9. GM1 is active in signal transduction and protein binding. CD9 is the most important membrane component in sperm penetration. The density and arrangement of the GM1 microdomains at the site of sperm contact influence the penetration of the sperm into the human oocyte. Sperm can attach to these GM1 points and penetrate with CD9 domains (Elder & Dale, 2020).

Plasma membrane fusion of two gametes leading to cell-cell adhesion is the final step in the interaction of gametes leading to oocyte activation and zygote formation. Although its mechanism remains unclear, lipid rafts and associated transmembrane proteins, including Izumo 1, Juno, and CD9, play a fundamental role during fusion (Wassarman, 1990). Immediately after fusion, the plasma membrane of the sperm integrates with the plasma membrane of the oocyte (Elder & Dale, 2020; Johnson, 2018).

Izumo 1 is a spermatozoal transmembrane protein that interacts with Juno, a receptor located on the surface of the unfertilized oocyte. Juno is a member of the Folr4 family of folate receptors and binds to glycophosphatidylinositol (GPI). Juno quickly disappears from the oocyte surface after fertilization; Juno Izumol interaction appears to be an essential adhesion step for gametes rather than a membrane fusion event. Juno is rapidly lost from the surface of the oocyte after fertilization; Juno-Izumo 1 interaction appears to be a necessary adhesion step for gametes, rather than a membrane fusion event. Fusion is considered to require other membrane proteins such as EEF-1 (Eukaryotic Elongation Factor 1) and myomaker. Sperm binding strength can be increased by local clustering of Juno on the oocyte membrane, organized by tetraspanin CD9. This protein has an obvious role in sperm-oocyte fusion; however, the corresponding sperm ligand remains unknown. Members of the CRISP (cysteine-rich secretory proteins) family are also known to be involved in the capacitation process and mammalian sperm-ZP interactions (Wassarman, 2014).

Sperm-Oocyte Fusion

The level of free intracellular calcium in the oocyte increases dramatically within 1 to 5 minutes after the union of the oocyte and the sperm, mostly as a result of the release of calcium from internal reserves. This elevation, which lasts about two to three minutes, spreads over the oocyte in waves starting at the place where the spermatozoa enter, rather than happening all at once. A succession of calcium spikes, each lasting 1-2 minutes, follow this initial surge. These spikes grow increasingly synchronous throughout the oocyte and occur every 3 to 15 minutes, depending on the specific oocyte. (Figure 4.2). This spiking activity can last for several hours.

Fusion of the spermatozoon with an oocyte triggers calcium release through the effect of a spermatozoal enzyme that passes into the oocyte after fusion. This enzyme is defined as a specific spermatozoal phospholipase Cζ (zeta). PLCζ stimulates the release of the second messengers inositol triphosphate (IP3) and diacylglycerol (DAG) to produce its effects. The first of these then promotes calcium release, while the latter stimulates protein phosphorylation by activating protein kinase C (PKC) (Wassarman, 2014; Johnson, 2018).

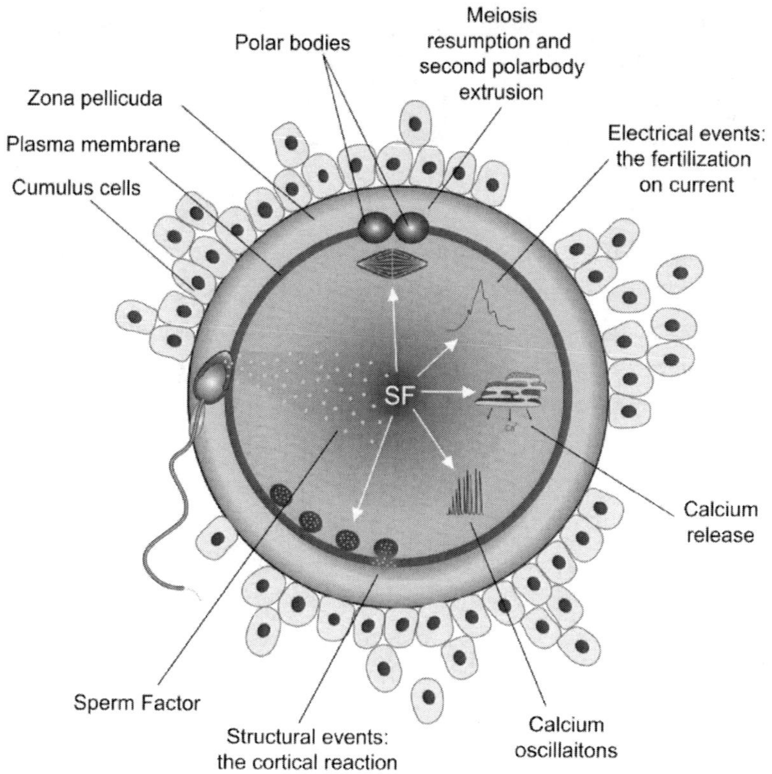

Figure 4.2 Release of sperm factor (SF) after sperm entry and changes in the oocyte (Created by the author).

Fertilization

The first week of development begins with fertilization (oocyte-sperm fusion). Fertilization is the process that involves the fusion of two mature germ cells, an egg, and a spermatozoon (haploid cells) to form a single cell, the zygote (diploid cell). The usual fertilization site is the ampulla of the fallopian tube. Sperm must penetrate the three barriers around the secondary oocyte (corona radiata, ZP, and vitelline membrane) to achieve fertilization. Only the nucleus and tail of the sperm enter the cytoplasm of the oocyte (ooplasm), leaving the body and the cytoplasm behind. After fertilization, the secondary oocyte completes the second meiotic division. The male haploid pronucleus (23) and the female haploid pronucleus (23) fuse to form a diploid zygote (46) (Sontakke, 2018).

Biochemistry of Fertilization

As mentioned above, PLCζ, a sperm protein transported into the oocyte during gamete fusion, is often regarded as the protein component responsible for the beginning of oocyte activation. PLCζ is a cytosolic sperm protein that enters the oocyte after fertilization and causes oocyte activation by releasing intracellular Ca2+ ions from endoplasmic reticulum storage (Figure 4.2). The PLCζ signal is activated with the diffusion of PLCζ from the sperm into the ooplasm. PLCζ hydrolyses PIP2-containing vesicles, producing InsP3 and DAG, thus stimulating the phosphoinositide signaling pathway. InsP3 then binds to InsP3 receptors (InsP3R) located on the surface of the endoplasmic reticulum and induces Ca^{2+} release, while DAG activates the PKC pathway to transform Ca^{2+} signals into cellular responses. The PLCζ protein translocates from the cytosol to the pronucleus when the calcium oscillations stop and the pronucleus forms. Furthermore, it has been demonstrated that this protein is rereleased into the cytosol during the first mitotic division of the embryo during the moment of nuclear envelope collapse, as well as during the second mitotic division. This suggests that calcium oscillations are involved in not just oocyte activation but also early embryonic development (Elder & Dale, 2020).

In summary, the formation of calcium spikes is essential for the completion of successful fertilization. Calcium is a secondary messenger that regulates different events during fertilization, such as cell cycle progression from arrest in metaphase II to dissociation of the chromatid, second polar body extrusion, and completion of the second meiosis, as well as cortical granule exocytosis (Jones, 2005).

Fertilization Results

After completion of fertilization, single cell embryos progress to the uterus by peristalsis and ciliary movements of the oviduct, while the zygote rapidly undergoes five or six mitotic cell divisions, but does not increase in total volume (Figure 4.3). After fertilization, a series of events occur in the embryo, including the formation of maternal and paternal pronuclei (2PN) on day 1 and the cleavage stage between day 1.5 and day 3 (Elder & Dale, 2020). The term "zygote cleavage" refers to recurrent mitotic divisions of the zygote that result in a fast increase in the number of cells (blastomeres). Approximately 30 hours after fertilization, cleavage begins, followed by subsequent divisions that eventually generate smaller blastomeres. The zygote differentiates into two blastomeres, and then these two cells divide into four blastomeres and finally eight blastomeres (Figure 4.3) (Stricker, 1999).

The blastomeres form a cluster up to the eighth cell stage. Following the third cleavage, their interaction with each other is maximized, resulting in compaction, a compact cluster of cells (Yanagida, 2004).

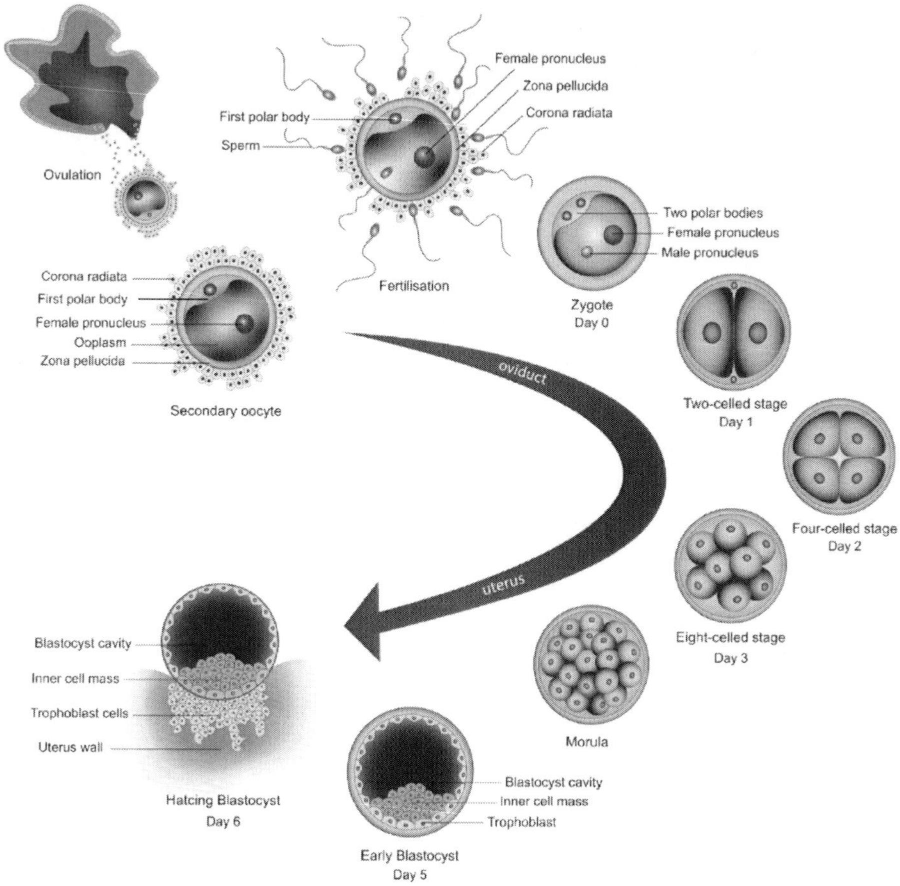

Figure 4.3 Embryonic developmental stages. Ovarian oocytes (OV). Fertilization (F). Morula (M). Blastocyst (B). Uterus (U). Endometrium (E). Implantation (I) (Created by the author).

Pronucleus Development and Syngamy

The cytoplasmic contents of the sperm cell membrane are transferred into the oocyte cytoplasm during oocyte-sperm union and second polar body ejection. The nuclear membrane of the spermatozoa breaks down, causing the highly condensed chromatin to expand and release filamentous strands of chromatin into the cytoplasm. Protamines that are present in such compacted chromatin are released and replaced by regular histones. 4 to 7 hours after fusion, each of the two haploid chromosome pairs is surrounded by a membrane and two pronuclei appear (Figure 4.3) (Tesarik & Kopecny, 1989). The male pronucleus is often larger. Both pronuclei contain a number of nucleoli. 4 to 7 hours after fusion, each of the two haploid chromosome pairs is surrounded by a membrane and two pronuclei appear (Fig. 3) (Tesarik & Kopecny, 1989). Then, the pronuclei gradually come from the subcortical region to the central area and move to the adjacent position. These haploid chromosomes are prepared for the first mitotic division by DNA synthesis approximately 18-24 hours after fusion. The pronuclear membranes then rupture, the mitotic metaphase spindle is formed, and the chromosomes line up in the equatorial plane. Now the final stage of fertilization has been reached: Syngamy (combination of gamete chromosomes) has occurred. The first mitotic anaphase and telophase are completed quickly. Then the cleavage stage is passed, and it evolves from a single-celled zygote to a two-celled formation (Johnson, 2018; Gardner et al., 2020).

When the zygote's two pronuclei form, structures known as nucleolar precursor bodies (NPBs) emerge. Spermatozoal nucleoli are lost during spermatogenesis. The nucleolar material of the oocyte is involved in the reassembly of the nucleoli in male and female pronuclei. The oocyte nucleolus originates from the germinal vesicle, and its structure may change during the maturation phase of the oocyte. The nucleoli of the two pronuclei are of maternal origin only (Elder & Dale, 2020).

Development of Zygote and Preimplantation

During syngamy, pronuclear fusion occurs and fertilization is complete. The resulting zygote now has a diploid chromosome. The first mitotic division occurs and continues its development by dividing through successive mitoses into smaller cells known as blastomeres. After all these steps, the embryo becomes a blastocyst. In humans, the first divisions of the embryo before implantation occur in the oviduct (Figure 4.3). The blastocyst grows as the cells divide and the cavity expands, where it "hatches" from ZP to implant in the endometrium. Oogenesis is the period in which the cell enters a period of growth without replication or division, while early embryo division is the period in which there is no growth, which includes intense DNA replication and cell division. As the cleavage stage progresses, the embryo becomes polarized and differences arise between the blastomeres. In this differentiation, the uneven distribution of predetermined cytoplasmic components in the oocyte during oogenesis or alterations in blastomeres induced by the transcription of new embryonic genes during development play a role. In conclusion, with the initiation of zygote gene activation, blastomeres perform their specific developmental stages (Elder & Dale, 2020; Dale, 2018).

Cleavage

Cleavage is characterized by multiple mitotic divisions of the zygote, which results in a fast increase in the number of blastomeres. These divisions begin approximately 30 h after fertilization and are not accompanied by cell growth. The blastomeres shrink with each cleavage division. The zygote is still surrounded by ZP during cleavage. After the eighth cell stage, the blastomeres change form and firmly align opposite one another (i.e., compaction). This phenomenon may be induced by cell surface adhesion glycoproteins and the formation of adherent junctions. Compaction allows for greater cell-to-cell interaction and is a precondition for separation of the internal cells that form the inner cell mass. This also leads to the development of polarization of each blastomere with an apical and a basolateral region. In the presence of 12 to 32 blastomeres, the conceptus is termed a morula (Moore et al., 2020). As the morula develops, these blastomeres divide into two types of cells: (i) the inner cell mass (ICM), which gives rise to the embryo tissues, or the inner cells of the morula, and (ii) the surrounding cells, which form the external cell mass (trophectoderm, TE), which contributes to the formation of the placenta. The blastocyst's metabolism occurs in two distinct locations: in trophectoderm (TE) cells, where glucose intake occurs and half is converted to lactate, and in ICM cells, where glycolysis occurs (Schoenwolf et al., 2020; Gardner, 2001).

Compaction

At about the third cleavage, a significant increase in RNA and protein synthesis occurs. The embryo undergoes compression called compaction to form a morula. Transcription takes place first in the zygote genome, and this process is calcium dependent. With compaction, the blastomeres come back to back in a printed form. It begins to form a connection between each blastomere and the boundaries of the blastomeres disappear. Tight junctions and desmosomes, composed of various integral and peripheral proteins such as cingulin (ZO-1) and occludin, are responsible for adhesion between blastomeres and form an epithelial barrier between cells that hinders permeability. Gap junction-type connections provide electrical flow and various molecule conduction between blastomeres (Elder & Dale, 2020; Sontakke, 2018).

Cavitation

A second morphological change, known as cavitation, occurs between the 16 and 32 cell stage. The first cell group to differentiate after genome activation in the zygote is the trophectoderm. This group of polarized blastomeres becomes compact and forms a complex that can carry ions and water. Fluid filling then takes place in the blastocoelic space.

In this process, activation of the Na+-K+ ATPase enzyme in trophectoderm cells is the first step. Active transport of sodium to the center of the embryo takes place. This event is followed by the passive osmotic movement of water into the blastocelic space. Trophectoderm cells sit on a basement membrane. It forms a continuous line between trophectoderm cells of tight junctions. All of these formations constitute the main mechanism that prevents the leakage of small ions in the blastocelic fluid.

Blastocele is very important for the differentiation of ICM. The inner cell matrix contains many proteins and protein factors for cell differentiation and proliferation. Apoptosis can occur in ICM, mainly to remove unsuitable or faulty cells. Trophectoderm cells eventually give rise to the placenta and extraembryonic tissue (Schoenwolf et al., 2020).

Blastocyst Formation and Development

Shortly after the morula enters the uterus (approximately 4 days after fertilization), uterine fluid passes through ZP to form the blastocystic cavity inside the morula. As a result, the blastomeres are divided into two parts: (i) trophoblasts, which are the thin outer cells that make up the embryonic portion of the placenta, and (ii) embryoblasts, which are a distinct group of blastomeres that make up the embryo's primordium. The resulting structure is now termed a blastocyst. At this stage, the trophoblast creates the blastocyst's wall, while the embryoblast extends into the hollow. After the blastocyst floated in the uterine fluid for about two days, ZP degenerates. The loss of ZP allows for a rapid increase in the size of the blastocyst. About six days after fertilization, the blastocyst is anchored to the endometrial epithelium (Figure 4.3) (Moore et al., 2020).

Blastocyst Expansion and Hatching

In the early stages of development, the embryo is surrounded by ZP to hold the cells together and act as a protective barrier. Monozygotic (single) twins may emerge if ICM is divided at this early stage. On day 5, the blastocyst projects out of the clear ZP by enzymatically drilling a hole and squeezing out, resulting in hatching. In humans, the early blastocyst (day 4/5) initially shows little size elevation, while it does have a cavity that accounts for 30% of its volume. Subsequently, it increases during the next 1 to 2 days (days 5 to 6) by active fluid build-up in the central blastocoelic cavity, accounting for 70% of embryo volume (Huang et al., 2016).

A strong association with viability and implantation was observed, with strong contractions occurring during blastocyst expansion and subsequent hatching. Therefore, blastocyst expansion and more prominent hatching are the guiding steps in embryo selection (Elder & Dale, 2020).

Cell Differentiations

ICM cells in the interior of the morula maintain their pluripotency. The external ones, in contrast, evolve into extraembryonic trophectoderm, which will help the embryo grow in the uterus and influence the pregastrulation embryonic pattern via signaling processes. TE cells are involved in the formation of fluid accumulation in the blastocoele.

However, the role of TE cells in the early stages of the blastocyst stage is unclear. TE cells transform into extraembryonic tissue, such as the placenta, with sequential changes. Moreover, TE cells are believed to play a role in the process of implantation of the blastocyst into the uterus. TE cells also produce cellular factors involved in the embryo implantation process. Along with the actin microfilament stabilizing protein ezrin, the $Ca2+$-dependent E-cadherin molecule is involved in the formation of blastomere polarity during division. Cdx2 transcription factor is necessary for the attachment of outer cells to the trophoblast (Elder & Dale, 2020).

Conclusion

Both male and female gametes undertake an extraordinarily long and complex journey involving biochemical, behavioral, endocrine, physiological, and genetic components. The purpose of this whole journey is to reach the fertilization stage and complete the embryological stage after fertilization perfectly. Oogenesis, spermiogenesis, embryogenesis, implantation, and fetal development mechanisms represent an embryological summary of all these stages. Some steps of this process can go wrong and result in infertility. Assisted reproductive technology (ART) has enabled new research in in vitro preimplantation of the transition from gametogenesis to the blastocyst stage. Total fertilization failures (TFF) of ICSI (intracytoplasmic sperm injection) are one of the consequences of ART. This has led embryologists to study the physiology of oocyte activation, the electrical properties of gamete membranes, and ion currents. Understanding the genesis and development of human blastocysts, as well as their physiology and morphology, will help to uncover the cause of the high rate of embryo implantation failure.

References

Barroso, G., Valdespin, C., Vega, E., Kershenovich, R., Avila, R., Avendaño, C., & Oehninger, S. (2009). Developmental sperm contributions: fertilization and beyond. *Fertility and sterility, 92*(3), 835-848. https://doi.org/10.1016/j.fertnstert.2009.06.030

Dale, B. (2018). *Fertilization The Beginning of Life.* Cambridge University Press. https://doi.org/10.1017/9781316650318.008

Dozortsev, D., Sutter, P. D., & Dhont, M. (1994). Fertilization and early embryology: Behaviour of spermatozoa in human oocytes displaying no or one pronucleus after intracytoplasmic sperm injection. *Human Reproduction, 9*(11), 2139-2144. https://doi.org/10.1093/oxfordjournals.humrep.a138406

Elder, K., & Dale, B. (2020). Gametes and Gametogenesis. In *In-Vitro Fertilization* (pp. 53–76). Cambridge University Press. https://doi.org/10.1017/9781108611633.004.

Forman H, Fissore R (2015) Fertilization in mammals. In: Plant TM, Zelezni AJ (eds.) *Knobil and Neill's Physiology of Reproduction* (4th ed., pp. 149–196). Elsevier, New York.

Gardner, D. K., Weissman, A., Howles, C. M., & Shoham, Z. (Eds.). (2020). *Textbook of assisted reproductive techniques: Clinical perspectives* (4th edt). CRC Press.

Gardner, R. L. (2001). Specification of embryonic axes begins before cleavage in normal mouse development. *Development, 128*(6), 839-847. https://doi.org/10.1242/dev.128.6.839

Gur Y, Breitbart H (2006) Mammalian sperm translate nuclear-encoded proteins by mitochondrial-type ribosomes. *Genes and Development, 20*(4), 411–416. https://doi.org/10.1101/gad.367606

Holubcová, Z., Howard, G., & Schuh, M. (2013). Vesicles modulate an actin network for asymmetric spindle positioning. *Nature cell biology, 15*(8), 937-947. https://doi.org/10.1038/ncb2802

Huang, T. T. F., Chinn, K., Kosasa, T., Ahn, H. J., & Kessel, B. (2016). Morphokinetics of human blastocyst expansion in vitro. *Reproductive BioMedicine Online, 33*(6), 659-667. https://doi.org/10.1016/j.rbmo.2016.08.020

Johnson, M. H. (2018). *Essential Reproduction* (8th ed.). Wiley Blackwell.

Jones, K. T. (2005). Mammalian egg activation: from Ca2+ spiking to cell cycle progression. *Reproduction, 130*(6), 813-823. https://doi.org/10.1530/rep.1.00710

Moore, K., Persaud, T. V., & Torchia, M. (2020). *Before We are Born* (10th ed.). Elsevier.

Schoenwolf, G. C., Bleyl, S. B., Brauer, P. R., & Francis-West, P. H. (2020). *Larsen's human embryology E-book* (5th ed.). Elsevier Health Sciences.

Sontakke, Y. (2018). *Textbook of Human Embryology with Clinical Cases and 3D Illustrations* (1st ed.). CBS Publishers & Distributors.

Stricker, S. A. (1999). Comparative biology of calcium signaling during fertilization and egg activation in animals. *Developmental biology, 211*(2), 157-176. https://doi.org/10.1006/dbio.1999.9340

Tesarik, J., & Kopecny, V. (1989). Developmental control of the human male pronucleus by ooplasmic factors. *Human Reproduction, 4*(8), 962-968. https://doi.org/10.1093/oxfordjournals.humrep.a137021

Wakai, T., Vanderheyden, V., Yoon, S. Y., Cheon, B., Zhang, N., Parys, J. B., & Fissore, R. A. (2012). Regulation of inositol 1, 4, 5-trisphosphate receptor function during mouse oocyte maturation. *Journal of cellular physiology, 227*(2), 705-717. https://doi.org/10.1002/jcp.22778

Wassarman, P. M. (2014). Sperm protein finds its mate. *Nature, 508*(7497), 466-467. https://doi.org/10.1038/nature13227

Wassarman PM, Liu C, Litscher ES (1996) Constructing the mammalian egg zona pellucida: some new pieces of an old puzzle. *Journal of Cell Science, 109*, 2001–2004. https://doi.org/10.1242/jcs.109.8.2001

Wassarman, P. M. (1990). Profile of a mammalian sperm receptor. *Development, 108*(1), 1-17. https://doi.org/10.1242/dev.108.1.1

Yanagida, K. (2004). Complete fertilization failure in ICSI. *Human Cell, 17*(4), 187-193. https://doi.org/10.1111/j.1749-0774.2004.tb00042.x

Yanagimachi, R. (1981). Mechanisms of fertilization in mammals. In *Fertilization and embryonic development in vitro* (pp. 81-182). Springer, Boston, MA. https://doi.org/10.1007/978-1-4684-4016-4_6

Chapter 5

Implantation and Early Stages of Fetal Development

Damla Gül Fındık, MD*
Department of Medicine, Bilecik Şeyh Edebali University, Bilecik, Turkiye

Abstract

Embryo implantation is a three-step process; apposition, adhesion, and invasion. The physiological and molecular pathways during the implantation process are complex and highly organized. The complex multisteps of implantation are initiated when the developing embryo first makes contact with the epithelial cells of the uterus. The outcome of pregnancy depends on the implantation of the embryo in a receptive endometrium. After successful implantation, the embryonic period that begins with fertilization ends in the 9th week. The fetal period begins at the beginning of the 9th week. During this period, the growth rate of the head has slowed compared to the rest of the body. Fetal length growth occurs especially in the third, fourth, and fifth months; and weight gain begins to be mainly observed in the last two months of pregnancy. In this headline, the previously mentioned stages are comprehensively discussed.

Key Words: Embryo, Fetus, Implantation

* Corresponding Author's E-mail: damla.findik@bilecik.edu.tr

In: Holistic Approach to Assisted Reproductive Technology
Editor: Kenan Demir and Rümeysa Yılmaz Göç
ISBN: 979-8-89113-017-3
© 2023 Nova Science Publishers, Inc.

Introduction

Implantation

Implantation of the Blastocyst

On the 4th day of pregnancy, the blastocyst is free in the fluid that fills the uterine cavity. During this period, as a result of estrogen and progesterone derived from ovarian cells, the uterine receptivity required for implantation and increased vascular permeability are generated at the implantation site (Kierszenbaum & Tres, 2020). On the 5th day of pregnancy, the blastocyst that separated from the zona pellucida attaches from the embryoblast pole to the upper and posterior wall of the uterus via trophoblasts (Kierszenbaum & Tres, 2020; Kim & Kim, 2017).

Implantation Window

Uterine sensitivity to implantation can be observed in three separate phases (Table 5.1) (Cha et al., 2012; Namiki et al., 2018; Sehring et al., 2022);

1. Prereceptive phase: It appears in the first 7 days after ovulation in the early luteal phase.
2. Receptive phase: Endometrial receptivity is triggered in the midluteal phase (~7-10 days after ovulation). Only during the receptive phase is it possible for embryos to implant in the uterine epithelium. This specific period of time is called the implantation window. The genes comprised in the endometrial receptivity process are Homeobox (HOX), Forkhead box O1 (FOXO1), Bone morphogenetic protein 2 (BMP2) and Wnt.
3. Refractory phase: The uterus proceeds into this phase in the remaining part of the cycle (late luteal phase), until menstruation.

Table 5.1 Phases of uterine sensitivity to implantation (Cha et al., 2012).

Uterine Phases	Duration
Pre-receptive phase	7 days after ovulation
Receptive phase (Implantation window)	~7-10 days after ovulation
Refractory phase	Until menstruation

Stages of Implantation

Implantation consists of three stages (Kierszenbaum & Tres, 2020; Kim & Kim, 2017);

1. Apposition: The blastocyst contacts the implantation site. Unstable adhesion of the blastocyst to the endometrium is called apposition.
2. Adhesion: Trophoblasts at the blastocyst embryoblast pole attach to the receptive endometrial epithelium with stable adhesion.
3. Invasion: Invasive trophoblast cells cross the endometrial epithelial basement membrane and invade the endometrial stroma.

Implantation is a pro-inflammatory reaction that involves increased vascular permeability at the attachment site through prostaglandins derived from cyclooxygenase (COX) (Kim & Kim, 2017). During apposition, this generalized stromal edema leads to the interaction of numerous pinopodes on the receptive endometrium with microvilli on the outer surface of the blastocyst (Figure 5.1) (Paul et al., 2019). Protrusions of the apical surface of uterine epithelial cells called pinopodes are partial morphometric indicators of uterine receptivity

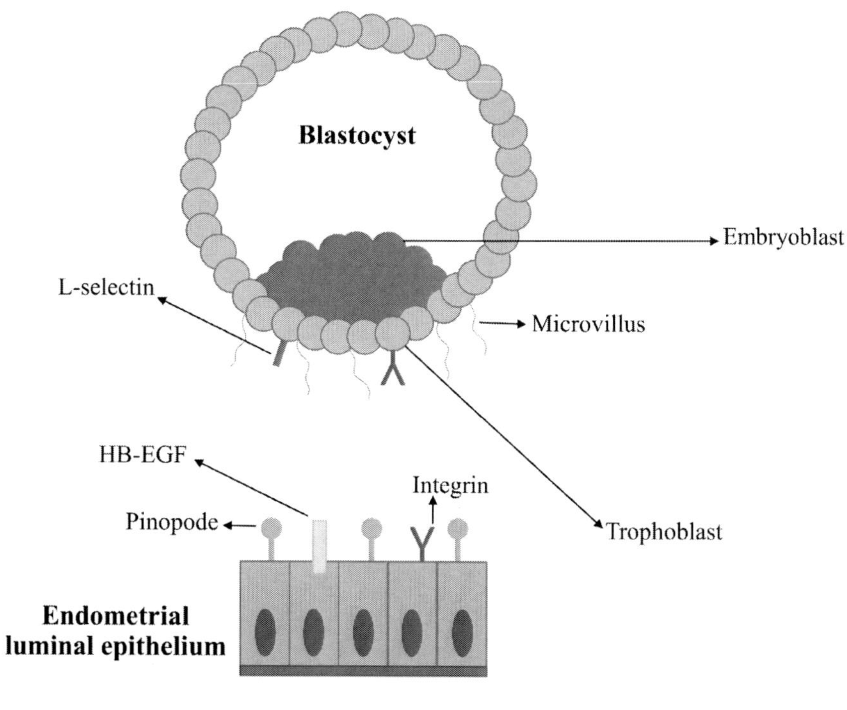

Figure 5.1 Schematic diagram of communication between the blastocyst and the endometrium (Created by the author).

(Murphy, 2000). Pinopodes are progesterone dependent and actively re-absorb the fluid of the uterine secretory phase (Elder & Dale, 2020). The embryo rolls along the uterine lumen through an interaction between L-selectin on the blastocyst and oligosaccharide ligands within the uterine glycocalyx to determine the implantation site. Current researches suggest that mucin (MUC1) is a barrier to implantation. Local depletion of MUC1 allows appropriate apposition and attachment of the embryo (Sehring et al., 2022). The embryo overcomes the glycocalyx barrier through enzymatic cleavage of extracellular glycoproteins or binding of receptors expressed by the embryo and subsequent cleavage of mucins (Elder & Dale, 2020). After apposition, the adhesion stage is a firm attachment mediated by integrins (Sehring et al., 2022). At this stage, osteopontin also regulates embryo implantation through binding $\alpha v\beta 3$ integrin (Davidson & Coward, 2016). Furthermore, heparin-binding EGF-like growth factor (HB-EGF) expressed by the receptive endometrium is a significant molecule for embryo-uterus communication. HB-EGF interacts with ErbB1 and/or ErbB4 on the blastocyst (Cao et al., 2020). The embryo adheres to the endometrium on the 6th to 7th day after ovulation (Elder & Dale, 2020). In the implantation process, leukemia inhibitory factor (LIF) is an important cytokine that is responsible for promoting the development of pinopode, supporting blastocyst attachment, invasion, and decidualization (Mrozikiewicz et al., 2021). During invasion, trophoblast cells penetrate the endometrial epithelium and invade the underlying endometrial stroma to reach maternal blood vessels (Ochoa-Bernal & Fazleabas, 2020). Trophoblast cells secrete matrix metalloproteinases (MMPs) to cleave the extracellular matrix (Ashary et al., 2018; Staun-Ram & Shalev, 2005).

Trophoblast Differentiation

After implantation, trophoblasts differentiate into two cell layers (2nd week) (Elder & Dale, 2020; Kierszenbaum & Tres, 2020);

1. Cytotrophoblasts: An inner layer with mitotically active mononucleated cells.
2. Syncytiotrophoblasts: An outer layer with multinucleated cells.

Multinucleated syncytiotrophoblasts are formed by fusion of villous cytotrophoblasts (VCT) (Tarrade et al., 2001). The proteases released by the syncytiotrophoblast erode the uterine blood vessels and generate lacunae filled with maternal blood within the cell mass of the syncytiotrophoblast. In this process, human chorionic gonadotropin (hCG) released by the syncytiotrophoblast ensures the

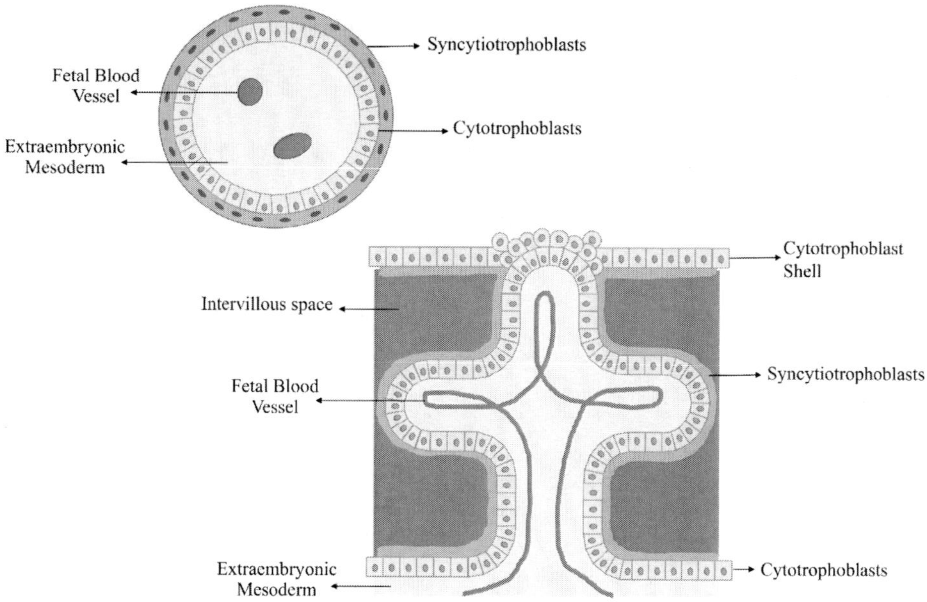

Figure 5.2 A schematic diagram of the tertiary villi with the transverse section of the structure (Created by the author).

continuity of the corpus luteum structure. The first step in the development of placental chorionic villi is primary villi formation (Day 10-13). The primary villus is a protrusion of cytotrophoblasts in the outer layer of the syncytiotrophoblast. In the early third week (Day 16), extraembryonic mesoderm into the primary villi forms the secondary villi structure (Kierszenbaum & Tres, 2020). At the end of the third week, tertiary villi consist of extraembryonic mesoderm, villous capillary, cytotrophoblast, and syncytiotrophoblast are formed (Figure 5.2) (Sadler, 2012). Further development of lacunae leads to the creation and expansion of intervillous space (Haram et al., 2020). At the tips of the villi, cytotrophoblasts make contact with the endometrium and extend laterally to form the cytotrophoblast shell (Elder & Dale, 2020). During pregnancy, villi extravillous cytotrophoblasts (EVCT) invade the maternal decidua and remodel spiral arteries to ensure vasodilation and supply adequate nutrients to the embryo (Figure 5.3) (Pollheimer et al., 2014). For remodeling, EVCT replaces the endothelium and tunica media of spiral arteries (Kierszenbaum & Tres, 2020). Cytotrophoblasts convert their adhesion molecules from epithelial cell type to vascular endothelial cell type. This transformation is necessary for the invasion of uterine spiral arterioles by cytotrophoblasts (Fisher, 2015). Invading cytotrophoblasts express endothelial adhesion markers such as VE-cadherin and $\alpha V\beta 3$ integrin (James et al., 2010). In pregnancy, physiological changes in spiral arteries extend to the myometrium (Burton et al., 2009). The invasion of

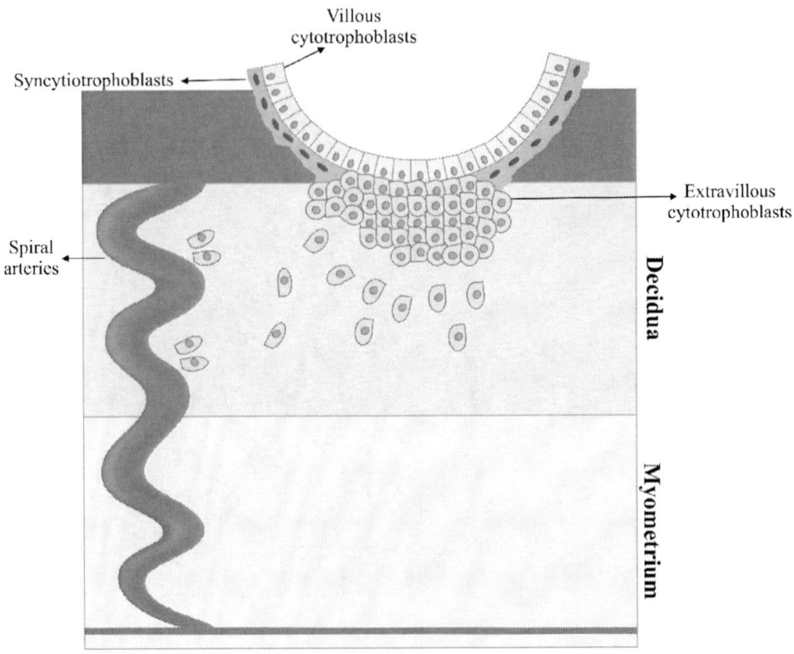

Figure 5.3 A schematic diagram of extravillous cytotrophoblast invasion (Created by the author).

EVCT is controlled by the tissue inhibitor of metalloprotease-1 (TIMP-1) and the type 1 plasminogen activator inhibitor (PAI-1) (Ye et al., 2017).

Decidualization

After implantation, the uterine stromal cells surrounding the implanting embryo transform into decidua through a process called decidualization (Ashary et al., 2018; Ochoa-Bernal & Fazleabas, 2020). The decidualized endometrium protects the embryo from maternal immunological rejection and provides nutritional support (Okada et al., 2018). Decidualization is triggered in the midsecretory phase of each menstrual cycle through elevated progesterone levels (Ochoa-Bernal & Fazleabas, 2020). In this process, elongated fibroblast-like mesenchymal cells in the uterine stroma differentiate into rounded epithelioid-like cells (Okada et al., 2018). Decidua include decidual stromal cells, macrophages, lymphocytes, and decidual natural killer (dNK)/ uterine natural killer (uNK) cells (Ochoa-Bernal & Fazleabas, 2020; Sojka, 2020). Maternal cells and fetal cells with foreign antigens coexist in the placental bed through immune regulation of the fetomaternal interface. In this immune tolerance, the human leukocyte antigen G (HLA-G) molecules that are expressed by EVCT are recognized by inhibitory receptors on dNK cells. This recognition leads to the inhibition of the cytotoxic effects of dNK in fetal trophoblast cells (Li et al., 2020). Whereas most somatic cells express HLA-A, HLA-B, HLA-C, and HLA-E, human trophoblast cells never express HLA-A and HLA-B (Elder & Dale, 2020). Furthermore, increased polarization ratios of Th2/Th1, Treg/Th17 and M2/M1 are significant mechanisms for maternal immune tolerance (Li et al., 2020).

Decidua regions are named according to their association with the implantation site (Bailey, 2014);
Decidua basalis: It lies between the embryo and stratum basalis of the uterus.
Decidua capsularis: It separates the embryo from the uterine cavity.
Decidua parietalis: It is the decidual part that remains in the uterine cavity.

Fetal Development

Prenatal development is divided into two periods. The embryonic period begins with fertilization and ends after 8 weeks (Tawfik et al., 2016). After an embryonic period, organogenesis is substantially complete (Carlson, 2018). The fetal period begins at the beginning of the 9th week and continues until delivery (Tawfik et al., 2016). This period is the time of growth and physiological maturation of organ systems (Carlson, 2018).

Estimation of the Fetal Age

Both crown-rump length (CRL) and crown-heel length (CHL) are used extensively during the fetal period for accurate determination of fetal age (O'rahilly & Müller, 1986). From the point of view of gestational age, the timeframe of the fetal period covers the 11th week and the following week. Gestational age (menstrual age) is the time elapsed between the first day of the last menstrual period and the day of delivery (Engle, 2004). CRL is the most crucial parameter for determining gestational age in the first trimester (Table 5.2) (Butt et al., 2014). The measurement of CRL is indicated as the minimum distance between the peak points of the cranial and caudal end in the straightest possible position of the fetus (Wladimiroff & Eik-Nes, 2009). In the second and third trimesters, gestational age is estimated using a combination of multiple biometric parameters (i.e., biparietal diameter, head circumference, abdominal circumference, and femur length). The biparietal diameter (BPD) is the axial plane through a symmetrical calvarium (Butt et al., 2014). Head circumference

Table 5.2 Crown rump length (CRL) during early pregnancy (Wladimiroff & Eik-Nes, 2009).

Gestational Age (week)	CRL (mm)
5	0-3
6	4-8
7	9-14
8	15-22
9	23-31
10	32-41
11	43-54

is commonly calculated from BPD and occipitofrontal diameter (OFD) using the formula for an ellipse (Wladimiroff & Eik-Nes, 2009). The abdominal circumference (AC) is the axial plane at the level of the bifurcation of the portal vein and the stomach (Butt et al., 2014).

Fetal Weight Estimation

There is no universally accepted formula for estimating fetal weight (Hammami et al., 2018). Current regression models to evaluate fetal weight are based on different combinations of ultrasound fetal biometrics (Melamed et al., 2009).

Developmental Changes during the Fetal Period

Fetal length growth occurs especially in the third, fourth and fifth months; and weight gain starts to be mainly observed in the last 2 months of pregnancy (Sadler, 2012). Ossification is first induced in the occipital bone and the primary centers of ossification of the head and long bones appear at the end of the 12th week (Moore et al., 2016; Wladimiroff & Eik-Nes, 2009). At the 9th week, the growth rate of the head, which is approximately equal to half of the fetus's CRL decreases. At the end of 12 weeks, the upper limbs reach their relative lengths and the CRL is almost doubled. The lower limbs are still slightly shorter than their final relative lengths (Moore et al., 2016). External genitalia also differentiate in the period between the 9th week and the 12th week (Sadler, 2012). Physiological umbilical herniation, which started in the 6th week, returns to the abdomen at the end of the 10th week (Conze et al., 2007).

By the 16th week, eyes facing the anterior lateral begin to localize anteriorly, and low-set ears approach their exact position (Moore et al., 2016). All movements with respect to the newborn have appeared in the fetus between the 16th and 18th weeks. At the end of the fourth month, the fetus begins activity periods, followed by periods of inactivity. Awareness of fetal movements by the mother starts at this time (Carlson, 2018).

Lanugo is the first silky and fine hair on the surface of the fetal skin in the 18th gestational week. After approximately the 33rd gestational week, lanugo starts to disappear. Vernix caseosa is a protective biofilm that covers the fetal skin. Vernix caseosa consists of secretions from the sebaceous glands and dead epidermal cells. The maturation of the sebaceous glands with the hair duct occurs when the first lanugo appears on the skin surface (Bystrova, 2009).

During the sixth month, the fetus lacks underlying connective tissue. Therefore, the skin is reddish and wrinkled. During the last 2 months, the fetus has developed well-rounded contours as a result of the deposition of subcutaneous fat (Sadler, 2012).

Digestive and Renal Function

Swallowing becomes detectable in the 10-11th gestational week. The swallowing reflex is followed by gastric peristalsis in the 12th week. The greenish meconium with shed intestinal cells, swallowed lanugo hairs, and secretions begins to fill the lower ileum and colon by the end of the fourth month. Non-coordinated precursor sucking movements at 16-18th weeks mature after the 36th week (Carlson, 2018).

Mesonephric kidneys are formed in the late 4th week and produce a small amount of very dilute urine (Carlson, 2018; Joseph & Vezina, 2018). After metanephric kidney formation, the mesonephros degenerates at the end of the third month. The tubules of the metanephric kidneys become functional between the 9th and 12th weeks of pregnancy (Carlson, 2018).

Pulmonary Function

Fetal breathing movements are detectable as early as 10 weeks of gestation (Plosa & Guttentag, 2018). The synthesis of pulmonary surfactant by type II alveolar cells begins in the 20th week. Stored surfactant is secreted after the 28-30th weeks (Kültürsay et al., 2014). The surfactant reduces surface tension, therefore, ensuring a reduction in the required inspiration force and preventing alveolar collapse during expiration (Carlson, 2018).

The summarized developmental changes during the fetal period are represented in Table 5.3.

Table 5.3 Developmental changes during the fetal period (Callahan, 2016; Moore et al., 2016).

9-12 weeks	
Length / weight	5 cm / 8 g - 8 cm / 45 g
Large head (Half of the fetus's CRL) Spontaneous fetal movements Eritrocytes production by liver/spleen The fetal heart sound can be detected by Doppler (10-12th week). Visible intestinal loops in the proximal end of the umbilical cord until the 11th week The well-formed and broad face Bile secretion Urine production Genital differentiation Developed urogenital duct Long limbs / legs are still shorter than arms Ossification begins in the skull and long bone / Primary ossification centers Eyes are widely spaced and fused The ears are set low and the progression into an adult shape starts Thyroid secretion Lymphoid development in the thymus	
13-16 weeks	
Length / weight	14 cm / 200 g (16th week)
Fetal movements Thumb sucking Embranchment of bronchial tubes Hard and soft palates Swallow amniotic fluid Meconium production Liver / Pancreas Secretions Gastric / intestinal glands Primordial follicles containing oogonia/primitive oocytes More muscle tissue development Ossification of the skeleton The lower limbs are longer than the upper limbs Lanugo hairs Transparent fetal skin Anteriorly facing eyes Fully formed, upward-migrated ears	

(Continued)

Table 5.3 (Continued)

17-20 weeks	
Length / weight	19 cm / 435 – 465 g (20th week)
Myelination of the spinal cord begins Primitive respiratory-type movements Terminal sacs are developing in the lung Sucking movements Peristalsis Subcutaneous brown fat / Fetal skin is less transparent Head hair / Eyebrows / Eyelashes Nails Awareness of fetal movements by the mother Vernix caseosa Bone marrow function	
21-24 weeks	
Length / weight	28 cm / 780 g (24th week)
Reflex hand grip Startle reflex Alveoli of lungs Surfactant secretion The testes descend to the inguinal ring Eyes open Sense of hearing Red and wrinkled skin	
25-29 weeks	
Length / weight	35-38 cm / 1200 g
Ended erythrocyte production by the spleen Lungs are capable of breathing air The testes descend into the scrotal sac Small labia majora / prominent clitoris Accumulation of adipose tissue	
30-34 weeks	
Length / weight	40 cm / 2000 g
Fingernails extend to the ends of the fingertips	
35-38 weeks	
Length / weight	46 cm / 2600 g (Term fetus 50 cm / 3000-3600 g)
Lanugo disappears Well-developed labia major Testes in the scrotum or palpable in the inguinal canal Fingernails extend beyond the fingertips	

Conclusion

In this section, fundamental points of embryo implantation and the main approaches for analyzing fetal parameters in the literature are discussed. In an orderly manner, the main points can be summarized as follows. The overall procedure related to ovarian-derived estrogen and progesterone before implantation results in uterine receptivity which is required for implantation and increased vascular permeability. The blastocyst begins to implant from the embryoblast pole to the upper and posterior walls of the uterus via trophoblasts. Implantation consists of three stages; apposition, adhesion, and invasion. After the embryonic period, the fetal period starts in the 9th week and is characterized by rapid growth. At the 9th week, the growth rate of the head, which makes up about half of the fetus's CRL decreases. Although CRL is the most crucial parameter to determine gestational age in the first trimester, gestational age is estimated through a combination of multiple biometric parameters in the second and third trimesters (i.e., biparietal diameter, head circumference, abdominal circumference, and femur length).

References

Ashary, N., Tiwari, A., & Modi, D. (2018). Embryo implantation: war in times of love. *Endocrinology*, 159(2), 1188-1198. https://doi.org/10.1210/en.2017-03082

Bailey, J. (2014). The placenta. In: Marshal J and Raynor M. (Eds.), *Myles Textbook for Midwives* (16th ed.) (pp. 101-123). Edinburgh: Churchill Livingstone.

Burton, G., Woods, A., Jauniaux, E., & Kingdom, J. (2009). Rheological and physiological consequences of conversion of the maternal spiral arteries for uteroplacental blood flow during human pregnancy. *Placenta*, 30(6), 473-482. https://doi.org/10.1016/j.placenta.2009.02.009

Butt, K., Lim, K., Bly, S., Cargill, Y., Davies, G., Denis, N., Hazlitt, G., Morin, L., Ouellet, A., & Salem, S. (2014). Determination of gestational age by ultrasound. *Journal of Obstetrics and Gynaecology Canada*, 36(2), 171-181. https://doi.org/10.1016/s1701-2163(15)30664-2

Bystrova, K. (2009). Novel mechanism of human fetal growth regulation: a potential role of lanugo, vernix caseosa and a second tactile system of unmyelinated low-threshold C-afferents. *Medical Hypotheses*, 72(2), 143-146. https://doi.org/10.1016/j.mehy.2008.09.033

Callahan, L. (2016). Fetal and Placental Development and Functioning. In S. Mattson, JE. Smith (Eds.), *Maternal-Newborn Nursing* (pp. 37-62). Elsevier.

Cao, D., Liang, J., Feng, F., Shi, S., Tan, Q., & Wang, Z. (2020). MiR-183 impeded embryo implantation by regulating Hbegf and Lamc1 in mouse uterus. *Theriogenology*, 158, 218-226. https://doi.org/10.1016/j.theriogenology.2020.09.005

Carlson, B. M. (2018). *Human embryology and developmental biology* (6th ed.). Elsevier Health Sciences.

Cha, J., Sun, X., & Dey, S. K. (2012). Mechanisms of implantation: strategies for successful pregnancy. *Nature medicine*, 18(12), 1754-1767. https://doi.org/10.1038/nm.3012

Conze, J., Prescher, A., Schlächter, M., & Schumacher, O. (2007). The umbilical hernia. In V. Schumpelick & R.J. Fitzgibbons (Eds.), *Recurrent Hernia* (pp. 359-364). Springer. https://doi.org/10.1007/978-3-540-68988-1_35

Davidson, L. M., & Coward, K. (2016). Molecular mechanisms of membrane interaction at implantation. *Birth Defects Research Part C: Embryo Today: Reviews*, 108(1), 19-32. https://doi.org/10.1002/bdrc.21122

Elder, K., & Dale, B. (2020). Implantation and Early Stages of Fetal Development. In Elder, K., & Dale, B (Eds.), *In-Vitro Fertilization* (pp. 120-134). Cambridge: Cambridge University Press. https://doi.org/10.1017/9781108611633.007

Engle, W. A. (2004). Age terminology during the perinatal period. *Pediatrics*, 114(5), 1362-1364. https://doi.org/10.1542/peds.2004-1915

Fisher, S. J. (2015). Why is placentation abnormal in preeclampsia? *Am J Obstet Gynecol*, 213(4 Suppl), S115-122. https://doi.org/10.1016/j.ajog.2015.08.042

Hammami, A., Mazer Zumaeta, A., Syngelaki, A., Akolekar, R., & Nicolaides, K. H. (2018). Ultrasonographic estimation of fetal weight: development of new model and assessment of performance of previous models. *Ultrasound in obstetrics & gynecology*, 52(1), 35-43. https://doi.org/10.1002/uog.19066

Haram, K., Mortensen, J. H., Myking, O., Roald, B., Magann, E. F., & Morrison, J. C. (2020). Early development of the human placenta and pregnancy complications. *The Journal of Maternal-Fetal & Neonatal Medicine*, 33(20), 3538-3545. https://doi.org/10.1080/14767058.2019.1578745

James, J. L., Whitley, G. S., & Cartwright, J. E. (2010). Pre-eclampsia: fitting together the placental, immune and cardiovascular pieces. *J Pathol*, 221(4), 363-378. https://doi.org/10.1002/path.2719

Joseph, D. B., & Vezina, C. M. (2018). Male Reproductive Tract: Development Overview. In M. K. Skinner (Eds.), *Encyclopedia of Reproduction* (pp. 248-255). Oxford: Academic Press. https://doi.org/10.1016/B978-0-12-801238-3.64366-0

Kierszenbaum, A. L., & Tres, L. (2020). *Histology and Cell Biology: an introduction to pathology* (5th ed.). Elsevier Health Sciences.

Kim, S. M., & Kim, J. S. (2017). A Review of Mechanisms of Implantation. *Dev Reprod*, 21(4), 351-359. https://doi.org/10.12717/dr.2017.21.4.351

Kültürsay, N., Uygur, Ö., & Yalaz, M. (2014). The use of surfactant in the neonatal period- the known aspects, those still under research and those which need to be investigated further. *Turk Pediatri Ars*, 49(1), 1-12. https://doi.org/10.5152/tpa.2014.963

Li, X., Zhou, J., Fang, M., & Yu, B. (2020). Pregnancy immune tolerance at the maternal-fetal interface. *International Reviews of Immunology*, 39(6), 247-263. https://doi.org/10.1080/08830185.2020.1777292

Melamed, N., Yogev, Y., Meizner, I., Mashiach, R., Bardin, R., & Ben-Haroush, A. (2009). Sonographic fetal weight estimation: which model should be used? *Journal of Ultrasound in Medicine*, 28(5), 617-629. https://doi.org/10.7863/jum.2009.28.5.617

Moore, K. L., Persaud, T. V. N., & Torchia, M. G. (2016). *The developing human: clinically oriented embryology* (10th ed.). Elsevier Health Sciences.

Mrozikiewicz, A. E., Ożarowski, M., & Jędrzejczak, P. (2021). Biomolecular markers of recurrent implantation failure—A review. *International Journal of Molecular Sciences*, 22(18), 10082. https://doi.org/10.3390/ijms221810082

Murphy, C. R. (2000). Understanding the apical surface markers of uterine receptivity: pinopods—or uterodomes? *Human Reproduction*, 15(12), 2451-2454. https://doi .org/10.1093/humrep/15.12.2451

Namiki, T., Ito, J., & Kashiwazaki, N. (2018). Molecular mechanisms of embryonic implantation in mammals: lessons from the gene manipulation of mice. *Reproductive Medicine and Biology*, 17(4), 331-342. https://doi.org/10.1002 %2Frmb2.12103

O'rahilly, R., & Müller, F. (1986). Human growth during the embryonic period proper. In F. Falkner & J.M. Tanner (Eds.), *Human growth* (pp. 245-253). Springer. https://doi.org/10.1007/978-1-4613-2101-9_13

Ochoa-Bernal, M. A., & Fazleabas, A. T. (2020). Physiologic events of embryo implantation and decidualization in human and non-human primates. *International Journal of Molecular Sciences*, 21(6), 1973. https://doi.org/10 .3390/ijms21061973

Okada, H., Tsuzuki, T., & Murata, H. (2018). Decidualization of the human endometrium. *Reproductive Medicine and Biology*, 17(3), 220-227. https://doi .org/10.1002%2Frmb2.12088

Paul, A., Sadek, S. T., & Mahesan, A. M. (2019). The role of microRNAs in human embryo implantation: a review. *Journal of assisted reproduction and genetics*, 36(2), 179-187. https://doi.org/10.1007%2Fs10815-018-1326-y

Plosa, E., & Guttentag, S. H. (2018). 42 - Lung Development. In C. A. Gleason & S. E. Juul (Eds.), *Avery's Diseases of the Newborn* (pp. 586-599.e582). Philadelphia: Elsevier. https://doi.org/10.1016/B978-0-323-40139-5.00042-5

Pollheimer, J., Fock, V., & Knöfler, M. (2014). the ADAM metalloproteinases–novel regulators of trophoblast invasion? *Placenta*, 35, S57-S63. https://doi.org/10 .1016/j.placenta.2013.10.012

Sadler, T. W. (2012). *Langman's medical embryology* (12th ed.). Lippincott Williams & Wilkins.

Sehring, J., Beltsos, A., & Jeelani, R. (2022). Human implantation: The complex interplay between endometrial receptivity, inflammation, and the microbiome. *Placenta*, 117, 179-186. https://doi.org/10.1016/j.placenta.2021.12.015

Sojka, D. K. (2020). Uterine natural killer cell heterogeneity: lessons from mouse models. *Frontiers in immunology*, 11, 290. https://doi.org/10.3389/fimmu.2020 .00290

Staun-Ram, E., & Shalev, E. (2005). Human trophoblast function during the implantation process. *Reproductive Biology and Endocrinology*, 3(1), 1-12. https://doi.org/10.1186/1477-7827-3-56

Tarrade, A., Lai Kuen, R., Malassiné, A., Tricottet, V., Blain, P., Vidaud, M., & Evain-Brion, D. (2001). Characterization of human villous and extravillous trophoblasts isolated from first trimester placenta. *Laboratory investigation*, 81(9), 1199-1211. https://doi.org/10.1038/labinvest.3780334

Tawfik, H. A., Abdulhafez, M. H., Fouad, Y. A., & Dutton, J. J. (2016). Embryologic and Fetal Development of the Human Eyelid. *Ophthalmic Plast Reconstr Surg*, 32(6), 407-414. https://doi.org/10.1097/iop.0000000000000702

Wladimiroff, J. W., & Eik-Nes, S. (2009). *Ultrasound in obstetrics and gynaecology* (1st ed.). Elsevier Health Sciences.

Ye, Y., Vattai, A., Zhang, X., Zhu, J., Thaler, C. J., Mahner, S., Jeschke, U., & von Schönfeldt, V. (2017). Role of Plasminogen Activator Inhibitor Type 1 in Pathologies of Female Reproductive Diseases. *Int J Mol Sci, 18*(8). https://doi.org/10.3390/ijms18081651

Chapter 6

Evaluation and Preparation of the Infertile Couple for couple In Vitro Fertilization

Zercan Kalı, MD*

Department of Obstetrics and Gynceology, Gözde Akademi Hospital Malatya, Turkey

Abstract

Infertility is defined as the absence of pregnancy even though having regular sexual intercourse for at least one year. Infertility affects 15% of couples of reproductive age. In preparations for IVF treatment, male and female factors must be evaluated individually in detail. Correct assessment affects treatment success. Evaluation should begin with the least invasive examinations. An evaluation of physical examination and reproductive, family, and medical story should be done. In the evaluation of female infertility, ovulation existence, function and structure of the genital system of the female should be evaluated. Semen analysis should also be evaluated in a male partner.

Key Words: In Vitro Fertilization, Evaluation, Female infertility, Male infertility

Introduction

Infertility is defined as the absence of pregnancy even though having regular sexual intercourse for at least one year (Vayena et al., 2002). Infertility affects 15% of couples of reproductive age. At the end of the 12th month, 80% of

* Corresponding Author's E-mail: zercankali@Jgmail.com

In: Holistic Approach to Assisted Reproductive Technology
Editor: Kenan Demir and Rümeysa Yılmaz Göç
ISBN: 979-8-89113-017-3
© 2023 Nova Science Publishers, Inc.

couples become pregnant (Gnoth et al., 2003; Wang et al., 2003). Male factor in 30-40% of all infertile couples and female factor in 40-50% detected. Pathologies of both male and female in 20-25% of couples observed together. In 15% of couples, the cause of infertility cannot be identified (unexplained infertility) (Gnoth et al., 2003).

The age range with the best fertility is between the ages of 20-25. There is a relative decrease between the ages of 30-32 and a rapid decline after the age of 40. Couples that should be examined without waiting 1 year are as follows:

- Women over 35 years old.
- Oligo/amenorrheic woman.
- Known or suspected uterine or tube disease or women with endometriosis.
- Abdominal and pelvic surgery women undergoing
- Known or suspected semen abnormality
- Men with a history of urogenital surgery and genital pathological findings
- Men with sexually transmitted disease

Evaluation of Male Infertility

In the evaluation of male infertility, the first examination to be performed is the semen analysis. It should be checked at least twice. There should be a minimum of 4-6 weeks between 2 examinations.3-6 days of sexual abstinence is required. It should be evaluated at the latest within 1 hour in the laboratory. According to the WHO final criteria, the sperm parameters should be as follows.

- Semen volume (ml) 1.5 (1.4-1.7)
- Total sperm count (106) 39 (33-46)
- Sperm concentration (106/ml) 15 (12-16)
- Total motility (PR+NP, %) 40 (38-42)
- Progressive motility (PR, %) 32 (31-34)
- Vitality (viable sperm, %) 58 (55-63)
- Sperm morfology (normal forms, %) 4 (3.0-4.0)
- pH >7.2
- Peroxidase-positive leukocytes (106 per ml) <50
- MAR TEST (Mixed Antiglobulin Reaction) test (%) <50
- Immunobead test (%) <50

If the values are normal according to WHO criteria, a single test should be considered sufficient. If abnormalities occur in the parameters, a further andrological evaluation is required. In the evaluation, first, a detailed anamnesis and physical examination should be performed. Pretesticular, testicular, and post-testicular causes of infertility should be investigated. If necessary, endocrinological, genetic, ultrasonographic and biopsy examinations should be performed. Oligozoospermia (<20 million spermatozoa/mL), asthenozoospermia (<50% motile spermatozoa), and teratozoospermia (<4% normal form).

Often, all three pathologies are seen together and are called OAT syndrome (oligo-astheno-teratozoospermia). Azoospermia is the absence of spermatozoa in standard microscopic examination. If there is severe OAT syndrome, (<1 million spermatozoa/mL), male genital tract obstruction and genetic defect must be investigated.

Although the prevalence of azoospermia in the community is 2%, this rate is 10-20% in the infertile group. The ethology and distribution of male infertility (%) are as follows.

- Sexual factors %1.7
- Urogenital infections %6.6
- Congenital anomalies % 2.1
- Varicocele % 12.3
- Endocrine disorders %0.6
- Immunological factors %3.1
- Other diseases %3.0
- Idiopathic semen disorders 75 (Van der Steeg et al., 2005)

Male infertility is analyzed under 3 main headings anatomically (Van der Steeg et al., 2005).

- <u>Pretesticular causes:</u> Chromosomal (Klinefelter syndrome, Kallman syndrome, Y microdeletion, Cystic Fibrosis), hormonal (hypogonadotropic hypogonadism, hyperprolactinemia), coital (erectile dysfunction, endocrine, neural, ejaculatory insufficiency (psychosexual, drug, surgical) causes are in this group.
- <u>Testicular causes:</u> Congenital (undescended testes, immotile cilia, absence of vas deferens), infection (orchitis), vascular (torsion, varicocele), antispermatogenic drugs (chemotherapy, x-ray), immunological, tumor (germ cell tumors, testicular microlithiasis), idiopathic reasons belong to this group.
- <u>Posttesticular causes:</u> Obstructive (epididymal, vasal) and accessory gland infections are included in this category.

Assessment of Female Interfility

The ethology and distribution of infertility for women are as follows.

- Ovulatory dysfunction ~40%
- Tubal and pelvic pathologies ~40%
- Uncommon causes (uterine, cervical pathologies) ~10%
- Unexplained infertility ~10%

Anamnesis

In anamnesis; infertility period, if any, previously used contraception methods, sexual history, frequency of coitus, if any previous pregnancies, menarche, and menstrual periods since the pattern and character of the menarche cycle, systemic diseases, previous operations, smoking, alcohol, or frequent use drugs, thyroid disease, androgenic skin changes, galactorrhea, presence of pelvic or abdominal pain, dysmenorrhea and dyspareunia, abnormal PAP smear results, family history of early menopause, infertility, and birth with anomalies should be questioned.

If there is a menstrual cycle in 21-25 days, if there is pain and swelling in the abdomen during the ovulation period, it shows that the woman is ovulatory with a probability of 99% (Chinta et al., 2020).

In a meta-analysis; long (32-35 days) and a short (21-27 days) menstrual cycle showed decreased ovarian reserve (Younis et al., 2020). Intermenstrual bleeding indicates problems such as polyps and chronic endometritis. Postcoital bleeding may indicate cervical polyps and cervical dysplasias, if there is menometrorrhagi, bleeding diathesis (Von Willebrand disease, etc.) adenomyosis and fibroid should be investigated. Severe dysmenorrhea dyspareunia and pelvic pain should suggest endometriosis (Lass, 1999).

Physical Examination

The weight and body mass index (BMI) should be determined (normal BMI range: 18.5-25 kg/m2), should be examined. Nodule and tenderness in the thyroid, presence of galactorrhea should be questioned (Wang et al., 2003). Secondary sex should be evaluated first in physical examination. Secondary sex character deficiency may be a sign of hypohypergonadism. Primary amenorrhea, short stature, square-shaped rib cage, may be a sign of Turner syndrome. The evaluation of hirsutismus should be performed with the Ferriman-Gallwey scoring score (Thurston et al., 2019).

Speculum examination should be performed in the pelvic examination. The vagina (in terms of septum, imperferatus of the hymen, Rokitanskty Küster Mayer syndrome) and the cervix (in terms of discharge, congenital cervical pathologies) should be examined in detail. A rectovaginal examination should always be performed.

Ovarian Reserve Test

The ovarian reserve is determined biochemically and sonographically. Biochemical tests are FSH, E2, and inhibin B, which are checked in the early follicular phase. Antimullerian hormone (AMH) measured on any day of the cycle. AMH is a glycoprotein. It is a member of the TGF-beta group. It is released by the preantral and antral follicles. In IVF treatments, the level of AMH is correlated with the number of oocytes to be obtained after OPU. But AMH is insufficient to predict live birth. Antral follicle count is the number of follicules measured in the size of 2-10 mm in USG. Although not a definite criterion, a low AFC <4 is considered as low ovarian reserve. According to medical recommendations, the serum level of FSH (>8.9 IU/L) level in the follicular phase shows a low ovarian reserve (Practice Committee of ASRM, 2020).

Imaging

Transvaginal and abdominal ultrasound helps in the differential diagnosis of uterine, endometrial, and adnexal pathologies. It is also frequently used in ovulation and follicle follow-up (Brannstorm et al., 1998). Uterine anomalies can be detected %16 with USG (Tur-Kaspal et al., 2006). USG is useful in the diagnosis of fibroids, polyps, and adenomyosis. USG is valuable, especially in intramural fibroids that cannot be diagnosed with HSG or hysteroscopy.

Evaluation of Ovulation:

Patients with PKOS (polycystic ovary syndrome), obesity, perimenopause, weight changes, excessive exercise, thyroid dysfunction, have an increased risk of ovulatory dysfunction (Practice Committee of ASRM, 2020). Evaluation of ovulation is also important in treatment. Ovulation tests can be used directly or indirectly divided into 2 groups.

- Direct methods: USG includes direct visualization of ovulation and laparoscopy.
- Indirect methods: Basal body temperature monitoring (Progesterone has a thermogenic effect. In the luteal phase, body temperature rises by 0.5°C and decreases again with the onset of menstruation, and a biphasic curve is formed). From the first day of menstruation, a sublingual regular body temperature measurement every morning gives information on ovulation (Bauman, 1981). Measurements of estrogen and LH (in blood, urine, or saliva), cervical mucus, measurement of midluteal progesterone give a clue. Midluteal progesterone measurement should be performed 1 week before the expected menstrual day. If there is a value greater than 3 ng/ml, it is evidence of ovulation (Wathen et al., 1984). But progesterone measurement changes up to 7 times in hours. Therefore, it cannot be considered as a definitive proof of ovulation. In the past, endometrial biopsies have been used to detect luteal phase defects (Duggan et al., 2001). But today its routine use is not recommended because it is an unnecessary and invasive procedure.

Evaluation of Tubal and Pelvic Pathologies

Methods are hysterosalpingography (HSG), hysteroscopy, son hysterography, and laparoscopy. The first preferred method is HSG. With HSG, both the tubal passage and the uterine cavity can be evaluated. The HSG gives an idea of the internal structure of the proximal, middle and distal tuba. Delayed peritoneal distribution of contrast in hsg suggests fimbria phimosis or peri tubal adhesion (Practice Committee of ASRM, 2020). The sensitivity of HSG for tubal pathologies is 65% and the specificity is 83%. Also, its success in proximal occlusion is less than in distal occlusion (Papaioannou et al., 2004).

If the damage is mild in distal tubal diseases, surgery can be tried. Because pregnancy rates after surgery can increase by 40-50%. However, it is more suitable for patients with severe distal tubal damage, so the choice should be IVF. If it occurs, the risk of ectopic pregnancy will increase by one-fifth. Unable to conceive a pregnancy within two years despite surgery, patients should be referred directly to IVF. Surgery is the most appropriate option for patients with hydrosalfenx because the inflammatory fluid in hydrosalpinx has a toxic effect on the embryo and endometrium. Pregnancy rates decrease 50% and abortion rates increase (Strandell & Lindhard, 2002). In the case of tubal damage, IVF should be the most appropriate option.

It provides very valuable information about intrauterine pathologies such as fibroids, endometrial polyps, intrauterine synechiae, and mullerian defects can also be defined. HSG is useful in determining the size and shape of the uterine cavity.

Diagnostic HSG has therapeutic effects. In subfertile patients, the pregnancy rate increased 3 times after HSG performed with oil-based media (Luttjeboer et al., 2007). Some clinicians also recommend the chlamydia antibody test (CAT) to evaluate the tubal pattern. If the antibody is positive, it means that there is a problem. Additional examinations should be performed.

Endometriosis

The mechanism by which endometriosis causes infertility is not yet clear. It is believed to suppress oocyte development and embryogenesis (Toya et al., 2000). The effect of mild or menial endometriosis on infertility is minimal. In stages 1 and 2 of endometriosis waiting, surgery, clomiphene citrate, or GnRH can be tried in patients with treatment and IUI can be tried. If pregnancy cannot be achieved with these treatments, IVF should be chosen. In stage 3 and 4 endometriosis, the option should be direct IVF.

Hysteroscopy is very useful for detecting intrauterine pathologies detected by HSG. but hysteroscopy cannot provide information on the myometrium, fallopian tube, and ovaries. It can be applied in office conditions. It can also be used as an operative hysteroscopy.

Laparoscopy is the last step in infertility examinations. It is important in the diagnosis and treatment of pelvic adhesions and endometriosis that cannot be diagnosed with other methods. Tubal patency can also be evaluated with transcervical methylene blue administered. It is possible to treat tubal phimosis and adhesions by laparoscopy (Thurston et al., 2019).

Evaluation of Cervical Factor

Cervical mucus examination; post-coital test and antisperm antibody investigation are used only in necessary cases today. It is not recommended in routine infertility research.

A karyotype should be requested in patients with phenotypic features of Turner syndrome, primary amenorrhea, amenorrhea due to hypergonadotropic hypogonodism. Patients with a familial history of early menopause (<40 years) should be evaluated for FragileX premutation. Oligospermia, Y-chromosome microdeletion, and azoospermia karyotyping must be checked for the male (Thurston et al., 2019).

Conclusion

In IVF preparation, TSH, PRL, Anti–HIV, Hbs Ag, Anti–HCV, Blood group, Rubella IgG, Complete blood count tests should be requested. In addition, hormones AMH or FSH, LH, E2 on the second or third day of menstruation are required at any time to assess ovaries reserve. If there is hirsutism, DHEAS, free testosterone hormones are checked. To evaluate ovulation, progesterone should be measured 7 days before menstruation.

Hysterosalpingography (HSG) is an examination in which the tubal factor is evaluated. It also provides information on uterine anomalies. If our IVF indication is male factor, HSG should not be performed routinely.

Semen analysis should be performed at least twice with an interval of 2-3 weeks. This analysis will be a test that illuminates almost half of the problems. If problems are detected in semen analysis, the research is widened. Following the examination by the urologist, scrotal ultrasound, transrectal ultrasound, genetic tests, FSH, LH, T-testosterone, PRL hormones should be evaluated. Anti– HIV, Hbs Ag, Anti–HCV should be requested from every patient who is scheduled for IVF.

References

Bauman, J. E (1981). Basal body temperature: unreliable method of ovulation detectio, *Fertil Steril*, 36(6), 729-733. https://doi.org/10.1016/s0015-0282(16)45916-9

Brannstorm, M., Zackrisson, U., Hagstrom, HG, Josefsson, B., Hellberg, Granberg, Collins, WP., & Bourne, T. (1998). Preovulatuar changes of blood flow in different regions of the human follicle. *Fertil Steril*, 69(3), 435-442. https://doi .org/10.1016/s0015-0282(97)00544

Chinta, P., Rebekah, G., Kunjummen, A., & Kamath, S. M. (2020), Revisiting the role of serum progesterone as a test of ovulation in eumenorrheic subfertile women: a prospective diagnostic accuracy study, *Fertil Steril,* 114(6), 1315-1321. https:// doi.org/10.1016/2020.06.030

Duggan, M.A., Brashert, P., Ostor, A., Scurry, J., Billson, V., Kneafsey,P., & Difrancesco, L. (2001). The accuracy and interobserver reproducibility of endometrial dating, *Pathology,* 33(3), 292-297. https://doi.org/10.1186/s12958-02

Gnoth, C., Godehardt, D., Godehardt, E., Frank-Herrmann, P., & Freundl, G. (2003). Time to pregnancy: results of the German prospective study and impact on the management of infertility. *Hum Reprod*, 18, 1959- 66. https://doi.org/10.1093/ humrep/deg366

Lass, A. (1999) The fertility potential of women with a single ovary. *Hum Reprod Update,* 5(5), 546-50. https://doi.org/10.1093/humupd/5.5.546

Luttjeboer, F., Harada, T., Hughes, E., Johnson, N., Lilford, R., & Mol, B.W. (2007). Tubal flushing for subfertility. *Cochrane Database Syst Rev,* 18(3), CD003718 https://doi:10.1002/14651858.CD003718

Papaioannou, S., Bourdrez, P., Varma, R., Afnan, M., Mol, B.W., & Coomarasamy, A. (2004). Tubal evaluation in the investigation of subfertility: a structured comparison of tests. *BJOG,* 111(12), 1313-21. https://doi.org/10.1111/j.1471-0528.2004.00403

Practice Committee of the ASRM (American Society for Reproductive Medicine) (2020). Testing and interpreting measures of ovarian reserve: a committee opinion. *Fertil Steril,* 114(6), 1151-7. https://doi.org/10.1016/j.fertnstert.2020.09.134

Strandell, A., Lindhard, A. (2002). Why does hydrosalpinx reduce fertility? The importance of hydrosalpinx fluid. *Hum Reprod*, 17, 1141-5. https://doi.org/10.1093/humrep/17.5.1141

Toya, M., Saito, H., Ohta, N., Saito, T., Kaneko, T. & Hiroi, M. (2000). Moderateand severe endometriosis is associated with alterations in the cell cycle of granulosa cells in patients undergoing in vitro fertilization and embryo transfer. *Fertil Steril,* 73, 344-50. https://doi.org/10.1016/s0015-0282(99)00507-5

Thurston, L., Abbara , A. & Dhillo, WS. (2019). Investigation and management of subfertility. *J Clin Pathol.* 72(9), 579-87. https://doi.org/10.1136/jclinpath-2018-205579

Tur-Kaspal, Gal, M., Hartman, M., Hartman, J., Hartman, A. (2006). A prospective evaluation of uterine abnormalities by saline infusion sonohysterography in 1,009 women with infertility or abnormal uterine bleeding. *Fertil Steril,* 86(6), 1731-5 https://doi.org10.1016/j.fertnstert.2006.05.044

Younis, J. S., Iskander, R., Fauser, BCJM. & Izhaki, I. (2020). Does an association exist between menstrual cycle length within the normal range and ovarian reserve biomarkers during the reproductive years? A systematic review and metaanalysis. *Hum Reprod Update,* 26(6), 904-28. https://doi.org/10.1093/humupd/dmaa013

Van der Steeg, JW., Steures, P., Hompes, PG., Eijkemans, MJ., van der Veen, F., & Mol, BW. (2005). Investigation of the infertile couple: a basic fertility work-up performed within 12 months of trying to conceive generates costs and complications for no particular benefit. *Hum Reprod*, 20, 2672 https://doi.org/10.1093/humrep/dei157

Vayena, E., Rowe, P., & Griffin, P. (2002, September 21). Current Practices and Controversies in Assisted Reproduction. Report of a meeting on Medical, Ethical and Social aspects of Assisted Reproduction held at WHO. https://apps.who.int/iris/handle/10665/42576

Wang, X., Chen, C., Wang, L., Chen, D., Guang, W., & French, J. (2003). Conception, early pregnancy loss, and time to clinical pregnancy: a population based prospective study. *Fertil Steril* 79, 577-84 https://doi.org/10.1016/s0015-0282(02)04694-0

Wathen, N.C., Perry, L., Lilford, R.J., & Chard, T. (1984). Interpretation of single progesterone measurement in diagnosis of anovulation and defective luteal phase: observations on analysis of the normal range. *Br Med J (Clin Res Ed)*, 288, 7-9. https://doi.org/10.1136/bmj.288.6410.7

Chapter 7

Evaluation and Management of Male Infertility

Mehmet Cetin[1], MD; Bahadir Sahin[2], MD and Gunes Ozdogan[3], MD*

[1,2]Department of Urology, Marmara University Pendik Training and Research Hospital, Istanbul, Turkiye

[3]Department of Obstetrics and Gynecology, Marmara University Pendik Training and Research Hospital, Istanbul, Turkiye

Abstract

Infertility is defined as the inability to conceive after at least 12 months of unprotected, regular sexual intercourse. It is estimated to affect 8-12 %of couples worldwide, and in approximately 50% of these cases, a male component is the primary or contributing factor. Congenital, acquired, and idiopathic factors can cause male infertility. In 30-50% of infertile men, no cause of infertility can be found. A thorough urological evaluation should be performed on all infertile males to detect and address modifiable risk factors. The medical history and physical examination are important for evaluating male infertility. Semen analysis is the gold standard for research in male infertility. To improve diagnosis and management, advanced diagnostic tests have been developed to examine sperm quality and function. There are various treatment modalities in the treatment of infertile men. The use of assisted reproductive technologies has significantly improved the ability of infertile couples to have children. The purpose of this chapter is to present a comprehensive overview of the evaluation and management of infertility in men.

Key Words: Male infertility, Hypogonadism, Evaluation, Azospermia, Testicular sperm extraction, Varicocele

---

* Corresponding Author's Email: gunesozdogan@gmail.com

In: Holistic Approach to Assisted Reproductive Technology
Editor: Kenan Demir and Rümeysa Yılmaz Göç
ISBN: 979-8-89113-017-3
© 2023 Nova Science Publishers, Inc.

Introduction

According to the WHO, infertility is the inability to become pregnant after at least a year of unprotected, regular sexual activity (Zegers-Hochschild et al., 2017).

Between 8 and 12% of reproductive age couples worldwide are estimated to be affected by infertility. Male factors are exclusively responsible for 20–30% of infertility cases and contribute to 50% of cases in general. However, these numbers vary according to regions of the world (Vander Borght & Wyns, 2018).

Although the development of assisted reproductive techniques has revolutionized male infertility, procedures in the evaluation of infertile patients continue to be important.

Production and distribution of male gametes require a harmonious work between the immune, endocrine, and nervous systems, passage through intact anatomy, appropriate gene expression and chromosomal sequences, and proper postnatal development of all systems (Partin et al., 2021).

Causes

Multiple risk factors and causes contribute to the increased incidence of male infertility, which can be classified as congenital, acquired, and idiopathic (Krausz, 2011).

Male fertility can be impaired as a result of;

- Acquired or congenital urogenital abnormalities
- Gonadotoxic exposure (e.g., radiotherapy or chemotherapy)
- Urogenital tract infections
- Malignancies
- Increased scrotal temperature (e.g., as a consequence of varicocele)
- Endocrine disorders
- Immunological factors, genetic abnormalities
- Genetic abnormalities; (Rowe & World Health, 2000)

Kallmann syndrome, congenital bilateral absence of the vas deferens associated with cystic fibrosis gene mutations, Y chromosome microdeletions that result in spermatogenic defects and chromosomal abnormalities leading to impaired testicular function, are the main known genetic causes of male infertility.

The most common and correctable cause of infertility in men is Varicocele, and its incidence in infertile men is 40% (Gul et al., 2020).

In 30-50% of infertile men, no cause can be found to cause infertility, which is called idiopathic male infertility (Chehab et al., 2015; Jungwirth et al., 2013). Although there is no history of any disease or hormonal disorder that may cause infertility in this group, there are abnormalities in the analysis of semen. It has been suggested that the etiology of idiopathic male infertility may be endocrine disorders due to chronic stress from environmental pollution, oxidative stress, and genetic disorders that have not yet been revealed by tests. Table 7.1 summarizes the main factors associated with male infertility (Nieschlag & Behre, 2001).

Evaluation

Evaluation and treatment of infertility is recommended for couples who cannot conceive naturally despite regular unprotected sexual intercourse for more than 12 months (Medicine, 2015). In couples which the female partner is older than 35 years, this period is six months. Male patients should always be evaluated. The evaluation of male patients should include a reproductive and medical history, physical examination, hormonal evaluation, and semen analysis.

Depending on the clinical characteristics and semen parameters, other investigations (e.g., genetic analysis and imaging) may be required.

Medical History

Obtaining a detailed history is the initial step in evaluating infertility. Whether infertility is primary or secondary, the duration of infertility, previous infertility treatments, and results should be questioned. The presence of erectile dysfunction, the use of lubricants, ejaculation disorder, the frequency and time of intercourse should also be learned.

The onset of puberty, history of undescended testes, testicular torsion or testicular trauma, presence of midline defects, systemic diseases such as diabetes mellitus and multiple sclerosis, urinary infection, presence of sexually transmitted diseases, history of epididymitis/orchitis, tuberculosis, history of febrile disease, renal failure, cancer, chemotherapy, radiotherapy history, orchiopexy, presence of retroperitoneal/pelvic surgery, vasectomy, bladder neck/prostate surgery history, systemic side effects drugs should be

Table 7.1 Causes and associated factors of male infertility and percentage of distribution in 10,469 patients (Nieschlag & Behre, 2001)

Diagnosis	Unselected patients (n = 12,945)	Azoospermic patients (n = 1,446)
All	%100	%11.2
Infertility of a known (possible) cause	42.6%	42.6%
Maldescended testes	8.4	17.2
Varicocele	14.8	10.9
Sperm autoantibodies	3.9	-
Testicular tumor	1.2	2.8
Others	5.0	1.2
Idiopathic infertility	30.0	13.3
Hypogonadism	10.1	16.4
Klinefelter syndrome (47, XXY)	2.6	13.7
XX male	0.1	0.6
Primary hypogonadism of unknown cause	2.3	0.8
Secondary (hypogonadotropic) hypogonadism	1.6	1.9
Kallmann syndrome	0.3	0.5
Idiopathic hypogonadotropic hypogonadism	0.4	0.4
Residual after pituitary surgery	< 0.1	0.3
Late-onset hypogonadism	2.2	-
Constitutional delay of puberty	1.4	-
Others	0.8	0.8
General/systemic disease	2.2	0.5
Cryopreservation due to malignant disease	7.8	12.5
Testicular tumor	5.0	4.3
Lymphoma	1.5	4.6
Leukemia	0.7	2.2
Sarcoma	0.6	0.9
Disturbance of erection/ejaculation	2.4	
Cystic fibrosis (congenital bilateral absence of vas deferens)	0.5	3.0
Obstruction	2.2	10.3
Vasectomy	0.9	5.3
Others	0.8	1.9

questioned. Exposure to gonadotoxins (heavy metal, peptides), smoking, and alcohol habits should also be questioned.

Numerous childhood conditions (e.g., postpubertal mumps orchitis, cryptorchidism, and trauma or testicular torsion) can result in decreased semen quality or testicular atrophy (Lewis & Kaplan, 2009).

Testicular torsion and trauma have been observed to decrease sperm motility by causing the formation of antisperm antibodies, as well as testicular atrophy (Shibahara, 2022).

In the presence of delayed puberty and anosmia, primary hypogonadotropic hypogonadism or Kallmann's syndrome is considered. Early puberty can be secondary to congenital adrenal hyperplasia.

Postpubertal mumbs can cause unilateral or bilateral orchitis, resulting in testicular damage. The effect of prepubertal mumps on fertility was not determined.

Urogenital tract infections of the male (epididymitis, orchitis, urethritis, or prostatitis) can cause male infertility (Kasturi et al., 2009). A common urogenital disease: prostatitis can have harmful effects on sperm parameters (Condorelli et al., 2017).

Among sexually active men older than 35 years, E coli is the predominant pathogen that causes epididymitis. The most common pathogens that cause epididymitis in sexually active men under 35 years of age are Chlamydia trachomatis and Neisseria gonorrhoeae. Leukocytospermia can occur in men with chronic prostatitis or epididymitis ($>1 \times 10^6$ WBC / ml) (Organization, 2021).

Lifestyle factors such as alcohol use, smoking, use of narvotic drug (e.g., opioids, cocaine, anabolic steroids and cannabis), and obesity can be the cause of male infertility (Sansone et al., 2018). Smoking affects sperm concentration, viability, motility, and morphology. It also negatively affects fertility by reducing the penetration potential of sperm. (Sharma et al., 2016) Cannabis inhibits the hypothalamic-pituitary-gonadal axis, spermatogenesis, sperm quality, and adversely affects male fertility (Gundersen et al., 2015).

Previous scrotal, inguinal, or retroperitoneal surgeries may cause obstruction or emission/ejaculation problems. After retroperitoneal lymphadenectomy in testicular cancer, anejaculation or retrograde ejaculation may be seen due to sympathetic nerve damage. Bladder neck surgery or prostatectomy can cause bladder neck insufficiency and cause retrograde ejaculation. Inguinal hernie repair with polypropylene mesh can cause inguinal vasal obstruction and obstructive azoospermia (Shin et al., 2005). Systemic diseases such as diabetes mellitus, multiple sclerosis, and spinal cord injuries can cause ejaculation disorder and erectile dysfunction. In patients with hypothyroidism and hyperthyroidism, both steroid hormone metabolism and sperm quality can be affected. Malignancies may cause disorders in spermatogenesis due to hormonal imbalances and immunological factors. Some malignancies, such as Hodgkin lymphoma disease, testicular germ cell tumors, may cause severe gonadotoxic effects. Testicular tumors can affect spermatogenesis by damaging both the parenchyma and increasing the temperature of the scrotum (Nalesnik et al., 2004). In addition, radiotherapy and chemotherapy may alter spermatogenesis by acting on germ cells (Ståhl et al., 2006).

Phyical Examination

Male infertility may be related to many genetic and systemic conditions; therefore, the general physical examination usually yields clues as to the cause of reproductive disorders. The female and male faces have different morphological features. Facial characteristics may suggest potential androgenization and sex chromosomal disorders (Veleminska et al., 2012).

Physical examination findings such as decreased body hair, absence of temporal baldness, euicoid body structure, and gynecomastia should suggest low serum testosterone, impaired estrogen/testosterone ratio, hyperprolactinemia, endocrinopathies such as adrenal dysfunction, and genetic syndromes such as Klinefelter syndrome (Oates & Lamb, 2009).

The phallus should be the first part of the genital examination. Penile plaques, penile curvature, hypospadias and epispadias, which can alter semen deposition in the vaginal vault, should be examined. The testicular examination should be performed in a non-cold room in both supine and standing positions. The testes should be examined by palpation for consistency, mass, and size.

Testicular sizes should be evaluated by orchidometer, calipers, or ultrasonographic methods. Scrotal ultrasonography can be useful, when the patient's body habitus or scrotal anatomy (dilated epididymis, hydrocele, or inguinal testes) is not suitable for measuring with a Prader orchidometer (Lotti & Maggi, 2015).

Testicular neoplasm is more common in men with infertility, therefore, testicular mass should be excluded (Walsh et al., 2009).

Since most of testicular volume is involved in sperm production, a decrease in testicular volume may indicate impaired spermatogenesis. The testes should be at least 4x3 cm in dimensions or 20 ml in volume for an adult male (Niederberger, 2011).

Examination of the epididymis should pay attention to induration or enlargements. Granulomatous changes in the epididymis can be associated with tuberculosis, sarcoidosis, or the treatment of Bacillus Calmette-Guérin. Small palpable lesions in the epididymis are usually spermatocele and do not often cause obstruction.

Enlargement of the epididymis at palpation may indicate distal obstruction. Bilateral or unilateral nonpalpable vas deferens with hypoplastic epididymis is consistent with vasal agenesis. Vasal agenezis can be related to renal or genetic abnormalities. Scars from previous operations should also be noted during physical examination. The spermatic cords should be examined in the standing and supine positions. Enlargement of the plexus pampiniformis within the spermatic cord is called a varicocele. Varicoceles are graded by size: palpable only by Valsalva maneuver called grade 1, palpable without valsalva maneuver is grade 2, and visible at rest is grade 3. Subclinic varicosele is nonpalpable or invisible varicocele detected by imaging methods (Agarwal et al., 2021). Digital rectal examination should be performed in men with low ejaculate volume. Rectal examination may be helpful in identifying Müller duct cysts and acute prostatitis. Induration and tenderness on examination suggest prostatitis. While the seminal vesicles are normally not palpable, they may become prominent in obstruction.

The sexual practices of the couple should be evaluated, such as the timing of coitus and erectile and ejaculatory function. Ovulation tracking methods should be used to establish that couples are effectively timing coitus. To maximize the possibility of fertilization, sexual intercourse is recommended every 48 hours during ovulation. The high frequency of sexual intercourse causes insufficient sperm storage in the epididymis. Furthermore, very infrequent sexual intercourse can lead to missed potential fertilization time (Tur-Kaspa et al., 1994). Vaginal lubricants, which many couples use, can be spermicidal (Mowat et al., 2014). Fertility-friendly lubricants (e.g., ING, Fertility, Pre-Seed, Spokane, USA, WA), raw egg white, and vegetable oil have the least spermicidal effects. (Agarwal et al., 2008; Goldenberg & White, 1975).

Semen Analysis

According to the World Health Organization (WHO) guidelines, the gold standard research in male infertility is semen analysis. Semen analysis is a key diagnostic test for the evaluation of spermatozoa, as well as seminal plasma and nonsperm cells. Before semen analysis, 2-7 days of sexual abstinence is required. A single test is sufficient if the semen analysis is normal. If the results are abnormal on at least two tests, further andrological examination is required. There should be at least 7 days between two semen analyzes. Semen should be examined within 1 hour of sample collection. Delays in examination can cause disturbances in sperm motility (Brown et al., 2006).

The major treatment decisions are based on the results of semen analysis, and most studies evaluate semen parameters as a main predictor of male fertility. However, a semen analysis cannot definitely differentiate infertile men from fertile men. (Boeri et al., 2021); for these reasons, it is necessary that laboratory work-up is standardized according to reference values.

Table 7.2 shows the lower reference limits for semen analysis according to the 2021 version of the WHO Manual.

Differentiating oligozoospermia (< 15 million spermatozoa / ml), asthenozoospermia (< 32% progressive motile spermatozoa), and teratozoospermia (< 4% normal forms) is important. Individual sperm parameters (e.g., morphology, motility, concentration) alone are not diagnostic for infertility. Usually, all three anomalies occur at the same time, which is defined as oligo-astheno-terato-zoospermia (OAT) syndrome. There is an increased incidence

Table 7.2 Lower reference limits (5th centiles and their 95% CIs) for semen characteristics

Parameter	2021 Lower reference limit (95% CI)
Semen volume (ml)	1.4 (1.3-1.5)
Total number of sperm (106 / ejaculate)	39 (35-40)
Sperm concentration (106 / ml)	16 (15-18)
Total motility (PR + NP, %)	42 (40-43)
Progressive motility (PR, %)	30 (29-31)
Vitality (live spermatozoa, %)	54 (50-56)
Sperm morphology (normal forms, %)	4 (3.9-4.0)
Other consensus threshold values	
pH	> 7.2
Peroxidase-positive leukocytes (106 / ml)	< 1.0
Function of the accessory gland	
Seminal zinc (µmol/ejaculate)	> 2.4
Seminal fructose (µmol / ejaculate)	> 13
Seminal neutral α-glucosidase (mU / ejaculate)	> 20

CIs = confidence intervals; MAR = mixed antiglobulin reaction; NP = non-progressive; PR = progressive (a+b motility).

** The distribution of the population data is presented with one-sided intervals (extremes of the data from the reference population data). The lower 5th percentile represents the level under which only results from 5% of the men in the reference population were found.*

of obstruction of the male genital tract and genetic abnormalities in severe cases of oligozoospermia (spermatozoa < 5 million / ml) (Grimes & Lopez, 2007). In azoospermia, there are no spermatozoa in the semen after centrifugation. The semen analysis may present with normal ejaculate volume in azoospermia. The recommended method for semen centrifugation is centrifugation of semen at 3,000 g for 15 minutes and a comprehensive microscopic examination with phase contrast optics at x200 magnification of the pellet. All specimens can be stained and reexamined microscopically (Organization, 2021). This allows the detection of small amounts of sperm that could potentially be used for cytoplasmic sperm injection (ICSI); therefore, there is no need for surgical intervention.

Sperm DNA Fragmentation Index

Traditional semen parameters cannot detect defects related to the functional aspects of spermatozoa. (Wang & Swerdloff, 2014) It is now known that sperm DNA damage can occur in men with infertility. The accumulation of single- and double-strand DNA breaks and an increased level of fragmentation of sperm DNA reduce the chances of natural conception. Sperm DNA fragmentation assays provide a more comprehensive evaluation of overall fertility status than traditional semen parameters (Oleszczuk et al., 2011). Sperm DNA damage can be increased by various factors, including chronic infection, varicocele, hormonal abnormalities, and lifestyle factors (e.g., smoking) (Nicopoullos et al., 2019). Although there are no studies that directly and certainly test the effect of sperm DNA damage on the clinical management of infertile couples, it is known to be that sperm DNA damage is more common in infertile men and contributes significantly to male infertility. In conclusion; in the evaluation of couples with recurrent loss of pregnancy from ART and natural conception or men with unexplained infertility, sperm DNA fragmentation tests should be performed.

Hormonal Evaluation

Although international societies recommend limiting hormonal evaluation to particular groups of patients, which are men with impaired sexual function or men with a sperm concentration below 10×10^6 / ml or if endocrinopathy is suspected, some clinicians consider routine hormonal evaluation necessary for male patients with infertility (Medicine, 2015; Jarow et al., 2010).

Analysis of follicle stimulating hormone and total testosterone is recommended for hormonal evaluation. Gonadotropins and testosterone have a pulsatile release, and the testosterone level declines physiologically during the day. For this reason, it is recommended that the sample be taken before 10:00 for testosterone level measurement. If the total testosterone concentration is low, repetition of the total testosterone, luteinising hormone assay and prolactin analysis should be performed.

In patients with elevated levels of sex hormone-binding globulin (e.g., diabetes, thyroid disease, men older than 75 years), measuring total testosterone concentration alone could be insufficient. Free testosterone measurement is recommended in these patients.

Men with primary hypogonadism (hypergonadotropic hypogonadism) is usually have high levels of LH and FSH, with any levels of testosterone. FSH levels are generally negatively correlated with the number of spermatogonia (Matin-du-Pan & Bischof, 1995). When spermatogonia are significantly decreased or absent, the FSH level is usually elevated; when the number of spermatogonia is average, but there is maturation arrest at the spermatid or spermatocyte level, the FSH is generally normal (Matin-du-Pan & Bischof, 1995).

In men with hypogonadotropic hypogonadism (e.g., Kallman's syndrome) is generally present with low levels of LH and FSH. In these patients, a complete pituitary evaluation should be performed, including measurements of thyroid stimulating hormone, adrenocorticotropic hormone, and growth hormone. Although inhibin-B levels are not routinely evaluated due to their cost and limited use, it can provide more reliable information on spermatogenesis than the FSH level. (Sussman et al., 2008)

The role of prolactin in male infertility is unclear. Mild elevations in prolactin levels are not important. Severe hyperprolactinemia could be associated with decreased total testosterone levels, which consequently affects male sexual function and spermatogenesis (Lotti et al., 2013).

Table 7.3 reports on the hormonal problems related to male infertility.

Genetic Testing

About 15% of men with infertility have genetic abnormalities (Krausz & Riera-Escamilla, 2018). Usually, severe oligozoospermia or azoospermia and increased aneuploidy are detected in Men with genetic abnormalities (Lipshultz & Lamb, 2007). Recurrent intracytoplasmic sperm injection failure, recurrent miscarriage, or vertical transmission of paternal genetic abnormalities can all

Table 7.3 Endocrine profiles of infertile men

Diagnosis	FSH	LH	Testosteron	Prolactin
Normal	Normal	Normal	Normal	Normal
Obstruction	Normal	Normal	Normal	Normal
Primary testicular failure	High	Normal/High	Low	Normal
Klinefelter syndrome	High	High	Low	Normal
Hyperprolactinemia	Low/Normal	Low	Low	High
Hypogonadotropic hypogonadism	Low	Low	Low	Normal

FSH: Follicle-stimulating hormone, LH: Luteinising hormone

be caused by genetic mutations in embryos. Determining genetic abnormalities is essential for accurate diagnosis and counseling prior to intracytoplasmic sperm injection.

Chromosomal analysis (karyotyping) can find structural or numerical chromosomal errors. The most prevalent type of genetic defect is a karyotype anomaly, present in 12–15% of cases of azoospermia, 5% of cases of severe oligozoospermia, and fewer than 1% of cases of normal semen. Therefore, men with azoospermia or oligozoospermia (spermatozoa 10 million / ml), karyotype analysis is recommended (Vincent et al., 2002).

The most common sex chromosomal aberration and karyotype defect is Klinefelter syndrome (47,XXY). Adult men with Klinefelter syndrome typically exhibit firm and tiny testes, as well as primary hypogonadism-related characteristics. Patients with Klinefelter syndrome are at increased risk of developing breast cancer, non-Hodgkin lymphoma, and extragonadal mediastinal germ cell tumor. Men with Klinefelter syndrome occasionally exhibit germ cell presence and sperm production, which is more common in mosaicism, 46,XY/47,XXY. In 0.9% and 7.0% of men with Klinefelter mosaicism, 24,XY sperm production has been reported (Chevret et al., 1996; Martini et al., 1996) and in 1.32–25% of males with the somatic karyotype 47,XXY (Cozzi et al., 1994; Guttenbach et al., 1997). TESE or mTESE are therapeutic options for patients with azoospermia, as spermatozoa can be retrieved in up to 50% of cases (Corona et al., 2017).

For patients with azoospermia or oligozoospermia and a sperm count less than 5×10^6/mL, Y chromosome microdeletion analysis is recommended. Azoospermia factor (AZF) a, b, or c in the long arm of the Y chromosome are affected by microdeletion of the Y chromosome. Complete deletions that comprise the AZFa and AZFb areas have a poor prognostic value for extracting sperm during TESE, and sperm is not detected in these patients. TESE should not be tried on these patients as a result (Hopps et al., 2003; Park et al., 2013). AZFc causes a multitude of phenotypes, from azoospermia to oligozoospermia. In 50–75% of men with AZFc microdeletions, sperm can be retrieved after TESE (Abur et al., 2019).

The congenital bilateral absence of vas deferens, which affects 1% of infertile men and up to 6% of men with obstructive azoospermia, is present in most cystic fibrosis patients. These patients will have azoospermia with a semen volume less than 0.5 ml due to seminal vesicle atrophy or hypoplasia, in addition to vas agenesis, and acidic pH ($pH < 6.5$) due to the inability to buffer prostate secretions. Around two thirds of men with congenital bilateral vas deferens have mutations in the CF transmembrane conductance regulator (CFTR) gene without experiencing any additional symptoms of cystic fibrosis. Since spermatogenesis is normal in these patients, successful pregnancies can be obtained with sperm extraction methods.

Infertility is associated with several hereditary diseases (e.g., Prader-Willi syndrome, Bardet-Biedl syndrome, Noonan's syndrome, autosomal dominant polycystic kidney disease, myotonic dystrophy, 5 α-reductase deficiency, etc.). Genetic testing prior to implantation may be required to enhance the success of ART in men with autosomal chromosomal abnormalities (Luo et al., 2019).

Imaging

Radiological examinations are not necessary in most patients. But still, in some cases, imaging could be used to evaluate a man with infertility. Due to its non-invasive nature, safety, and low cost, scrotal ultrasound is a preferred imaging modality.

Testicular neoplasms and varicocele are some of the disorders that can be diagnosed by scrotal ultrasound. Physical examination is the mainstay of the clinical management of varicocele. Measurement of venous reflux and diameter with scrotal color Doppler US is helpful, venous reflux flow during Valsalva maneuver or spermatic vein diameters greater than 3 mm support the diagnosis of varicocele.

Abdominal ultrasonography can be used in the diagnosis of accompanying renal abnormalities in patients with vas deferens agenesis.

Transrectal US provides detailed information about the ejaculatory duct, the vas deferens ampulla, the seminal vesicles, and the prostate. It is used in patients with suspected obstruction of the ejaculatory duct. They are usually azoospermia with less than 1 ml of semen, with an acid pH in the semen analysis and negative semen fructose. A seminal vesicle A-P diameter greater than

12-15 mm or greater than 2.3 mm in diameter in the ejaculatory duct suggests obstruction (Smith et al., 2008).

The gold standard test for detecting disorders of the ductus deferens is Vasography. It is an invasive imaging technique to determine whether the ejaculatory duct or vas deferens is obstructed, generally performed only as a component of definitive reconstructive surgery (Ammar et al., 2012).

Management

Azoospermia

Azoospermia is the inability to identify spermatozoa in semen after centrifugation at a magnification of 400. Semen analyzes must be performed at least twice (Medicine, 2015). There should be at least two weeks between the two tests. Around 10% of infertile men and %1 of all men have azoospermia. When the volume of semen is low, spermatozoa in the urine that follows ejaculation must be examined. The lack of spermatozoa and immature germ cells in the semen pellet suggests that the seminal duct is completely blocked.

Azolospermia can have a pretesticular, testicular, or post-testicular etiology.

Endocrine issues related to the hypothalamic-pituitary-gonad axis are among the pretesticular causes of azoospermia. It can occur due to congenital (Kallman syndrome) or acquired hypogonadotropic hypogonadism. In order to stimulate fertility in patients with hypogonadotropic hypogonadism, the combination of human menopausal gonadotropin and human chorionic gonadotropin is frequently used in clinical practice as an alternative to follicle-stimulating hormone and luteinizing hormone. After treatment, 16–57% of men with congenital hypogonadotropic hypogonadism reported successful pregnancies (Young et al., 2019).

The testicular causes of azoospermia include pathologies that cause primary testicular failure and the most common reason for azoospermia. Pathologies that result in primary testicular failure are among the testicular causes of azoospermia, which are the most frequent cause. Pathologies leading to primary testicular failure can be listed as anorchia, undescended testis, genetic anomalies, testicular torsion, trauma, drugs, infections, systemic diseases, testicular tumors, varicocele, surgeries that cause testicular atrophy by disrupting the blood supply of the testes.

Post-testicular causes of azoospermia include pathologies that cause ejaculatory dysfunction and obstructions of the genital tract. Obstructive

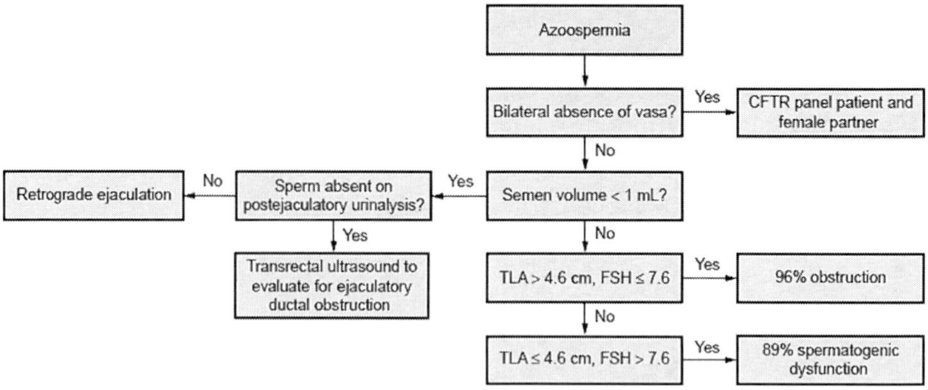

Figure 7.1 Algorithm for evaluation of azoospermia. *CFTR,* Cystic fibrosis transmembrane conductance regulator; *FSH,* follicle-stimulating hormone; *TLA,* testis longitudinal axis measured by caliper orchidometer (Partin et al., 2021).

azoospermia(OA) occurs in 20-40% of men with azoospermia (Medicine, 2018). Patients with obstructive azoospermia usually have normal FSH, normal-sized testes, and enlarged epididymis. In primary infertile males, obstruction is more usually found at the epididymal level. Vas deferens obstruction after a vasectomy is the most common type of acquired obstruction. Vasal obstruction may also occur after hernia repair. In addition to testicular biopsy, cryopreservation requires testicular sperm extraction (TESE). It is recommended that testicular biopsies (including fine needle aspiration) not be performed without concurrent sperm retrieval for therapeutic purposes because, after biopsy, this would require another surgery. Males with obstructive azoospermia have a variety of alternatives, such as surgical reconstruction or collection of sperm from testicles or epididymis for intracytoplasmic injection (Niederberger, 2020).

Men with obstructive azoospermia have a greater rate of successful testicular sperm retrieval than men with non-obstructive azoospermia (NOA) (Figure 7.1).

Varicosele

Varicoceles are enlargements of the pampiniform plexus veins that drain blood away from the testicles. Almost 15% of the normal male population, 25% of males with abnormal semen analysis, and 35–40% of men with infertility have varicocele (Jensen et al., 2017). The exact relationship between varicocele and decreased male fertility is unclear. Due to increased overall survival and DNA damage, elevated scrotal temperature, hypoxia, and toxic metabolite reflux could result in testicular dysfunction and infertility A meta-analysis revealed that among males with aberrant parameters, improvements in semen parameters are typically seen after surgical repair (Baazeem et al., 2011). In oligospermic men, varicocelectomy can increase pregnancy and live birth rates, and in men with non-obstructive azoospermia (NOA), varicocelectomy can increase pregnancy and sperm retrieval rates (Esteves et al., 2016; Kirby et al., 2016). In males with NOA, treatment of a clinical varicocele (grade 2/3) can promote sperm production and increase surgical sperm retrieval success rates (Esteves et al., 2016; Sajadi et al., 2019). In males with subclinical varicosele, varicosele treatment did not improve the likelihood of a spontaneous pregnancy (Yamamoto et al., 1996). The rate of spontaneous pregnancies increased when varicoceles were treated in the presence of unexplained subfertility (Kroese et al., 2012). After varicocelectomy, it usually takes two spermatogenic cycles for the semen parameters to improve (Machen et al., 2020). Recognizing the possibility of delays in surgical sperm retrieval methods and assisted reproductive technology (ART) is important.

Because most adolescents with varicocele have no trouble getting pregnant later in life, there is a major risk of overtreating them. Only in cases with known testicular growth degradation, determined by repeated clinical or Doppler US tests and/or abnormal semen analysis, is prophylactic treatment recommended (Silay et al., 2019).

In conclusion; in order to increase fertility rate, it is advised to treat infertile men who have clinical varicocele, abnormal semen parameters, or other unexplained infertility in a couple where the female partner has a healthy ovarian reserve.

The most effective varicocelectomy procedure, according to current research, is microsurgical varicocelectomy (Ding et al., 2012).

Although they have higher recurrence rates than microscopic varicocelectomy (4–27%), radiological procedures (sclerotherapy and embolization) are minimally invasive and are often used approaches.

Idiophatic Male Infertility

No male-associated cause is discovered to explain the deterioration of sperm parameters in 30–40% of cases and was previously known as idiopathic male infertility. Idiopathic male infertility (IMI) can be caused by endocrine disruption caused by pollution, the generation of reactive oxygen species (ROS)/ sperm DNA damage, or genetic and epigenetic abnormalities. The definition of IMI generally refers to idiopathic oligo-astheno-teratozoospermia (OAT). Oligo-astheno-teratozoospermia (OAT) is a clinical condition characterized by a decrease in the number of spermatozoa in the ejaculate, as well as a decrease in sperm motility and morphology; OAT syndrome (OATS) is a term that is frequently used. OATS can be caused by a variety of conditions, with the etiology unknown in a significant number of cases (Tournaye et al., 2017).

Non-Invasive Male Infertility Management

Weight loss, physical exercise, smoking cessation, and alcohol cessation all improve sperm parameters and should be recommended because they may improve the overall health of the male partner. Specific or empirical treatments are recommended. The main purpose of treatment is to improve the quality of semen.

Abnormal sperm parameters have been shown to be associated with increased levels of seminal reactive oxygen species (ROS). The most commonly used empirical medical therapy is oral antioxidants. The effects of empirical antioxidant therapy in the treatment of male infertility have been the subject of several investigations. A Cochrane systematic review and meta-analysis of 61 studies using various antioxidant compounds were conducted with 6,264 infertile men aged 18-65 years. Antioxidant therapy was found to improve live-birth and pregnancy rates in infertile couples undergoing ART cycles (Smits et al., 2019). More recently, the Men, Antioxidants and Infertility (MOXI) trial demonstrated that among infertile men with male factor infertility, antioxidants did not increase DNA integrity or semen parameters compared to placebo. Furthermore, at 6 months, the cumulative live birth rate did not differ between the antioxidant and placebo groups (15% vs. 24%) (Steiner et al., 2020). There were no clear conclusions about the antioxidants to use or therapeutic regimens to improve sperm parameters and pregnancy rate.

Selected estrogen receptor modulators and aromatase inhibitors are the most commonly used empirical hormonal therapies. Selective modulators of estrogen receptors, especially clomiphene citrate, were associated with a much higher conception rate and were also associated with a markedly improved sperm and hormonal profile (Cannarella et al., 2019). It should be noted that the quality of the included articles was low and that only a small number of studies were placebo controlled. The use of SERMs in men with idiopathic infertility has produced some promising results, but because the quality of the evidence is so poor, no clear recommendations can be offered. Furthermore, SERM-related side effects such as venous thrombosis and a counterintuitive drop in blood testosterone were underreported.

Due to its ability to prevent spermatogenesis, exogenous testosterone should not be used to treat male infertility in men (Mulhall et al., 2018).

Gonadotropins are well known for their usage in secondary hypogonadism. According to a meta-analysis, 75% of NOA patients with hypogonadotropic hypogonadism produced spermatozoa in their ejaculate when given human chorionic gonadotropin with or without FSH (Rastrelli et al., 2014).

The recommendations for non-invasive therapy for male infertility are listed in Table 7.4 of the EAU guidelines.

Table 7.4 The recommendations of the European Association of Urology guideline for noninvasive treatments for male infertility

Recommendation	Strength rating
In men with idiopathic oligo-astheno-teratozoospermia, lifestyle changes, including weight loss and increased physical activity, smoking cessation, and reduction of alcohol intake can improve sperm quality and the chances of conception.	Weak
No clear recommendation can be made for the treatment of patients with idiopathic infertility using antioxidants, although the use of antioxidants can improve semen parameters.	Weak
No conclusive recommendations on the use of selective oestrogen receptor modulators in men with idiopathic infertility can be drawn.	Weak
No conclusive recommendations on the use of either steroidal (testolactone) or nonsteroidal (anastrozole and letrozole) aromatase inhibitors in men with idiopathic infertility can be drawn, even before testis surgery.	Weak
Hypogonadotropic hypogonadism (secondary hypogonadism), including congenital causes, should be treated with combined human chorionic gonadotropin (hCG) and follicle stimulating hormone (FSH) (recombinant FSH; highly purified FSH) or pulsed Gonadotropinreleasing hormone (GnRH) via pump therapy to stimulate spermatogenesis.	Strong
In men with hypogonadotropic hypogonadism, induce spermatogenesis by effective drug therapy (hCG; human menopausal gonadotropins; recombinant FSH; highly purified FSH).	Strong
Do not use testosterone therapy for the treatment of male infertility.	Strong
Provide testosterone therapy for symptomatic patients with primary and secondaryhypogonadism who are not considering parenthood.	Strong

FSH = follicle stimulating hormone; GnRH = gonadotropin releasing hormone; hCG = human chorionic gonadotropin. A table amended from the European Association of Urology guidelines on sexual and reproductive health

Invasive Management of Male Infertility

Obstructive azoospermia

Obstructive azoospermia (OA) is not an aberration of spermatogenesis, but rather the absence of sperm in the ejaculate as a result of a blockage in the sperm conduit. It is often classified based on where the impediment is located anatomically (intratesticular, epididymal, vasal, ejaculatory duct, or functional obstruction of the distal seminal ducts). The treatment of OA depends on the cause. Only TESE allows sperm retrieval in men with intratesticular obstruction. Men with epididymal obstruction or inguinal vasal obstruction can be offered microsurgical reconstruction (such as vasoepidydostomy) or sperm retrieval using microsurgical epididymal sperm aspiration (MESA), percutaneous epididymal sperm aspiration (PESA), testicular sperm aspiration (TESA) or testicular sperm extraction (TESE). The etiology of the obstruction and the source of sperm used for ICSI in cases of OA had no effect on the result in terms of rates of fertilization, pregnancy, or miscarriage (Esteves et al., 2013).

Reversal of the microsurgical vasectomy is necessary following vas deferens obstruction caused by the vasectomy. The period of patency ranges from 1.7 to 4.3 months on average, and late failures are rare (0–12%) (Farber et al., 2019).

Transurethral ejaculatory duct resection (TURED) is a treatment option for ejaculatory duct obstruction caused by post-inflammatory or cystic obstruction. Part of the verumontanum may be removed during resection. An incision, unroofing, or aspiration of the cyst is necessary when a midline intraprostatic cyst is the cause of obstruction (Avellino et al., 2019). This method is safer when intraoperative TRUS is used. Installing methylene blue dye in the seminal vesicles (chromotubation) can help confirm intraoperative opening of the ducts if the distal seminal tract examination is performed at the time of the procedure. Epididymitis, UTI, macroscopic hematuria, hematospermia, azoospermia (in patients with partial distal ejaculatory duct occlusion), urine reflux into the ejaculatory ducts, and seminal vesicles are complications that could result from TURED (Avellino et al., 2019). Nevertheless, the female partner's ovarian reserve must be addressed while assessing treatment choices (e.g., sperm retrievel and ICSI) in all OA cases for whom surgical reconstruction is being explored.

Non-obstructive azoospermia

Non-obstructive azoospermia (NOA) is described as the lack of sperm in the centrifuged semen analysis with commonly a normal ejaculate volume. The primary goal of surgical treatment for NOA is direct removal of vital sperm from the testicles. This procedure is typically included in ART regimens, such as IVF cycles with ICSI.

A prognostic method called fine needle aspiration (FNA) mapping is used to choose patients who have NOA for TESE and ICSI (Beliveau & Turek, 2011). Comparison of mTESE with and without testicular mapping has not been performed in RCTs. FNA requires a subsequent therapeutic surgical strategy, raising the possibility of testicular destruction. As a result, FNA mapping cannot be suggested as the main therapy strategy for men with NOA.

Conventional TESE (cTESE) includes the execution of random testicular biopsies to extract sperm. An overall success rate of 35% has been recorded for sperm retrieval using this technique (Bernie et al., 2015).

Micro testicular extraction of sperm (mTESE) involved using an operational optical microscope to examine seminiferous tubules at a magnification of 20 to 25x and extract those that were larger, dilated, and opaque as these were more likely to harbor sperm. The purpose of this procedure is to increase the chances of sperm retrieval while requiring less tissue and providing a reduced risk of complications. The surgical sperm retrieval rates were similar between mTESE and cTESE, according to a meta-analysis that compared cTESE and mTESE in patients with NOA (Giovanni et al., 2019). In 46.5% of the patients in a study evaluating the efficacy of salvage mTESE after a previous failure of cTESE or TESA, the sperm was successfully retrieved (Kalsi et al., 2015).

In conclusion, mTESE is the best method for surgical sperm retrieval treatments in patients with NOA.

Conclusion

Male infertility is important for the patient's health and its consequences must be properly considered for the welfare of society. For the purpose of identifying and treating any modifiable risk factors that affect fertility, the male partner in infertile couples should have a thorough urological evaluation. Male patients should be evaluated with a reproductive and medical history, physical examination, hormonal evaluation, and semen analysis. Depending on clinical features and semen parameters, further research (e.g., genetic analysis and imaging) may be required. Semen analysis is a key diagnostic test for the evaluation of infertile males. Major treatment decisions are based on the results of semen analysis. Men with sexual dysfunction or a sperm concentration below 10×10^6 / ml or suspected endocrinopathy should undergo hormonal evaluation. Before intracytoplasmic sperm injection, determining genetic abnormalities is critical for accurate diagnosis and counseling. First of all, lifestyle changes should be recommended to infertile men. Oral anti-oxidants are the most commonly used empirical medical therapy. Selected estrogen receptor modulators and aromatase inhibitors can also be used in empirical therapy. The use of empirical treatments and interventions currently used in clinical practice is supported by low quality data; the effectiveness of these treatments must be confirmed in large-scale randomized controlled studies. Specific treatment options can be determined according to the underlying cause of infertility. OA management depends on the cause, surgical methods to eliminate obstruction can be preferred or ICSI can be performed after sperm retrieval methods. mTESE is the best method for surgical sperm retrieval treatments in patients with NOA. At the genetic, molecular and cellular levels, technological advancements make it easier to diagnose and treat male infertility. Considering technological advances, future treatments for male infertility could increasingly combine andrology with artificial intelligence, employing machine learning.

References

Abur, U., Gunes, S., Ascı, R., Altundag, E., Akar, O. S., Ayas, B., Karadag Alpaslan, M., & Ogur, G. (2019). Chromosomal and Y-chromosome microdeletion analysis in 1,300 infertile males and the fertility outcome of patients with AZFc microdeletions. *Andrologia*, *51*(11), e13402. https://doi.org/10.1111/and.13402

Agarwal, A., Baskaran, S., Parekh, N., Cho, C.-L., Henkel, R., Vij, S., Arafa, M., Selvam, M. K. P., & Shah, R. (2021). Male infertility. *The Lancet*, *397*(10271), 319-333. https://doi.org/10.1016/S0140-6736(20)32667-2

Agarwal, A., Deepinder, F., Cocuzza, M., Short, R. A., & Evenson, D. P. (2008). Effect of vaginal lubricants on sperm motility and chromatin integrity: a prospective comparative study. *Fertility and sterility*, *89*(2), 375-379. https://doi.org/10.1016/j.fertnstert.2007.02.050

Ammar, T., Sidhu, P., & Wilkins, C. (2012). Male infertility: the role of imaging in diagnosis and management. *The British journal of radiology*, *85*(special_issue_1), S59-S68. https://doi.org/10.1259/bjr/31818161

Avellino, G. J., Lipshultz, L. I., Sigman, M., & Hwang, K. (2019). Transurethral resection of the ejaculatory ducts: etiology of obstruction and surgical treatment options. *Fertility and sterility*, *111*(3), 427-443. https://doi.org/10.1016/j.fertnstert.2019.01.001

Baazeem, A., Belzile, E., Ciampi, A., Dohle, G., Jarvi, K., Salonia, A., Weidner, W., & Zini, A. (2011). Varicocele and male factor infertility treatment: a new meta-analysis and review of the role of varicocele repair. *European urology*, *60*(4), 796-808. https://doi.org/10.1016/j.eururo.2011.06.018

Beliveau, M. E., & Turek, P. J. (2011). The value of testicular 'mapping'in men with non-obstructive azoospermia. *Asian Journal of Andrology*, *13*(2), 225. https://doi.org/10.1038/aja.2010.178

Bernie, A. M., Mata, D. A., Ramasamy, R., & Schlegel, P. N. (2015). Comparison of microdissection testicular sperm extraction, conventional testicular sperm extraction, and testicular sperm aspiration for nonobstructive azoospermia: a systematic review and meta-analysis. *Fertility and sterility*, *104*(5), 1099-1103.e1093. https://doi.org/10.1016/j.fertnstert.2015.07.1136

Boeri, L., Belladelli, F., Capogrosso, P., Cazzaniga, W., Candela, L., Pozzi, E., Valsecchi, L., Papaleo, E., Viganò, P., & Abbate, C. (2021). Normal sperm parameters per se do not reliably account for fertility: A case–control study in the real-life setting. *Andrologia*, *53*(1), e13861. https://doi.org/10.1111/and.13861

Brown, D. J., Hill, S., & Baker, H. (2006). Male fertility and sexual function after spinal cord injury. *Progress in brain research*, *152*, 427-439. https://doi.org/10.1016/S0079-6123(05)52029-6

Cannarella, R., Condorelli, R. A., Mongioì, L. M., Barbagallo, F., Calogero, A. E., & La Vignera, S. (2019). Effects of the selective estrogen receptor modulators for the treatment of male infertility: a systematic review and meta-analysis. *Expert Opinion on Pharmacotherapy*, *20*(12), 1517-1525. https://doi.org/10.1080/14656566.2019.1615057

Chehab, M., Madala, A., & Trussell, J. (2015). On-label and off-label drugs used in the treatment of male infertility. *Fertility and sterility*, *103*(3), 595-604. https://doi.org/10.1016/j.fertnstert.2014.12.122

Chevret, E., Rousseaux, S., Monteil, M., Usson, Y., Cozzi, J., Pelletier, R., & Sèle, B. (1996). Increased incidence of hyperhaploid 24, XY spermatozoa detected by three-colour FISH in a 46, XY/47, XXY male. *Human genetics*, *97*(2), 171-175. https://doi.org/10.1007/BF02265260

Condorelli, R., Russo, G. I., Calogero, A., Morgia, G., & La Vignera, S. (2017). Chronic prostatitis and its detrimental impact on sperm parameters: a systematic review and meta-analysis. *Journal of Endocrinological Investigation*, *40*(11), 1209-1218. https://doi.org/10.1007/s40618-017-0684-0

Corona, G., Pizzocaro, A., Lanfranco, F., Garolla, A., Pelliccione, F., Vignozzi, L., Ferlin, A., Foresta, C., Jannini, E. A., & Maggi, M. (2017). Sperm recovery and ICSI outcomes in Klinefelter syndrome: a systematic review and meta-analysis. *Human Reproduction Update*, *23*(3), 265-275. https://doi.org/10.1093/humupd/dmx008

Cozzi, J., Chevret, E., Rousseaux, S., Pelletier, R., Benitz, V., Jalbert, H., & Sele, B. (1994). Achievement of meiosis in XXY germ cells: study of 543 sperm karyotypes from an XY/XXY mosaic patient. *Human genetics*, *93*(1), 32-34. https://doi.org/10.1007/BF00218909

Ding, H., Tian, J., Du, W., Zhang, L., Wang, H., & Wang, Z. (2012). Open non-microsurgical, laparoscopic or open microsurgical varicocelectomy for male infertility: a meta-analysis of randomized controlled trials. *BJU international*, *110*(10), 1536-1542. https://doi.org/10.1111/j.1464-410X.2012.11093.x

Esteves, S. C., Lee, W., Benjamin, D. J., Seol, B., Verza Jr, S., & Agarwal, A. (2013). Reproductive potential of men with obstructive azoospermia undergoing percutaneous sperm retrieval and intracytoplasmic sperm injection according to the cause of obstruction. *The Journal of urology*, *189*(1), 232-237. https://doi.org/10.1016/j.juro.2012.08.084

Esteves, S. C., Roque, M., & Agarwal, A. (2016). Outcome of assisted reproductive technology in men with treated and untreated varicocele: systematic review and meta-analysis. *Asian Journal of Andrology*, *18*(2), 254. https://doi.org/10.4103/1008-682X.163269

Farber, N. J., Flannigan, R., Li, P., Li, P. S., & Goldstein, M. (2019). The kinetics of sperm return and late failure following vasovasostomy or vasoepididymostomy: a systematic review. *The Journal of urology*, *201*(2), 241-250. https://doi.org/10.1016/j.juro.2018.07.092

Giovanni, C., Suks, M., Aleksander, G., Carlo, B., Marij, D.-S., Gert, D., Ferdinando, F., Ates, K., Sabine, K., & Zsolt, K. (2019). Sperm recovery and ICSI outcomes in men with non-obstructive azoospermia: a systematic review and meta-analysis. *Human Reproduction Update*, *25*, 733-757. https://doi.org/10.1093/humupd/dmz028

Goldenberg, R. L., & White, R. (1975). The effect of vaginal lubricants on sperm motility in vitro. *Fertility and sterility*, *26*(9), 872-873. https://doi.org/10.1016/s0015-0282(16)41350-6

Grimes, D. A., & Lopez, L. M. (2007). "Oligozoospermia," "azoospermia," and other semen-analysis terminology: the need for better science. *Fertility and sterility*, *88*(6), 1491-1494. https://doi.org/10.1016/j.fertnstert.2007.04.013

Gul, M., Carvajal, A., Serefoglu, E. C., Minhas, S., & Salonia, A. (2020). European association of urology guidelines for sexual and reproductive health 2020: What is new? *International Journal of Impotence Research*, *32*(5), 477-479. https://doi.org/10.1038/s41443-020-0335-4

Gundersen, T. D., Jørgensen, N., Andersson, A.-M., Bang, A. K., Nordkap, L., Skakkebæk, N. E., Priskorn, L., Juul, A., & Jensen, T. K. (2015). Association between use of marijuana and male reproductive hormones and semen quality: a study among 1,215 healthy young men. *American journal of epidemiology*, *182*(6), 473-481. https://doi.org/10.1093/aje/kwv135

Guttenbach, M., Michelmann, H., Hinney, B., Engel, W., & Schmid, M. (1997). Segregation of sex chromosomes into sperm nuclei in a man with 47, XXY Klinefelter's karyotype: a FISH analysis. *Human genetics*, *99*(4), 474-477. https://doi.org/10.1007/s004390050391

Hopps, C., Mielnik, A., Goldstein, M., Palermo, G., Rosenwaks, Z., & Schlegel, P. (2003). Detection of sperm in men with Y chromosome microdeletions of the AZFa, AZFb and AZFc regions. *Human reproduction*, *18*(8), 1660-1665. https://doi.org/10.1093/humrep/deg348

Jarow, J., Sigman, M., Kolettis, P., Lipshultz, L., Mcclure, R., & Nangia, A. (2010). *The optimal evaluation of the infertile male: AUA best practice statement.* American Urological Association Education and Research.

Jensen, C. F. S., Østergren, P., Dupree, J. M., Ohl, D. A., Sønksen, J., & Fode, M. (2017). Varicocele and male infertility. *Nature Reviews Urology*, *14*(9), 523-533. https://doi.org/10.1038/nrurol.2017.98

Jungwirth, A., Diemer, T., Dohle, G., Giwercman, A., Kopa, Z., Tournaye, H., & Krausz, C. (2013). EAU guidelines on male infertility. *Eur Urol*, *7*. https://doi.org/10.1016/j.eururo.2012.04.048

Kalsi, J. S., Shah, P., Thum, Y., Muneer, A., Ralph, D. J., & Minhas, S. (2015). Salvage micro-dissection testicular sperm extraction; outcome in men with non-obstructive azoospermia with previous failed sperm retrievals. *BJU international, 116*(3), 460-465. https://doi.org/10.1111/bju.12932

Kasturi, S. S., Osterberg, C., Tannir, J., & Brannigan, R. E. (2009). The effect of genital tract infection and inflammation on male infertility. In (pp. 295-330): Cambridge University Press Cambridge. https://doi.org/10.1017/CBO9780511635656.018

Kirby, E. W., Wiener, L. E., Rajanahally, S., Crowell, K., & Coward, R. M. (2016). Undergoing varicocele repair before assisted reproduction improves pregnancy rate and live birth rate in azoospermic and oligospermic men with a varicocele: a systematic review and meta-analysis. *Fertility and sterility, 106*(6), 1338-1343. https://doi.org/10.1016/j.fertnstert.2016.07.1093

Krausz, C. (2011). Male infertility: pathogenesis and clinical diagnosis. *Best practice & research Clinical endocrinology & metabolism, 25*(2), 271-285. https://doi .org/10.1016/j.beem.2010.08.006

Krausz, C., & Riera-Escamilla, A. (2018). Genetics of male infertility. *Nature Reviews Urology, 15*(6), 369-384. https://doi.org/10.1038/s41585-018-0003-3

Kroese, A. C., de Lange, N. M., Collins, J., & Evers, J. L. (2012). Surgery or embolization for varicoceles in subfertile men. *Cochrane Database of Systematic Reviews*(10). https://doi.org/10.1002/14651858.CD000479.pub5

Lewis, J. M., & Kaplan, W. E. (2009). Anatomy and embryology of the male reproductive tract and gonadal development. *Lipshultz LI Howards SS Niederberger CS Infertility in the male. 4th edn. Cambridge University Press, New York*, 1-13. https://doi.org/10.1017/CBO9780511635656

Lipshultz, L. I., & Lamb, D. J. (2007). Risk of transmission of genetic diseases by assisted reproduction. *Nature clinical practice Urology, 4*(9), 460-461. https:// doi.org/10.1038/ncpuro0879

Lotti, F., Corona, G., Maseroli, E., Rossi, M., Silverii, A., Degl'Innocenti, S., Rastrelli, G., Forti, G., & Maggi, M. (2013). Clinical implications of measuring prolactin levels in males of infertile couples. *Andrology, 1*(5), 764-771. https://doi.org/10 .1111/j.2047-2927.2013.00114.x

Lotti, F., & Maggi, M. (2015). Ultrasound of the male genital tract in relation to male reproductive health. *Human Reproduction Update, 21*(1), 56-83. https://doi.org /10.1093/humupd/dmu042

Luo, K., Lan, Y., Xie, P., Gong, F., Xiong, B., Tan, Y., Zhou, S., Yang, Z., Lin, G., & Hu, L. (2019). Next-generation sequencing analysis of embryos from mosaic patients undergoing in vitro fertilization and preimplantation genetic testing. *Fertility and sterility, 112*(2), 291-297. e293. https://doi.org/10.1016/j.fertnstert.2019.03.035

Machen, G. L., Johnson, D., Nissen, M. A., Naber, E., & Sandlow, J. I. (2020). Time to improvement of semen parameters after microscopic varicocelectomy: When it occurs and its effects on fertility. *Andrologia, 52*(2), e13500. https://doi.org/10 .1111/and.13500

Martini, E., Geraedts, J. P. M., Liebaers, I., Land, J., Capitanio, G. L., Ramaekers, F. C. S., & Hopman, A. H. N. (1996). Genetics: Constitution of semen samples from XYY and XXY males as analysed by in-situ hybridization. *Human reproduction, 11*(8), 1638-1643. https://doi.org/10.1093/oxfordjournals.humrep .a019461

Matin-du-Pan, R., & Bischof, P. (1995). Increased follicle stimulating hormone in infetile men: Is increased plasma FSH always due to damaged germinal epithelium? *Human reproduction, 10*(8), 1940-1945. https://doi.org/10.1093/oxfordjournals.humrep.a136211

Medicine, P. C. o. t. A. S. f. R. (2015). Diagnostic evaluation of the infertile male: a committee opinion. *Fertility and sterility, 103*(3), e18-e25. https://doi.org/10.1016/j.fertnstert.2014.12.103

Medicine, P. C. o. t. A. S. f. R. (2018). Management of nonobstructive azoospermia: a committee opinion. *Fertility and sterility, 110*(7), 1239-1245. https://doi.org/10.1016/j.fertnstert.2018.09.012

Mowat, A., Newton, C., Boothroyd, C., Demmers, K., & Fleming, S. (2014). The effects of vaginal lubricants on sperm function: an in vitro analysis. *Journal of assisted reproduction and genetics, 31*(3), 333-339. https://doi.org/10.1007/s10815-013-0168-x

Mulhall, J. P., Trost, L. W., Brannigan, R. E., Kurtz, E. G., Redmon, J. B., Chiles, K. A., Lightner, D. J., Miner, M. M., Murad, M. H., & Nelson, C. J. (2018). Evaluation and management of testosterone deficiency: AUA guideline. *The Journal of urology, 200*(2), 423-432. https://doi.org/10.1016/j.juro.2018.03.115

Nalesnik, J. G., Sabanegh Jr, E. S., Eng, T. Y., & Buchholz, T. A. (2004). Fertility in men after treatment for stage 1 and 2A seminoma. *American journal of clinical oncology, 27*(6), 584-588. https://doi.org/10.1097/01.coc.0000135736.18493.dd

Nicopoullos, J., Vicens-Morton, A., Lewis, S. E., Lee, K., Larsen, P., Ramsay, J., Yap, T., & Minhas, S. (2019). Novel use of COMET parameters of sperm DNA damage may increase its utility to diagnose male infertility and predict live births following both IVF and ICSI. *Human reproduction, 34*(10), 1915-1923. https://doi.org/10.1093/humrep/dez151

Niederberger, C. (2011). *An introduction to male reproductive medicine.* Cambridge University Press. https://doi.org/10.1017/CBO9780511736254

Niederberger, C. (2020). Re: The Management of Obstructive Azoospermia. *Journal of Urology, 203*(1), 16-17. https://doi.org/10.1097/01.JU.0000605040.50060.d2

Nieschlag, E., & Behre, H. M. (2001). *Andrology: male reproductive health and dysfunction.* Springer Science & Business Media. ISBN : 978-3-662-04493-3

Oates, R. D., & Lamb, D. J. (2009). Genetic aspects of infertility. *Infertility in the Male*, 251. https://doi.org/10.1017/CBO9780511635656.016

Oleszczuk, K., Giwercman, A., & Bungum, M. (2011). Intra-individual variation of the sperm chromatin structure assay DNA fragmentation index in men from infertile couples. *Human reproduction, 26*(12), 3244-3248. https://doi.org/10.1093/humrep/der328

Organization, W. H. (2021). *WHO laboratory manual for the examination and processing of human semen.* World Health Organization. https://doi.org/10.1016/j.fertnstert.2021.12.012

Park, S. H., Lee, H. S., Choe, J. H., Lee, J. S., & Seo, J. T. (2013). Success rate of microsurgical multiple testicular sperm extraction and sperm presence in the ejaculate in korean men with y chromosome microdeletions. *Korean journal of urology, 54*(8), 536-540. https://doi.org/10.4111/kju.2013.54.8.536

Partin, A. W., Dmochowski, R. R., Kavoussi, L. R., Peters, C., Walsh, P. C., & Wein, A. J. (2021). *Campbell-Walsh-Wein urology* (Twelfth edition. ed.). Elsevier. ISBN: 9780323672276

Rastrelli, G., Corona, G., Mannucci, E., & Maggi, M. (2014). Factors affecting spermatogenesis upon gonadotropin-replacement therapy: a meta-analytic study. *Andrology*, *2*(6), 794-808. https://doi.org/10.1111/andr.262

Rowe, P. J., & World Health, O. (2000). *WHO manual for the standardized investigation, diagnosis and management of the infertile man*. Cambridge University Press. ISBN: 9780521774741

Sajadi, H., Hosseini, J., Farrahi, F., Dadkhah, F., Sepidarkish, M., Sabbaghian, M., Eftekhari-Yazdi, P., & Gilani, M. A. S. (2019). Varicocelectomy may improve results for sperm retrieval and pregnancy rate in non-obstructive azoospermic men. *International Journal of Fertility & Sterility*, *12*(4), 303. https://doi.org/10.22074/ijfs.2019.5344

Sansone, A., Di Dato, C., de Angelis, C., Menafra, D., Pozza, C., Pivonello, R., Isidori, A., & Gianfrilli, D. (2018). Smoke, alcohol and drug addiction and male fertility. *Reproductive biology and endocrinology*, *16*(1), 1-11. https://doi.org/10.1186/s12958-018-0320-7

Sharma, R., Harlev, A., Agarwal, A., & Esteves, S. C. (2016). Cigarette smoking and semen quality: a new meta-analysis examining the effect of the 2010 World Health Organization laboratory methods for the examination of human semen. *European urology*, *70*(4), 635-645. https://doi.org/10.1016/j.eururo.2016.04.010

Shibahara, H. (2022). Production of Anti-sperm Antibody (ASA) in Men. In *Gamete Immunology* (pp. 127-142). Springer. https://doi.org/10.1002/rmb2.12477

Shin, D., Lipshultz, L. I., Goldstein, M., Barmé, G. A., Fuchs, E. F., Nagler, H. M., McCallum, S. W., Niederberger, C. S., Schoor, R. A., & Brugh III, V. M. (2005). Herniorrhaphy with polypropylene mesh causing inguinal vasal obstruction: a preventable cause of obstructive azoospermia. *Annals of surgery*, *241*(4), 553-558. https://doi.org/10.1097/01.sla.0000157318.13975.2a

Silay, M. S., Hoen, L., Quadackaers, J., Undre, S., Bogaert, G., Dogan, H. S., Kocvara, R., Nijman, R. J., Radmayr, C., & Tekgul, S. (2019). Treatment of varicocele in children and adolescents: a systematic review and meta-analysis from the European Association of Urology/European Society for Paediatric Urology Guidelines Panel. *European urology*, *75*(3), 448-461. https://doi.org/10.1016/j.eururo.2018.09.042

Smith, J. F., Walsh, T. J., & Turek, P. J. (2008). Ejaculatory duct obstruction. *Urologic Clinics of North America*, *35*(2), 221-227. https://doi.org/10.1016/j.ucl.2008.01.011

Smits, R. M., Mackenzie-Proctor, R., Yazdani, A., Stankiewicz, M. T., Jordan, V., & Showell, M. G. (2019). Antioxidants for male subfertility. *Cochrane Database of Systematic Reviews*(3). https://doi.org/10.1002/14651858.CD007411.pub4

Ståhl, O., Eberhard, J., Jepson, K., Spano, M., Cwikiel, M., Cavallin-Ståhl, E., & Giwercman, A. (2006). Sperm DNA integrity in testicular cancer patients. *Human reproduction*, *21*(12), 3199-3205. https://doi.org/10.1093/humrep/del292

Steiner, A. Z., Hansen, K. R., Barnhart, K. T., Cedars, M. I., Legro, R. S., Diamond, M. P., Krawetz, S. A., Usadi, R., Baker, V. L., & Coward, R. M. (2020). The effect of antioxidants on male factor infertility: the Males, Antioxidants, and Infertility (MOXI) randomized clinical trial. *Fertility and sterility*, *113*(3), 552-560. e553. https://doi.org/10.1016/j.fertnstert.2019.11.008

Sussman, E. M., Chudnovsky, A., & Niederberger, C. S. (2008). Hormonal evaluation of the infertile male: has it evolved? *Urologic Clinics of North America*, *35*(2), 147-155. https://doi.org/10.1016/j.ucl.2008.01.010

Tournaye, H., Krausz, C., & Oates, R. D. (2017). Novel concepts in the aetiology of male reproductive impairment. *The lancet Diabetes & endocrinology*, *5*(7), 544-553. https://doi.org/10.1016/S2213-8587(16)30040-7

Tur-Kaspa, I., Maor, Y., Levran, D., Yonish, M., Mashiach, S., & Dor, J. (1994). How often should infertile men have intercourse to achieve conception? *Fertility and sterility*, *62*(2), 370-375. https://doi.org/10.1016/s0015-0282(16)56893-9

Vander Borght, M., & Wyns, C. (2018). Fertility and infertility: Definition and epidemiology. *Clinical biochemistry*, *62*, 2-10. https://doi.org/10.1016/j.clinbiochem.2018.03.012

Veleminska, J., Bigoni, L., Krajicek, V., Borsky, J., Smahelova, D., Caganova, V., & Peterka, M. (2012). Surface facial modelling and allometry in relation to sexual dimorphism. *Homo*, *63*(2), 81-93. https://doi.org/10.1016/j.jchb.2012.02.002

Vincent, M. C., Daudin, M., DE MAS, P., Massat, G., Mieusset, R., Pontonnier, F., Calvas, P., Bujan, L., & BOURROUILLOU, G. (2002). Cytogenetic investigations of infertile men with low sperm counts: a 25-year experience. *Journal of andrology*, *23*(1), 18-22. https://doi.org/10.1002/j.1939-4640.2002.tb02597.x

Walsh, T. J., Croughan, M. S., Schembri, M., Chan, J. M., & Turek, P. J. (2009). Increased risk of testicular germ cell cancer among infertile men. *Archives of internal medicine*, *169*(4), 351-356. https://doi.org/10.1001/archinternmed.2008.562

Wang, C., & Swerdloff, R. S. (2014). Limitations of semen analysis as a test of male fertility and anticipated needs from newer tests. *Fertility and sterility*, *102*(6), 1502-1507. https://doi.org/10.1016/j.fertnstert.2014.10.021

Yamamoto, M., Hibi, H., Hirata, Y., Miyake, K., & Ishigaki, T. (1996). Effect of varicocelectomy on sperm parameters and pregnancy rate in patients with subclinical varicocele: a randomized prospective controlled study. *The Journal of urology*, *155*(5), 1636-1638. https://doi.org/10.1016/S0022-5347(01)66149-4

Young, J., Xu, C., Papadakis, G. E., Acierno, J. S., Maione, L., Hietamäki, J., Raivio, T., & Pitteloud, N. (2019). Clinical management of congenital hypogonadotropic hypogonadism. *Endocrine reviews*, *40*(2), 669-710. https://doi.org/10.1210/er.2018-00116

Zegers-Hochschild, F., Adamson, G. D., Dyer, S., Racowsky, C., De Mouzon, J., Sokol, R., Rienzi, L., Sunde, A., Schmidt, L., & Cooke, I. D. (2017). The international glossary on infertility and fertility care, 2017. *Human reproduction*, *32*(9), 1786-1801. https://doi.org/10.1093/humrep/dex234

Chapter 8

Testing Ovarian Reserve

Emine Ahu Koç, MD*

Department of Obstetrics and Gynecology, Samsun Training and Research Hospital, Samsun, Turkiye

Abstract

The decrease in fertility with advanced age in women has been shown in various scientific trials. Many factors such as genetics, environmental factors, and treatment processes affect reproductive function. The ovarian reserve is defined as the oocyte sufficiency needed to sustain the ovarian reproductive function. In the diagnosis of infertility and the planning of treatment, the evaluation of this reserve is notably essential in terms of increased clinical success and the prevention of economic losses. It is possible to evaluate the ovaries by biochemical tests and ultrasonographic imaging. However, there is still no evaluation test that can be the gold standard.

Key Words: Advanced age, Fertility, Ovarian reserve

Introduction

Two duties of the ovaries are the sustainability of ovulatuar functions with the maturation of oocytes and the production of steroid hormones (Gougeon, 1996). The number of oocytes in the ovaries increases with mitosis division and reaches the highest number, which is 5-7 million, in the 16-20th weeks of fetal life. From this period, production stops and the decrease process begin.

---

* Corresponding Author's Email: emineahu52dr@hotmail.com

In: Holistic Approach to Assisted Reproductive Technology
Editor: Kenan Demir and Rümeysa Yılmaz Göç
ISBN: 979-8-89113-017-3
© 2023 Nova Science Publishers, Inc.

Depending on apoptosis, this number decreases to 1-2 million at birth and 500,000 at puberty. With puberty, the decrease, continuing with both the apoptosis and ovulation pathways, accelerates in the mid-30s. At the end of the 30s, the total number of oocytes falls below 50.000 (Peck et al., 2016; Hansen et al., 2008). Furthermore, the reproduction potential also decreases. In addition to advanced age, many factors, such as genetics and environmental factors, also affect reproduction potential (Peck et al., 2016; Tal & Seifer, 2017). Therefore, the reserve and reproductive potential of the ovary are different in every woman, even if they are the same ages (Practice Committee of the American Society for Reproductive Medicine, 2015; de Marcillac et al., 2017).

Generally, age is insufficient, although it is an important and basic way to obtain information on ovarian reserve. Therefore, different identifiers have been studied (Hendriks et al., 2005a). The ovarian reserve can be determined by measuring hormone levels and imaging the ovaries by ultrasonography. These tests are screening tests that are used to detect women with the risk of decreased ovarian reserve (DOR). As in all screen tests, ovarian reserve screen tests should have features such as simple, trustworthy, reproducible, and high prognosis rate.

The aim of this chapter is to define ovarian reserve and ovarian reserve tests and to inform about the clinical benefits and predictive capabilities of these tests.

Ovarian Reserve Tests

Ovarian reserve is a term used to define the number of oocytes in the ovaries or their quantity. The quality of the oocyte is a term for the fertilized oocyte that can result in live birth and is different from the quantity term (Practice Committee of the American Society for Reproductive Medicine, 2015). In practice, these two terms are closely related to each other and can be classified as a biological and clinical reserve (Ulrich & Marsh, 2019). The tests used for evaluating the ovarian reserve reveal the biological reserve of ovaries; however, they are poor predictors of the clinical reserve. Age is still the best predictor of oocyte quality (Bishop et al., 2017).

Today, with the postponement of pregnancy and childbearing age,the growing need for assisted reproduction technology requires evaluating the ovarian reserve correctly. Ovarian reserve tests are screening tests based on evaluation of the ovaries by biochemical and ultrasonographic methods. The main purpose here is to detect women with the possibility of DOR. Therefore, the necessity of assisted reproduction therapy is detected and a treatment plan can be implemented in a correct and reliable way (Practice Committee of the American Society for Reproductive Medicine, 2015). An

Table 8.1 Indications for the Evaluation of the Ovarian Reserve

1- History of infertility over the age of 35 and for more than 6 months
2- Family history of early menopause
3- History of previous ovarian surgery, chemotherapy, or pelvic radiotherapy
4- Unexplained infertility
5- Those who are planned to be treated with assisted reproduction technology

ideal ovarian reserve test should be inexpensive, noninvasive, reproducible, and rapidly interpretable. It should vary with minimal alteration between the menstrual cycle and have high sensitivity and specificity (Toner & Seifer, 2013). Guidance on assisted reproduction therapy should not be the only criterion because there are certain limitations in all ovarian reserve tests. Furthermore, decreased ovarian reserve should not mean a barrier to conception. Women with DOR possibility can be summarized in Table 8.1 (Sharara et al., 1998; Azhar et al., 2015).

Ovarian reserve tests;

1. Static tests: Follicle stimulating hormone (FSH), estradiol (E2), inhibin B, antimullerian hormone (AMH).
2. Dynamic tests: Clomiphene citrate challenge test (CCCT), GnRH agonist stimulation test (GAST), Exogenous FSH ovarian reserve test (EFORT)
3. Ultrasonographic identifiers: Antral follicle count (AFC), Ovarian volume, Ovarian stromal blood flow

Can be seen as three titles.

Baseline serum FSH

The baseline serum FSH value measured in the early follicular phase has been the most commonly used test to evaluate the ovarian reserve for a long time. Women with normal ovarian reserve have a low FSH value that is measured on the 2nd-4th days of the cycle based on inhibition of inhibin B and E2 (Schuh-Huerta et al.,2012; Steiner et al., 2017). As the follicular pool decreases, sufficient pressure cannot occur and the FSH value increases. For this reason, a high FSH value is closely related to a decreased ovarian reserve. However, its wide variability within and between cycles limits its trustworthiness (Practice Committee of the American Society for Reproductive Medicine, 2015; Abdalla & Thum, 2006). When the FSH cutoff value is taken at 10-20 IU/L, it has high specificity (45-50%) in predicting a poor response to ovarian stimulation, but its sensitivity is low (11-86%). The prognosis of conception has also high specificity (50-100%), but its sensitivity is lower (3-65%) (Esposito et al., 2002; Broekmans et al., 2006). Evaluation together with FSH and E2 measurements increases trustworthiness. In women over 40 years of age, one-time high FSH value may not be sufficient in a poor response to stimulation or the prognosis of conception (Ramalho de Carvalho et al., 2012).

Baseline serum E2

The baseline serum E2 value taken on days 2-4 of the cycle should not be used solely to assess an ovarian reserve and should be interpreted with FSH. A high value of E2 (60-80 pg/ml) in the early follicular phase is a characteristic finding of reproductive aging. It causes suppression of FSH and normal measurement of the hormone that is originally high (Practice Committee of the American Society for Reproductive Medicine, 2015; Ramalho de Carvalho et al., 2012). If the FSH value is normal but the E2 value is high, this situation may be associated with decreased ovarian reserve (Evers et al., 1998).

Baseline serum Inhibin B

Inhibin B is released from the granulosa cells of small antral follicles during the follicular phase and inhibits the production of FSH (Speroff & Fritz, 2005; Klein et al., 1996). Serum level varies greatly during the menstrual cycle and between cycles. Inhibin B is generally not accepted as a reliable indicator of ovarian reserve (Knauff et al., 2009; Hee et al., 1993). Despite that those with decreased ovarian reserve have a low level of it, it has a specificity of 64-90% and a sensitivity of 40-80% in predicting poor response to stimulation even at a low threshold value of 40-45 pg/ml (Speroff & Fritz, 2005).

AMH

Released from granulosa cells of preantral and small antral follicles, AMH is a glycoprotein structure hormone belonging to the transforming growth factor-Beta (TGF-B) family (La Marca et al., 2010). It starts to produce in the 36th week of fetal life and increases until it peaks at 25 years of age (Rajpert-De Meyts et al., 1999). After that, it decreases with age and becomes undetectable before menopause. The release of AMH release is independent of gonadotrophins; therefore, it does not show variability in and between cycles (Hehenkamp et al., 2006; La Marca et al., 2006; Tsepelidis et al., 2007). Although there are studies that indicate that AMH shows variability, these are limited to young women and those who have high AMH levels

(Sowers et al., 2010; Kissell et al., 2014; Overbeek et al., 2012). Birth control drugs, body mass index, and vitamin D may affect AMH values (Van den Berg et al., 2010; Moslehi et al., 2018; Dennis et al., 2017). AMH is more sensitive than FSH in evaluating ovarian reserve and has commonly replaced FSH and E2 (Practice Committee of the American Society for Reproductive Medicine, 2015). When the cut-off value is taken as 0.1-1.66 ng/ml, it has high specificity and sensitivity rates in predicting poor ovarian response and when taken as 3.36-5.0 ng/ml, excessive ovarian response (La Marca et al., 2010). However, its prognosis for conception is poor (Broer et al., 2009).

Clomiphene Citrate Challenge Test

The clomiphene citrate challenge test (CCCT) is a dynamic test based on FSH measurement on the 3rd and 10th days before and after oral administration of clomiphene citrate on the 5th-9th days of the cycle (Tanbo et al., 1992; Scott et al., 1993). When the ovarian reserve is sufficient, the increase in the value of FSH in response to clomiphene is suppressed by the released E2 and inhibin B. After clomiphene administration, high value of FSH on 10th day can increase sensitivity in the detection of low ovarian reserve (Hendriks et al., 2005b). However, the FSH values on day 10 after CCCT are not superior in predicting a decrease in ovarian reserve and pregnancy after ART compared to baseline serum FSH or antral follicle count (AFC) (Hendriks et al., 2006; Yanushpolsky et al., 2003).

GnRH Stimulation Test

GAST is based on the evaluation of the difference between the E2 values measured on the second and third day of the cycle, after subcutaneous administration of 1 mg of GnRH agonists. E2 release increases from the ovaries after the flare-up effect of GnRH agonists and pituitary gonadotrophin (Padilla et al., 1990; Winslow et al., 1991). An increase in the E2 value is related to the ovarian reserve. If the ovarian reserve is low, the increase will also decrease (Ranieri et al., 1998). In studies, it has been shown that GAST has limited benefit in determining a decreased ovarian reserve with normal ovarian response and in predicting pregnancy.

Exogenous FSH Ovarian Reserve Test

EFORT compares baseline serum FSH and E2 values with increase in E2 value 24 hours after intramuscular 300 IU FSH administration (Fanchin et al., 1994). Limited studies have detected that there are incorrectly high positivity rates (Broekmans et al., 2006).

Antral Follicle Count

AFC defines total follicle numbers with an average diameter of 2-10mm, which are detected by transvaginal ultrasonography in both ovaries in the early follicular phase (Practice Committee of the American Society for Reproductive Medicine, 2015). It reflects the number of the primordial follicle in ovaries, in other words, ovarian reserve (Scheffer et al., 1999; Kevenaar et al., 2006). When the threshold value for total AFC in both ovaries is taken as 3-4, specificity is high, but the sensitivity is low for DOR. The sensitivity to pregnancy prediction is even lower (Tal & Seifer, 2017, Broer et al., 2011; Jayaprakasan et al., 2008). This situation can be due to the fact that the ultrasonographic image of antral follicles that are more than 2mm in diameter sensitive to gonadotropins and follicles that do not respond to gonadotropins in early or advanced stages of atresia are the same (Gougeon, 1986; Westergaard et al., 1986).

The variability of AFC on cycle to cycle is quite low compared to the average ovarian volume and the baseline value of FSH and is a clinically neglected level (Bancsi et al., 2004). Additionally, the variability between individuals is at a minimal level with experienced hands at it (Hansen et al., 2003; Scheffer et al., 2002).

In summary, AFC is a valid criterion for detecting ovarian reserve; however, it should not be used as the only criterion in ART administration.

Ovarian Volume

With advanced age, the volume of the ovary decreases in parallel with the decrease in the follicle pool and the stromal blood flow in the ovaries (Kupesic et al., 2003). Ovarian volume smaller than 3cm3 is a high-specificity predictor of DOR, but is not successful in the prognosis of conception (Lass et al., 1997). In evaluating ovarian reserve, ovarian volume measurement has no superiority over AFC and has not been used in routine evaluation (Broekmans et al., 2006).

Ovarian Stromal Blood Flow

There has been detected that there is a positive correlation between ovarian stromal blood flow and follicular response and the maximum systolic rate is lower in those with DOR in the early follicular phase (Zaidi et al., 1995). However, the ovarian stromal veins are thin and convoluted, requiring time and experience to properly evaluate with the correct insonation angle (Kupesic et al., 2003). It should not be used in the routine evaluation.

Which Test Should Be Preferred?

AMH and AFC are more sensitive than baseline serum FSH in predicting ovarian reserve (Toner & Seifer, 2013). A decrease in the AMH value is a finding that occurs much earlier than an increase in the FSH value. AMH is released in the early stages of folliculogenesis and shows a higher correlation with the primordial follicle than the inhibin B and E2 released during late folliculogenesis and the indirect marker FSH (Tal & Seifer, 2017). Studies comparing AFC and AMH have shown that both have similar predictive values (Broekmans et al., 2006; 37,59). However, four prospective multicenter trials show that AMH is better than AFC in predicting the number of retrieved oocytes and low and high responses to stimulation (Andersen et al., 2011; Arce et al., 2013; Polyzos et al., 2013; Nelson et al., 2015). The different results from trials may be caused by factors such as the ultrasonography devices used and the experience of the person performing the ultrasonography.

Comparing baseline tests, dynamic tests do not have an additional benefit in DOR, ART after pregnancy, or nonassisted predicting pregnancy. They are not the tests of choice today. The most trustworthy and sensitive choices for today's two tests are AMH and AFC.

It has been shown that there is no additional benefit when multiple tests are used instead of a single test to increase the predictive value of ovarian reserve tests (Tal et al., 2018; Jirge, 2011; Jayaprakasan et al., 2010). When combining AMH, inhibin B, AFC, and ovarian volume, the predictive value obtained has been shown to be less than the predictive value obtained independently of each test (Lorusso et al., 2007). Similarly, when combining AMH and AFC, the results obtained are not superior to the result of each test alone (Broer et al., 2013).

Conclusion

Ovarian reserve tests are quite beneficial in predicting a poor or excessive response to ovarian stimulation in women who are planned assisted reproduction therapy and in the safe individualization of treatment protocols. It enables women to be informed about their reproductive potential and can guide their future plans. It is helpful in determining the gonadotoxic pretreatment management strategy. However, there is a weak relationship between ovarian reserve test and oocyte quality, and between clinic pregnancy rates and live birth rates. Ovarian reserve tests should not be used as a prognosis of conception, including a low value of AMH, and should not affect the decision on admission of the patient to assisted reproductive therapy.

References

Abdalla, H., & Thum, M. Y. (2006). Repeated testing of basal FSH levels has no predictive value for IVF outcome in women with elevated basal FSH. *Human Reproduction*, *21*(1), 171-174.

Andersen, A. N., Witjes, H., Gordon, K., & Mannaerts, B. (2011). Predictive factors of ovarian response and clinical outcome after IVF/ICSI following a rFSH/GnRH antagonist protocol with or without oral contraceptive pre-treatment. *Human reproduction*, *26*(12), 3413-3423. https://doi.org/10.1093/humrep/der318

Arce, J. C., La Marca, A., Klein, B. M., Andersen, A. N., & Fleming, R. (2013). Antimüllerian hormone in gonadotropin releasing-hormone antagonist cycles: prediction of ovarian response and cumulative treatment outcome in good-prognosis patients. *Fertility and sterility*, *99*(6), 1644-1653. https://doi.org/10.1016/j.fertnstert.2012.12.048

Azhar, E., Seifer, D. B., Melzer, K., Ahmed, A., Weedon, J., & Minkoff, H. (2015). Knowledge of ovarian reserve and reproductive choices. *Journal of Assisted Reproduction and Genetics*, *32*, 409-415.

Bancsi, L. F., Broekmans, F. J., Looman, C. W., Habbema, J. D. F., & te Velde, E. R. (2004). Impact of repeated antral follicle counts on the prediction of poor ovarian response in women undergoing in vitro fertilization. *Fertility and sterility*, *81*(1), 35-41. https://doi.org/10.1016/j.fertnstert.2003.06.011

Bishop, L. A., Richter, K. S., Patounakis, G., Andriani, L., Moon, K., & Devine, K. (2017). Diminished ovarian reserve as measured by means of baseline follicle-stimulating hormone and antral follicle count is not associated with pregnancy loss in younger in vitro fertilization patients. *Fertility and sterility*, *108*(6), 980-987.

Broekmans, F. J., Kwee, J., Hendriks, D. J., Mol, B. W., & Lambalk, C. B. (2006). A systematic review of tests predicting ovarian reserve and IVF outcome. *Human reproduction update*, *12*(6), 685-718.

Broer, S. L., Dólleman, M., Opmeer, B. C., Fauser, B. C., Mol, B. W., & Broekmans, F. J. M. (2011). AMH and AFC as predictors of excessive response in controlled ovarian hyperstimulation: a meta-analysis. *Human reproduction update*, *17*(1), 46-54. https://doi.org/10.1093/humupd/dmq034

Broer, S. L., Mol, B. W. J., Hendriks, D., & Broekmans, F. J. (2009). The role of antimullerian hormone in prediction of outcome after IVF: comparison with the antral follicle count. *Fertility and sterility*, *91*(3), 705-714.

Broer, S. L., van Disseldorp, J., Broeze, K. A., Dolleman, M., Opmeer, B. C., Bossuyt, P., Eijkemans, M. J., Mol, B. W., & Broekmans, F. J. (2013). Added value of ovarian reserve testing on patient characteristics in the prediction of ovarian response and ongoing pregnancy: an individual patient data approach. *Human reproduction update*, *19*(1), 26-36. https://doi.org/10.1093/humupd/dms041

de Marcillac, F. D., Pinton, A., Guillaume, A., Sagot, P., Pirrello, O., & Rongieres, C. (2017). What are the likely IVF/ICSI outcomes if there is a discrepancy between serum AMH and FSH levels? A multicenter retrospective study. *Journal of Gynecology Obstetrics and Human Reproduction*, *46*(8), 629-635.

Dennis, N. A., Houghton, L. A., Pankhurst, M. W., Harper, M. J., & McLennan, I. S. (2017). Acute supplementation with high dose vitamin D3 increases serum anti-Müllerian hormone in young women. *Nutrients*, *9*(7), 719.

Esposito, M. A., Coutifaris, C., & Barnhart, K. T. (2002). A moderately elevated day 3 FSH concentration has limited predictive value, especially in younger women. *Human Reproduction*, *17*(1), 118-123.

Evers, J. L., Slaats, P., Land, J. A., Dumoulin, J. C., & Dunselman, G. A. (1998). Elevated levels of basal estradiol-17β predict poor response in patients with normal basal levels of follicle-stimulating hormone undergoing in vitro fertilization. *Fertility and sterility*, *69*(6), 1010-1014.

Fanchin, R., de Ziegler, D., Olivennes, F., Taieb, J., Dzik, A., & Frydman, R. (1994). Endocrinology: exogenous follicle stimulating hormone ovarian reserve test (EFORT): a simple and reliable screening test for detecting 'poor responders' in in-vitro fertilization. *Human Reproduction*, *9*(9), 1607-1611. https://doi.org/10.1093/oxfordjournals.humrep.a138760

Gougeon, A. (1986). Dynamics of follicular growth in the human: a model from preliminary results. *Human reproduction*, *1*(2), 81-87. https://doi.org/10.1093/oxfordjournals.humrep.a136365

Gougeon, A. (1996). Regulation of ovarian follicular development in primates: facts and hypotheses. *Endocrine reviews*, *17*(2), 121-155.

Hansen, K. R., Knowlton, N. S., Thyer, A. C., Charleston, J. S., Soules, M. R., & Klein, N. A. (2008). A new model of reproductive aging: the decline in ovarian non-growing follicle number from birth to menopause. *Human reproduction*, *23*(3), 699-708.

Hansen, K. R., Morris, J. L., Thyer, A. C., & Soules, M. R. (2003). Reproductive aging and variability in the ovarian antral follicle count: application in the clinical setting. *Fertility and sterility*, *80*(3), 577-583. https://doi.org/10.1016/S0015-0282(03)00741-6

Hee, J., MacNaughton, J., Bangah, M., & Burger, H. G. (1993). Perimenopausal patterns of gonadotrophins, immunoreactive inhibin, oestradiol and progesterone. *Maturitas*, *18*(1), 9-20.

Hehenkamp, W. J., Looman, C. W., Themmen, A. P., de Jong, F. H., Te Velde, E. R., & Broekmans, F. J. (2006). Anti-Mullerian hormone levels in the spontaneous menstrual cycle do not show substantial fluctuation. *The Journal of Clinical Endocrinology & Metabolism*, *91*(10), 4057-4063.

Hendriks, D. J., Broekmans, F. J. M., Bancsi, L. F. J. M. M., De Jong, F. H., Looman, C. W. N., & Te Velde, E. R. (2005b). Repeated clomiphene citrate challenge testing in the prediction of outcome in IVF: a comparison with basal markers for ovarian reserve. *Human reproduction*, *20*(1), 163-169.

Hendriks, D. J., Broekmans, F. J., Bancsi, L. F. J. M. M., Looman, C. W. N., De Jong, F. H., & Te Velde, E. R. (2005a). Single and repeated GnRH agonist stimulation tests compared with basal markers of ovarian reserve in the prediction of outcome in IVF. *Journal of Assisted Reproduction and Genetics*, *22*, 65-74.

Hendriks, D. J., Mol, B. W. J., Bancsi, L. F., te Velde, E. R., & Broekmans, F. J. (2006). The clomiphene citrate challenge test for the prediction of poor ovarian response and nonpregnancy in patients undergoing in vitro fertilization: a systematic review. *Fertility and sterility*, *86*(4), 807-818.

Jayaprakasan, K., Campbell, B., Hopkisson, J., Clewes, J., Johnson, I., & Raine-Fenning, N. (2008). Establishing the intercycle variability of three-dimensional ultrasonographic predictors of ovarian reserve. *Fertility and sterility*, *90*(6), 2126-2132. https://doi.org/10.1016/j.fertnstert.2007.10.028

Jayaprakasan, K., Campbell, B., Hopkisson, J., Johnson, I., & Raine-Fenning, N. (2010). A prospective, comparative analysis of anti-Müllerian hormone, inhibin-B, and three-dimensional ultrasound determinants of ovarian reserve in the prediction of poor response to controlled ovarian stimulation. *Fertility and sterility*, *93*(3), 855-864. https://doi.org/10.1016/j.fertnstert.2008.10.042

Jirge, P. R. (2011). Ovarian reserve tests. *Journal of human reproductive sciences*, *4*(3), 108. https://doi.org/10.4103/0974-1208.92283

Kevenaar, M. E., Meerasahib, M. F., Kramer, P., van de Lang-Born, B. M., de Jong, F. H., Groome, N. P., Themmen, A. P. N., & Visser, J. A. (2006). Serum anti-mullerian hormone levels reflect the size of the primordial follicle pool in mice. *Endocrinology*, *147*(7), 3228-3234. https://doi.org/10.1210/en.2005-1588

Kissell, K. A., Danaher, M. R., Schisterman, E. F., Wactawski-Wende, J., Ahrens, K. A., Schliep, K., Perkins, N.J., Sjaarda, L., Weck, J., & Mumford, S. L. (2014). Biological variability in serum anti-Müllerian hormone throughout the menstrual cycle in ovulatory and sporadic anovulatory cycles in eumenorrheic women. *Human reproduction*, *29*(8), 1764-1772.

Klein, N. A., Illingworth, P. J., Groome, N. P., McNeilly, A. S., Battaglia, D. E., & Soules, M. R. (1996). Decreased inhibin B secretion is associated with the monotropic FSH rise in older, ovulatory women: a study of serum and follicular fluid levels of dimeric inhibin A and B in spontaneous menstrual cycles. *The Journal of Clinical Endocrinology & Metabolism*, *81*(7), 2742-2745.

Knauff, E. A., Eijkemans, M. J., Lambalk, C. B., ten Kate-Booij, M. J., Hoek, A., Beerendonk, C. C., Laven JS, Goverde AJ, Broekmans FJ, Themmen AP, de Jong FH, Fauser BC & Dutch Premature Ovarian Failure Consortium. (2009). Anti-Mullerian hormone, inhibin B, and antral follicle count in young women with ovarian failure. *The Journal of Clinical Endocrinology & Metabolism*, *94*(3), 786-792.

Kupesic, S., Kurjak, A., Bjelos, D., & Vujisic, S. (2003). Three-dimensional ultrasonographic ovarian measurements and in vitro fertilization outcome are related to age. *Fertility and sterility*, *79*(1), 190-197. https://doi.org/10.1016/S0015-0282(02)04567-3

La Marca, A., Sighinolfi, G., Radi, D., Argento, C., Baraldi, E., Artenisio, A. C., Stabile, G., & Volpe, A. (2010). Anti-Müllerian hormone (AMH) as a predictive marker in assisted reproductive technology (ART). *Human reproduction update*, *16*(2), 113-130.

La Marca, A., Stabile, G., Artenisio, A. C., & Volpe, A. (2006). Serum anti-Mullerian hormone throughout the human menstrual cycle. *Human reproduction*, *21*(12), 3103-3107.

Lass, A., Skull, J., McVeigh, E., Margara, R., & Winston, R. (1997). Measurement of ovarian volume by transvaginal sonography before ovulation induction with human menopausal gonadotrophin for in-vitro fertilization can predict poor response. *Human Reproduction (Oxford, England)*, *12*(2), 294-297. https://doi .org/10.1093/humrep/12.2.294

Lorusso, F., Vicino, M., Lamanna, G., Trerotoli, P., Serio, G., & Depalo, R. (2007). Performance of different ovarian reserve markers for predicting the numbers of oocytes retrieved and mature oocytes. *Maturitas*, *56*(4), 429-435. https://doi.org /10.1016/j.maturitas.2006.11.007

Moslehi, N., Shab-Bidar, S., Tehrani, F. R., Mirmiran, P., & Azizi, F. (2018). Is ovarian reserve associated with body mass index and obesity in reproductive aged women? A meta-analysis. *Menopause*, *25*(9), 1046-1055.

Nelson, S. M., Klein, B. M., & Arce, J. C. (2015). Comparison of antimüllerian hormone levels and antral follicle count as predictor of ovarian response to controlled ovarian stimulation in good-prognosis patients at individual fertility clinics in two multicenter trials. *Fertility and Sterility*, *103*(4), 923-930. https:// doi.org/10.1016/j.fertnstert.2014.12.114

Overbeek, A., Broekmans, F. J., Hehenkamp, W. J., Wijdeveld, M. E., van Disseldorp, J., van Dulmen-den Broeder, E., & Lambalk, C. B. (2012). Intra-cycle fluctuations of anti-Müllerian hormone in normal women with a regular cycle: a re-analysis. *Reproductive biomedicine online*, *24*(6), 664-669.

Padilla, S. L., Bayati, J., & Garcia, J. E. (1990). Prognostic value of the early serum estradiol response to leuprolide acetate in in vitro fertilization. *Fertility and sterility*, *53*(2), 288-294.

Peck, J. D., Quaas, A. M., Craig, L. B., Soules, M. R., Klein, N. A., & Hansen, K. R. (2016). Lifestyle factors associated with histologically derived human ovarian non-growing follicle count in reproductive age women. *Human Reproduction*, *31*(1), 150-157.

Polyzos, N. P., Tournaye, H., Guzman, L., Camus, M., & Nelson, S. M. (2013). Predictors of ovarian response in women treated with corifollitropin alfa for in vitro fertilization/intracytoplasmic sperm injection. *Fertility and sterility*, *100*(2), 430-437. https://doi.org/10.1016/j.fertnstert.2013.04.029

Practice Committee of the American Society for Reproductive Medicine. (2015). Testing and interpreting measures of ovarian reserve: a committee opinion. *Fertility and sterility*, *103*(3), e9-e17.

Rajpert-De Meyts, E., Jørgensen, N., Græm, N., Müller, J., Cate, R. L., & Skakkebæk, N. E. (1999). Expression of anti-Mullerian hormone during normal and pathological gonadal development: association with differentiation of Sertoli and granulosa cells. *The Journal of Clinical Endocrinology & Metabolism*, *84*(10), 3836-3844.

Ramalho de Carvalho, B., Gomes Sobrinho, D. B., Vieira, A. D. D., Resende, M. P. S., Barbosa, A. C. P., Silva, A. A., & Nakagava, H. M. (2012). Ovarian reserve assessment for infertility investigation. *International Scholarly Research Notices, 2012*.

Ranieri, D. M., Quinn, F., Makhlouf, A., Khadum, I., Ghutmi, W., McGarrigle, H., Davies, M., & Serhal, P. (1998). Simultaneous evaluation of basal follicle-stimulating hormone and 17β-estradiol response to gonadotropin-releasing hormone analogue stimulation: an improved predictor of ovarian reserve. *Fertility and sterility*, *70*(2), 227-233. https://doi.org/10.1016/S0015-0282(98)00159-9

Scheffer, G. J., Broekmans, F. J. M., Bancsi, L. F., Habbema, J. D. F., Looman, C. W. N., & Te Velde, E. R. (2002). Quantitative transvaginal two-and three-dimensional sonography of the ovaries: reproducibility of antral follicle counts. *Ultrasound in Obstetrics and Gynecology: The Official Journal of the International Society of Ultrasound in Obstetrics and Gynecology*, *20*(3), 270-275. https://doi.org/10.1046/j.1469-0705.2002.00787.x

Scheffer, G. J., Broekmans, F. J., Dorland, M., Habbema, J. D., Looman, C. W., & te Velde, E. R. (1999). Antral follicle counts by transvaginal ultrasonography are related to age in women with proven natural fertility. *Fertility and sterility*, *72*(5), 845-851. https://doi.org/10.1016/S0015-0282(99)00396-9

Schuh-Huerta, S. M., Johnson, N. A., Rosen, M. P., Sternfeld, B., Cedars, M. I., & Reijo Pera, R. A. (2012). Genetic variants and environmental factors associated with hormonal markers of ovarian reserve in Caucasian and African American women. *Human reproduction*, *27*(2), 594-608.

Scott, R. T., Leonardi, M. R., Hofmann, G. E., Illions, E. H., Neal, G. S., & Navot, D. (1993). A prospective evaluation of clomiphene citrate challenge test screening of the general infertility population. *Obstetrics & Gynecology*, *82*(4 Part 1), 539-544.

Sharara, F. I., Scott Jr, R. T., & Seifer, D. B. (1998). The detection of diminished ovarian reserve in infertile women. *American journal of obstetrics and gynecology*, *179*(3), 804-812.

Sowers, M., McConnell, D., Gast, K., Zheng, H., Nan, B., McCarthy, J. D., & Randolph, J. F. (2010). Anti-Müllerian hormone and inhibin B variability during normal menstrual cycles. *Fertility and sterility*, *94*(4), 1482-1486.

Speroff, L., & Fritz, M. A. (Eds.). (2005). *Clinical gynecologic endocrinology and infertility*. Lippincott Williams & Wilkins.

Steiner, A. Z., Pritchard, D., Stanczyk, F. Z., Kesner, J. S., Meadows, J. W., Herring, A. H., & Baird, D. D. (2017). Association between biomarkers of ovarian reserve and infertility among older women of reproductive age. *Jama*, *318*(14), 1367-1376.

Tal, R., & Seifer, D. B. (2017). Ovarian reserve testing: a user's guide. *American journal of obstetrics and gynecology*, *217*(2), 129-140.

Tal, R., Seifer, D. B., Wantman, E., Baker, V., & Tal, O. (2018). Antimüllerian hormone as a predictor of live birth following assisted reproduction: an analysis of 85,062 fresh and thawed cycles from the Society for Assisted Reproductive Technology Clinic Outcome Reporting System database for 2012–2013. *Fertility and sterility*, *109*(2), 258-265. https://doi.org/10.1016/j.fertnstert.2017.10.021

Tanbo, T., Dale, P. O., Lunde, O., Norman, N., & Åbyholm, T. (1992). Prediction of response to controlled ovarian hyperstimulation: a comparison of basal and clomiphene citrate-stimulated follicle-stimulating hormone levels. *Fertility and sterility*, *57*(4), 819-824.

Toner, J. P., & Seifer, D. B. (2013). Why we may abandon basal follicle-stimulating hormone testing: a sea change in determining ovarian reserve using antimüllerian hormone. *Fertility and sterility*, *99*(7), 1825-1830.

Tsepelidis, S., Devreker, F., Demeestere, I., Flahaut, A., Gervy, C., & Englert, Y. (2007). Stable serum levels of anti-Müllerian hormone during the menstrual cycle: a prospective study in normo-ovulatory women. *Human reproduction*, *22*(7), 1837-1840.

Ulrich, N. D., & Marsh, E. E. (2019). Ovarian reserve testing: a review of the options, their applications, and their limitations. *Clinical obstetrics and gynecology*, *62*(2), 228.

Van den Berg, M. H., Van Dulmen-den Broeder, E., Overbeek, A., Twisk, J. W. R., Schats, R., Van Leeuwen, F. E., Kaspers, G. J. & Lambalk, C. B. (2010). Comparison of ovarian function markers in users of hormonal contraceptives during the hormone-free interval and subsequent natural early follicular phases. *Human Reproduction*, *25*(6), 1520-1527.

Westergaard, L., Christensen, I. J., & McNatty, K. P. (1986). Steroid levels in ovarian follicular fluid related to follicle size and health status during the normal menstrual cycle in women. *Human Reproduction*, *1*(4), 227-232. https://doi.org /10.1093/oxfordjournals.humrep.a136390

Winslow, K. L., Toner, J. P., Brzyski, R. G., Oehninger, S. C., Acosta, A. A., & Muasher, S. J. (1991). The gonadotropin-releasing hormone agonist stimulation test—a sensitive predictor of performance in the flare-up in vitro fertilization cycle. *Fertility and sterility*, *56*(4), 711-717.

Yanushpolsky, E. H., Hurwitz, S., Tikh, E., & Racowsky, C. (2003). Predictive usefulness of cycle day 10 follicle-stimulating hormone level in a clomiphene citrate challenge test for in vitro fertilization outcome in women younger than 40 years of age. *Fertility and sterility*, *80*(1), 111-115.

Zaidi, J., Campbell, S., Pittrof, R., Kyei-Mensah, A., Shaker, A., S. Jacobs, H., & Tan, S. L. (1995). Contraception: Ovarian stromal blood flow in women with polycystic ovaries—a possible new marker for diagnosis?. *Human Reproduction*, *10*(8), 1992-1996. https://doi.org/10.1093/oxfordjournals.humrep.a136222

Chapter 9

Basics of Ovarian Stimulation and Oocyte Retrieval

Mehmet Güçlü, MD*

Marmara University Department of Obstetrics and Gynecology, Istanbul, Turkiye

Abstract

Oocyte retrieval and ovarian stimulation procedures were covered in this chapter. The formation of several follicles and the retrieval of an adequate number of oocytes, necessary for laboratory procedures, are made possible by ovarian stimulation for in vitro fertilization (IVF). During the follicular phase of the cycle, exogenous injection of FSH causes the formation of numerous follicles, which raises E2 levels above physiological levels. High levels ofE2 might cause premature LH surges that can negatively affect oocyte maturation, fertilization, endometrial receptivity, and eventually pregnancy rates. Prestimulation management and baseline hormone tests were discussed. Then, based on the patients' responses, we categorize the ovarian stimulation procedures (poor, normal, and high response). GnRH antagonist treatments are recommended for patients who respond well. GnRH antagonist treatments are also recommended for normal responders. Both GnRH agonists and antagonists are recommended for patients who are expected to respond poorly. GnRH antagonist therapy is advised in GnRH agonist protocols, based on our discussion on LH suppression regimens. Lastly, in this chapter, we cover the fundamentals of oocyte retrieval.

Key Words: Ovarian stimulation, Oocyte retrieval, Ovarian stimulation protocols

---

* Corresponding Author's E-mail: drmguclu@gmail.com

In: Holistic Approach to Assisted Reproductive Technology
Editor: Kenan Demir and Rümeysa Yılmaz Göç
ISBN: 979-8-89113-017-3

© 2023 Nova Science Publishers, Inc.

Introduction

Pharmacological therapy used to stimulate ovarian follicle growth is known as ovarian stimulation. It has two uses that can be put to: 1) for timed insemination or insemination; 2) for multiple oocyte aspiration during assisted reproductive technology (ART) (Zegers-Hochschild et al., 2017).

Response to ovarian stimulation is often divided into three categories: poor, normal, and excessive. Although this word may possibly stigmatize or traumatize patients. Therefore, according to the ESHRE Guidelines they use the terminology low, normal, and high response to categorize (predicted) response to OS for future reference (ESHRE Reproductive Endocrinology Guideline Group, 2019).

-A high ovarian response is an excessive reaction to ovarian stimulation using standard methods (150–225 IU FSH), and it is defined by the existence of extra follicles or/and oocytes. (Griesinger et al., 2016). In general, a high response (Griesinger et al., 2016) is characterized by the collection of 18 or more oocytes and/or more than 18 follicles that are less than 11 mm on the day the oocyte maturation trigger occurs.

A small number of follicles and/or oocytes are indicative of a low ovarian response, which is a decreased response to conventional ovarian stimulation (Ferraretti et al., 2011). In general, a poor response is defined as having less than three follicles on the day the trigger for oocyte maturation occurs and/or three or more oocytes (ESHRE Reproductive Endocrinology Guideline Group, 2019).

Ovarian Stimulation

Ovarian Response Testing

Pre-Stimulation Management

Antral folicular count (AFC) has been investigated in patients stimulated with various doses and regimens of FSH, as well as in GnRH agonist and antagonist cycles. AFC has been shown to be more valuable than age alone for predicting the ovarian response. AMH has been studied in GnRH agonist and antagonist cycles, in people stimulated with various dosages of FSH, and during various FSH operations. AMH was an excellent predictor of ovarian response despite the fact that the definitions of poor and high response were inconsistent. To predict a high or low response to ovarian stimulation, the use of antral follicle count (AFC) or anti-Müllerian hormone (AMH) is recommended above other ovarian reserve assays.

Both AFC and AMH predict ovarian response categories with a high degree of precision (high or poor). It could be advised for clinical use, taking into account the false positive and negative rate of the test. The doctor can choose the best test for a given clinical situation.

A very high cut-off value must be used for a reliable prediction, despite the fact that basal FSH and inhibin B have some predictive value for the ovarian response. This suggests that a very small percentage of women will have FSH or inhibitory B test findings that are so abnormal. Since alternative tests are readily available with better accuracy, this has very little clinical relevance. Age also has some predictive relevance, although the classification of the ovarian response category by age alone is insufficiently precise. One cannot anticipate the ovarian response just based on BMI and basal estradiol levels. Therefore, to predict the ovarian response, we do not recommend using baseline FSH, inhibin B, basal oestradiol, age or BMI (ESHRE Reproductive Endocrinology Guideline Group, 2019).

Additional Hormonal Assessment at the Baseline

Baseline Oestradiol: In IVF/ICSI, measuring oestradiol at the beginning of stimulation is a common practice. An elevated level frequently indicates the presence of a simple follicular cyst, which is later confirmed by ultrasound. The E2 level at the beginning of stimulation has also been used to attempt to predict the results of stimulation. There is no advice that can be given due to the complete lack of evidence on the prognostic efficacy of baseline oestradiol in women who receive ovarian stimulation for IVF/ICSI (ESHRE Reproductive Endocrinology Guideline Group, 2019).

Progesterone: Progesterone levels in menstruation are high in some cycles. Reduced pregnancy rates may be associated with elevated progesterone levels at the time when ovarian stimulation is supposed to begin.

The proportion of patients with progesterone levels >1.6 ng/ml on cycle day 2 was 4.9 percent (95 percent CI 3.2-7.4) in a cohort study by Kolibianakis et al. and 6.2 percent (95 percent CI 4-9) in a cohort study by Blockeel et al., respectively (Kolibianakis et al., 2004; Stanger& Yovich, 1985).A more recent study found that 13.3% (95% confidence interval [CI] 8–20] of the patients had progesterone levels greater than 1.5 ng/ml. According to Faulisi et al. (Faulisi et al., 2017), progesterone levels were present on cycle day 3 in 0.3% (95 percent confidence interval [CI] 0.01-1.15) of individuals (Hamdine et al., 2014). Given the low incidence, it does not seem appropriate to take this study question into account for progesterone levels >1.6 ng/ml on cycle day 3. Checking progesterone on cycle day 2, when ovarian stimulation starts, is generally not a good idea. The recommendation is not available to patients older than 39 years (ESHRE Reproductive Endocrinology Guideline Group, 2019).

Pretreatment Therapies

Prior to gonadotrophin stimulation in IVF cycles, pretreatment medications seek to inhibit or diminish LH and/or FSH release. They are used by physicians for a variety of purposes, including coordinating follicular growth, preventing early large follicles or spontaneous LH surges, and minimizing cyst formation. To organize IVF cycles in a way that is beneficial to patients, medical personnel, and lab personnel, pretreatment is also used. It makes it possible to spread IVF operations over several weeks or months, skipping work on weekends and vacations (ESHRE Reproductive Endocrinology Guideline Group, 2019).

Estrogen Pretreatment: In a Cochrane meta-analysis on the pretreatment of estrogen for ovarian stimulation protocols for women undergoing assisted reproductive technologies, four randomized controlled trials (RCTs) were combined that included 744 women (ART). In GnRH antagonist protocols, the estrogen pretreatment and nontreatment groups did not vary in the frequency of live births/ongoing pregnancy (2 RCT, OR 0.79, 95% CI 0.53-1.17, 502 women), or clinical pregnancy (4 RCT, OR 0.91, 95% CI 0.66-1.24, 688 women) (Farquhar et al., 2017). Significantly more oocytes were recovered in the estrogen-treated group using the GnRH antagonist regimen than in the control group (2 RCT, MD 2.23, 95% CI 0.71 to 3.75, 139 women) (Farquhar et al., 2017). Pretreatment with estrogen prior to ovarian stimulation using the GnRH antagonist method is probably not indicated to improve effectiveness and safety (ESHRE Reproductive Endocrinology Guideline Group, 2019).

Progesterone Pretreatment: In 4 RCTs with 421 female participants, the previously mentioned Cochrane meta-analysis also looked at the effect of progesterone pretreatment for OS. There was no difference in live birth/ongoing pregnancy rate between the groups in GnRH agonist protocols (2 RCT, OR 1.35, 95% CI 0.69-2.65, 222 women) when pretreatment with progestogen was compared with no intervention. To increase efficacy and safety, pretreatment with progesterone before ovarian stimulation is probably not recommended (ESHRE Reproductive Endocrinology Guideline Group, 2019).

Combined Oral Contraceptive Pill (COCP) Pretreatment: Progesterone pretreatment for OS was also investigated in the previously mentioned Cochrane meta-analysis in 4 RCTs with 421 female participants. When progestogen pretreatment was compared with no intervention, there was no difference in live birth/ongoing pregnancy rate between the groups in GnRH agonist protocols (2 RCT, OR 1.35, 95 percent CI 0.69-2.65, 222 women). It is probably not advisable to administer progesterone as a pretreatment before ovarian stimulation to increase effectiveness and safety (ESHRE Reproductive Endocrinology Guideline Group, 2019).

Gnrh Antagonist Pretreatment: A small RCT involving 69 normogonadotropic women found no difference between the early follicular pretreatment with the GnRH antagonist (delayed start protocol) and no pre-treatment in the fixed antagonist protocol in terms of the ongoing pregnancy rate (42 vs 33%, 95% CI -13-3) or the number of oocytes (12.87.8 vs 9.94.9). (not PCOS, not poor responder) (Blockeel et al., 2011). In a delayed-start gonadotrophin operation, it is probably not indicated to administer a GnRH antagonist before ovarian stimulation (ESHRE Reproductive Endocrinology Guideline Group, 2019).

Ovarian Stimulation and LH Suppression

Ovarian Stimulation Protocols

High Responder

GnRH Antagonist vs Agonist: The live birth rate was comparable in both groups of women with PCOS who were randomly assigned to a prolonged treatment with an agonist or antagonist of GnRH, according to a meta-analysis (3 RCT, RR 0.90, 95% CI 0.69-1.19, 363 women) (Lambalk et al., 2017). Administration of the GnRH antagonist significantly reduced the risk of OHSS compared to the GnRH agonist regimen (9 RCT, RR 0.53; 95% CI 0.30-0.95; 1294 women) (Lambalk et al., 2017). According to ESHRE recommendations, the GnRH antagonist approach is indicated for women with PCOS due to improved safety and equal effectiveness. Regarding increased safety and equal effectiveness, the GnRH antagonist method is recommended for high-response projected participants (ESHRE Reproductive Endocrinology Guideline Group, 2019). There is evidence that the GnRH antagonist regimen is just as effective as the GnRH agonist regimen in reducing the risk of OHSS in PCOS women. According to the conclusion of the ESHRE GDG, the GnRH antagonist regimen should be recommended in these patient categories since it offers the best chances for the prevention of OHSS (ESHRE Reproductive Endocrinology Guideline Group, 2019).

Mild Stimulation: Using gonadotropins and/or other pharmacological agents, the ovaries are slightly stimulated during the IVF process to encourage the production of a few follicles. Modest stimulation is characterized differently in research and practice. Instead of the usual daily dose of 150-225 IU of FSH, a smaller dose or delayed start can be used to offer modest stimulation (ESHRE Reproductive Endocrinology Guideline Group, 2019).

Clomiphene Citrate: For projected high responders, adding Clomiphene Citrate to gonadotropins in stimulation protocols is probably not a good idea. Adding clomiphene citrate to gonadotropin stimulation in OS does not, according to cohort studies, result in better outcomes in terms of efficacy and safety. Due to the paucity of high-quality data, the guideline committee does not recommend using Clomiphene citrate in stimulation regimens for high-response expected patients (ESHRE Reproductive Endocrinology Guideline Group, 2019).

Aromatase Inhibitors: The present findings do not support the addition of letrozole to gonadotropin stimulation regimens for the high responders expected. According to the limited information from nonrandomized trials, the addition of letrozole to FSH for OS is not associated with any advantages in terms of effectiveness or safety. Due to the lack of high-quality data, the ESHRE GDG does not recommend utilizing letrozole in stimulation protocols for anticipated high responders. Letrozole is also used for off-label ovarian stimulation, and the teratogenic potential of the drug has raised safety concerns (ESHRE Reproductive Endocrinology Guideline Group, 2019).

Reduced Dose Protocol: It is suggested to use the GnRH antagonist regimen for patients with high predicted response rates. When using GnRH agonist regimens, a lower dose of gonadotropin is generally indicated to reduce the risk of OHSS. Recent studies suggest that safety can be improved by lowering the dose of gonadotropin in a GnRH agonist treatment. It is crucial to consider the combination of GnRH agonist and antagonist procedures, the permitted dosage adjustments in the second cycle, and the extremely high cycle cancelation rate among high responders when examining the available data. The lack of a freeze-all strategy, which may reflect actual clinical practice, raises more doubts about the potential negative consequences of standard dosage stimulation on the cumulative pregnancy rate and OHSS rates (ESHRE Reproductive Endocrinology Guideline Group, 2019).

Modified Natural Cycle:

A modified natural cycle (MNC) is an IVF technique in which one or more oocytes are extracted from the ovaries throughout a regular menstrual cycle. Only to stop the natural surge in LH and / or trigger the last stages of oocyte maturation are pharmaceuticals administered. There is no evidence to support the use of NC or MNC for OS in high responders (ESHRE Reproductive Endocrinology Guideline Group, 2019).

Normal Responder

GnRH Antagonist vs GnRH Agonist

Due to greater safety, the GnRH antagonist regimen is suggested for women with estimated normal response. Due to the equal live birth rates between the

GnRH antagonist and GnRH agonist protocols and the significant decrease in OHSS risk with the GnRH antagonist protocol in the general IVF population, the GnRH antagonist protocol is indicated in patients who are normal responders (ESHRE Reproductive Endocrinology Guideline Group, 2019).

Mild Stimulation

Clomiphene Citrate (CC): There is no evidence to support the suggestion that stimulation treatments for patients who are expected to respond normally should also contain clomiphene citrate.

The proof came from studies done on patients who were not predicted to react negatively. Therefore, participants in the study could be both normal and high responders. The only one that could be found was a pilot study that was not randomized. As a result, extrapolating the research findings proved impossible (ESHRE Reproductive Endocrinology Guideline Group, 2019).

Aromatase Inhibitors: Letrozole should probably not be added to gonadotropins in stimulation protocols for projected normal responders. Letrozole is not added to FSH in a GnRH antagonist approach to increase OS efficacy. The use of letrozole may reduce the risk of OHSS, but this was only proven in one limited RCT. Furthermore, letrozole cannot be used to stimulate ovarian function (ESHRE Reproductive Endocrinology Guideline Group, 2019).

Reduced Dose Protocol: A lower gonadotrophin dose is probably not recommended for anticipated normal responders over a usual gonadotrophin dose. Due to the improved safety offered by the GnRH agonist trigger option, the ESHRE GDG considers that the recommendation may also be applicable to GnRH antagonist protocols. The advice is based on research done on GnRH agonist protocols (ESHRE Reproductive Endocrinology Guideline Group, 2019).

Poor Responder

GnRH Antagonist vs GnRH Agonist

A recent RCT compared the brief treatment with the GnRH agonist strategy with the GnRH antagonist strategy and included 146 people with poor responses. The clinical pregnancy rate with the short GnRH agonist protocol was significantly higher compared to the long GnRH antagonist regimen (29.3% (22/75) vs. 14.1% (10/71)).

Patients who are expected to respond poorly are recommended to take both GnRH agonists and antagonists.

Both the GnRH agonist and GnRH antagonist protocols are equally safe and effective for use in women with limited ovarian response. The long GnRH agonist protocol is compared with the shorter treatment duration associated with the GnRH antagonist regimen (ESHRE Reproductive Endocrinology Guideline Group, 2019).

Mild Stimulation

Clomiphene Citrate (CC): The previously cited meta-analysis by Bechtejew et al. examined the interaction of CC with gonadotrophins in a GnRH antagonist protocol as well and discovered that it was not superior to gonadotrophins in a GnRH agonist protocol in terms of live birth rate (3 RCT, RR 0.88, 95% CI 0.62-1.26, 874 women) (Bechtejew et al., 2017).

Both gonadotropin stimulation alone and clomiphene citrate alone or in combination with gonadotrophins are equally suggested for patients who are expected to respond badly.

In women with a poor ovarian response, there were no discernible differences in terms of safety and efficacy between CC alone, CC combined with gonadotropins, or gonadotropin stimulation alone (ESHRE Reproductive Endocrinology Guideline Group, 2019).

Aromatase Inhibitors: Letrozole should not typically be administered to stimulation techniques involving gonadotropins for patients who are predicted to respond poorly.

Letrozole is not added to FSH in a GnRH antagonist approach to increase OS efficacy. There are no studies that compare the use of letrozole alone vs. gonadotropin stimulation alone for IVF / ICIS.

Off-label use of letrozole for ovarian stimulation has raised safety concerns due to the possible teratogenicity of the drug (ESHRE Reproductive Endocrinology Guideline Group, 2019).

Reduced Dose Protocol: There are no studies comparing conventional FSH stimulation in non-responders with a lower FSH dose (150 IU/day) (ESHRE Reproductive Endocrinology Guideline Group, 2019).

Higher Gonadotropin Dose

Patients who are predicted to respond poorly are encouraged to take more gonadotropin than 150 IU. There is evidence that gonadotropin doses above 150 IU increase the number of oocytes in weak responders and increase the probability of having an embryo for transfer.

It is not recommended to provide patients who are expected to respond poorly with a gonadotropin dose greater than 300 IU.

There is unlikely to be a major advantage with doses >300 IU daily, as comparisons with doses >300 IU did not indicate significant differences in the aforementioned preclinical results (ESHRE Reproductive Endocrinology Guideline Group, 2019).

Modified Natural Cycle

Modified natural cycles are probably not recommended over conventional stimulation for predicted poor responders. There are no high-quality controlled trials that support the use of modified natural cycle or natural cycle IVF in underachieving women (ESHRE Reproductive Endocrinology Guideline Group, 2019).

LH Suppression Regimens

GnRH Agonist Protocols

In the Cochrane meta-analysis there is no evidence of a difference in live birth rate between short and long protocols (Siristatidis et al., 2015). Also in the same meta-analysis the clinical pregnancy rate does not differ between short and long protocols (Frydman et al., 1988; Stanger & Yovich, 1985).

They compared long and ultrashort protocols and there is no difference in live birth rate (Siristatidis et al., 2015 ; Kingsland et al., 1992). There were no documented negative outcomes data. When ultrashort protocol compared to short protocol there was no difference between clinical pregnancy rate (Berker et al., 2010; Siristatidis et al., 2015). There were no documented negative outcomes data (ESHRE Reproductive Endocrinology Guideline Group, 2019).

Continuation vs. discontinuation at the beginning of long GnRH agonist therapy

When the GnRH agonist was terminated versus continued, there was no discernible change in the number of ongoing pregnancies with Ovarian Hyperstimulation syndrome (Siristatidis et al., 2015). The dose of the GnRH agonist should be maintained rather than decreased until the trigger.

Contrary to when the same amount of GnRH agonist was used, there are no signs that the pregnancy rate changed when the dose was decreased (Siristatidis et al., 2015). There were no documented negative outcomes data.

The long GnRH agonist regimen is probably recommended over the short or ultra-short GnRH agonist protocols if GnRH agonists are utilized.

Long-term treatment with the GnRH agonist has been shown to be quite effective in reducing the LH surge. Since its implementation, fewer cycles have been abandoned, more oocytes have been recovered, and pregnancy rates have increased. The comprehensive regimen is more effective than alternate GnRH agonist treatments and more evidence supports it.

The original purpose of the brief GnRH agonist treatment was to improve cycle results in patients with weak responses and older individuals. The evidence we now have indicates that this objective has not been achieved. The original purpose of the brief GnRH agonist treatment was to improve cycle results in patients with weak responses and older individuals. The evidence we now have indicates that this objective has not been achieved (ESHRE Reproductive Endocrinology Guideline Group, 2019).

GnRH Antagonist Protocol

73 RCTs were included in a Cochrane meta-analysis contrasting the extended GnRH agonist regimen with the GnRH antagonist treatment (Al-Inanyet al., 2016). There was no proof that the live birth rate changed after the GnRH antagonist versus the GnRH agonist (12 RCT, OR 1.02, 95% CI 0.85-1.23, 2303 women). However, there was evidence that women who received GnRH antagonist treatment had a lower OHSS rate than those who received GnRH agonist treatment (6% (290/4474) vs. 11% (396/3470); 36 RCT, OR 0.61, 95% CI 0.51-0.72, 7944 women) (Al-Inanyet al., 2016).

The comparable efficacy and improved safety in the general population of IVF / ICSI favor the GnRH antagonist regimen over the GnRH agonist protocols.

The development of GnRH antagonists allowed the severe negative effects of GnRH agonist treatments to be overcome. The GnRH antagonist regimen had to be implemented later due to the slightly but consistently lower pregnancy rates of the initial studies, although multiple sizable meta-analyses published in the last 5-7 years support comparable live birth rates (ESHRE Reproductive Endocrinology Guideline Group, 2019).

Progestin

It is a novel strategy that does not include GnRH analogs to use oral progestins to inhibit LH surge. Treatment with progestin during stimulation maintains pituitary control and has been shown to effectively suppress the LH surge. Due to the effect of progestins, the endometrium would not respond in a new cycle; therefore, the use of this method requires the preservation of all embryos and their transfer into a subsequent endometrial preparation cycle (ESHRE Reproductive Endocrinology Guideline Group, 2019).

The results of progestin LH suppression against alternative methods have been compared in three prospective cohort studies (Chen et al., 2017a; Kuang et al., 2015; Hamdi et al., 2018). Treatment with progestin and natural cycle had the same live birth rate (8.3% (10/102) vs. 3.92% (4/102) in 204 women, according to Chen et al (Chen et al., 2017a). However, after the progestin regimen, considerably more oocytes were recovered (1.09 (0.93-1.18) versus 0.76 (0.65-0.86)) (Chen et al., 2017b).

Progesterone is probably not recommended for LH peak suppression. Progestin can only be administered during nontransfer cycles.

Oral progestins are as effective at suppressing LH as the GnRH short-agonist protocol in terms of oocyte yield and pregnancy outcomes. This strategy is simple, affordable, and patient-friendly.

But there is not much evidence at this time. Additionally, this strategy can only be used for OS cycles when there is no planned fresh embryo transfer, including cycles for oocyte donation, freeze all, or fertility preservation (ESHRE Reproductive Endocrinology Guideline Group, 2019).

Oocyte Retrieval

Principles

The guiding principle behind any successful oocyte collection is to provide the embryologist with healthy oocytes. The aim is to retrieve the oocyte from each and every aspirated follicle, with the minimum risk of damage to the delicate cumulus–oocyte complex, and transfer them to the laboratory without a significant drop in temperature.

The procedure itself must be performed in a stable, comfortable and safe environment, with minimal risk of complications. To achieve this goal, a suitable facility with a procedure room attached to a laboratory is needed, equipped not only with the necessary instruments for vaginal oocyte retrieval but also with the appropriate safety apparatus to allow the delivery of sedation anesthesia with adequate resuscitation if necessary in anemergency. Additionally, as in any medical scenario, appropriately trained and competent staff must be available (Kovacs et al., 2019).

Equipment

Ultrasound

The first attempts at a transvaginal ultrasound-guided transvaginal approach to egg collection were described by Feichtinger in 1986 (Feichtinger & Kemeter, 1986), using a newly developed transvaginal transducer (Kretztechnik-Zipf, Austria), with a needle guide attached to the probe. Their technique involved using a spring-guided puncture device. Since those early days, both ultrasound technology and needle design have improved significantly. Although 3D ultrasound has been tried as a means of collecting to collect oocytes, with 3D puncture procedures performed in close to real-time ultrasound, there is a delay of approximately 5 seconds per follicle from coasting to resuming real-time ultrasound to allow volume calculation and precise location of the needle tip in the follicle (Feichtinger, 1998). Therefore, in most clinical situations where the ovaries are accessible transvaginally, conventional 2D transvaginal ultrasound probes are employed. Occasionally, where the ovaries are highly mobile, abdominal pressure may be required to push the ovaries closer to the vagina. In rare circumstances where this is not possible, a transabdominal, transvesical approach may still be used (Kovacs et al., 2019).

Needle Design

The aim is to collect the oocyte from the follicle into a suitable container to be passed to the scientist as quickly as possible without physical damage to mass of the cumulus – oocytes and significant loss of temperature. The needle must be long enough to pass safely through the vaginal wall into the ovary, but the dead space, representing the volume of the cylinder created by the cross-sectional interior area of the needle and its length (Rose, 2014), must be minimized, so collected oocytes pass through the collecting tube and do not remain in the tube. Historically, the diameter of the needle employed varies between 14 and 16gauge, giving internal diameters of between 1.6 and 1.194 mm, respectively (Lenz & Lauritzen, 1982;Lewin et al., 1986), with relatively short bevels (Aziz et al., 1993). Today, the most commonly used needles are 16 to 17 gauge, which have a dead space of 1.0–1.2 cc respectively. The needle must be as rigid as possible to ensure that it stays in the course of the guideline visible on the screen, and it is vital that the tip of the needle is visualized at all times (Kovacs et al., 2019).

Physics of Suction Aspiration

Before the onset of accurate monitored electrical pumps, the high aspiration pressures associated with handheld syringes were shown to negatively impact the zona pellucida (Lowe et al., 1988). A suction source with a graduated controlled aspiration pressure is required to drain the follicular fluid in a controlled manner, without exerting too much pressure. Aspiration pressure is determined to some extent by the Hagen–Poiseuille law, which determines the steady flow through the pipes (Lowe et al., 1988).

The pressure within an individual follicle is dependent on size, shape, and position within the ovary with increased pressure in bigger follicles (Lowe et al., 1988). The pressure within the follicle increases by approximately 60 mm Hg as the needle presses on the follicular wall, such that there is a risk that when the follicle is entered fluid escapes past the needle, unless the seal is tight. Potentially, this escape of follicular fluid could be avoided if the vacuum is applied before the follicle is entered, as the build-up in aspiration pressure has occurred outside the follicle, but this needs to be balanced by the fact that, in these circumstances, as the needle enters the follicle, the flow rate dramatically increases, causing turbulence within the tube, which may damage the oocyte. If suction is applied once the follicle is entered, the flow rates normally take one to two seconds to stabilize, with a rapid increase in the flow rate followed by a more stable gradual rise to maximum flow. Assuming a good seal around the needle tip, the flow remains constant until the follicle starts to collapse, and then the flow rate falls. If the vacuum is stopped too soon before the needle is removed from the follicle, there is a risk of back flow, which could leave the oocyte in the follicle. Again, the flow rate increases significantly as the needle is completely withdrawn from the ovary (Kovacs et al., 2019).

Damage to the Cumulus-Oocyte Complex

Damage to the oocyte cumulus complex can occur from turbulence, vacuum pressure or velocity, and it can occur in the needle, vacuum lines, or the follicle. There is a vacuum gradient through the collection system. The vacuum at the needle tip is only approximately 5% of that at the vacuum pump. The oocyte is exposed to ever-increasing vacuum pressures along the collection system. This may cause the oocyte to swell or the zona to crack. High velocities may cause the cumulus cells to detach. There will be a significant difference in the flow rate within the needle, with higher flow rates centrally (laminar flow). This may exert drag pressure on the cumulus cells. In a 17 gauge needle, the cumulus–oocyte complex (COC) will occupy25% of the diameter of the needle. Turbulence can scatter the oocyte around in the tube and cause the cell stripping of the cumulus or the zona pellucida to crack (Kovacs et al., 2019).

Follicular Flushing

Pregnancy rates are believed to be directly related to the number of retrieved oocytes (Sunkara et al., 2011). In most studies, the oocytes are recovered from approximately 80% of follicles aspirated. Originally, most oocyte collection needles used to be single channel; if an oocyte was not retrieved in the initial aspirate, flushing was required. This could result in the oocyte moving back and forward in the operating channel of the needle. Dual-channel needles were designed to allow follicular flushing by providing a second channel down which flush medium could be administered (Kovacs et al., 2019).

Temperature Control

The meiotic spindles of the human oocyte consist of microtubules and, like most mammals, are extremely sensitive to temperature fluctuation, both up and down. The spindle structure can dissemble relatively quickly upon cooling, but takes longer to recover on rewarming. The temperature drop and the length of time the oocyte is exposed to coolingwill determine whether the spindle will recover. Relatively minor drops in temperature from37° C to 33° C can be tolerated for less than 10 minutes, before rewarming, but greater drops in temperature for longer periods of time will result in permanent damage. This is very pertinent in assisted conception, as the oocyte is subject to temperature changes at the time of recovery of the oocyte and during manipulation in the laboratory. The meiotic spindles are responsible for chromosome alignment and separation of maternal chromosomes during fertilization. Therefore, any spindle disruption can lead to abnormal chromosome distribution, leading subsequently to failed fertilization or aneuploidy (Kovacs et al., 2019).

Complications of Transvaginal Oocyte Recovery

Transvaginal ultrasound-guided oocyte retrieval is a safe, well-tolerated procedure with a low risk of serious complications. The blood loss of the oocyte procedure is calculated using preoperative and postoperative hemoglobin measurements and is estimated to be approximately230 ml. The most at risk are those with multiple follicles to aspirate, such as women with PCOS. Occasionally, patients may bleed from the vaginal puncture sites, but in most cases this bleeding will settle with the application of pressure. Rarely can a haemostatic suture be required if bleeding persists. Rarely can more significant bleeding occur, with an incidence of 1–2 per 1000 cases. This is most likely to be ovarian, but could arise from a punctured iliac vessel. It is important to be vigilant, as most women who have oocyte retrieval are young and healthy, and tolerate a significant blood loss, decompensating later than expected. Often the bleeding site is difficult to identify, and simple over sowing of capsular puncture sites will be sufficient to control hemorrhage. Infection is the other significant complication that can occur in the first week after the oocyte collection procedure, but can be delayed up to six weeks. Pelvic infection with pyrexia and pelvic tenderness that required antibiotic therapy occurred in 9 cases in a large series of 2677 oocyte collection procedures, with 9 more significant infections with abscess formation giving an overall incidence of 0.6 percent, which is similar to the rate of pelvic tubo-ovarian abscess found in other large series. Those most at risk are those with endometrioma, although the risk is too small to justify routine removal of endometrioma before treatment. Other more unusual but extremely rare complications have been reported, such as ureteric injury, damage to the appendix, or vertebral osteomyelitis (Kovacs et al., 2019).

Conclusion

Compared to other predictors, AFC and AMH are reliable indicators of ovarian response. We discussed pretreatment therapies prior to ovarian stimulation. However, there are no suggestions on pretreatment therapies prior to beginning ovarian stimulation. In patients with high and normal responder levels, GnRH antagonist treatments are advised. Higher-dose protocols are advised for people with unsatisfactory responses. To prevent the surge of LH, extended GnRH agonist treatment has been shown to be quite effective. Oral progestins are as effective at suppressing LH as the GnRH short-agonist protocol in terms of oocyte yield and pregnancy outcomes. There is no difference in LH surge prevention between long and short GnRH agonist treatments. Before oocyte retrieval, transvaginal ultrasonography is the preferred ultrasound method for oocyte visualization. Today, physicians frequently use 16, 17, or 18 gauge needles to retrieve oocytes. When suctioning oocytes, it is important to consider the possibility of cumulus-oocyte complex destruction as well as the possibility of follicular flushing. Controlling temperature is yet another crucial aspect of oocyte retrieval. Potential complications issues are also crucial and should be handled properly.

References

Al-Inany, H. G., Youssef, M. A., Ayeleke, R. O., Brown, J., Lam, W. S., & Broekmans, F. J. (2016). Gonadotrophin-releasing hormone antagonists for assisted reproductive technology. *Cochrane Database of Systematic Reviews*, (4), 1-142. https://doi.org/10.1002/14651858.CD001750.pub4.

Aziz, N., Biljan, M. M., Taylor, C. T., Manasse, P. R., & Kingsland, C. R. (1993). Effect of aspirating needle calibre on outcome of in-vitro fertilization. *Human Reproduction*, *8*(7), 1098-1100.https://doi.org/10.1093/oxfordjournals.humrep.a138200.

Bechtejew, T. N., Nadai, M. N., Nastri, C. O., & Martins, W. P. (2017). Clomiphene citrate and letrozole to reduce follicle-stimulating hormone consumption during ovarian stimulation: systematic review and meta-analysis. *Ultrasound in Obstetrics & Gynecology*, *50*(3), 315-323.https://doi.org/10.1002/uog.17442.

Berker, B., Duvan, C. İ., Kaya, C., Aytaç, R., & Şatıroğlu, H. (2010). Comparison of the ultrashort gonadotropin-releasing hormone agonist-antagonist protocol with microdose flare-up protocol in poor responders: a preliminary study. *Journal of the Turkish German Gynecological Association*, *11*(4), 187.

Blockeel, C., Baumgarten, M., De Vos, M., Verheyen, G., & Devroey, P. (2011). Administration of GnRH antagonists in case of elevated progesterone at initiation of the cycle: a prospective cohort study. *Current Pharmaceutical Biotechnology*, *12*(3), 423-428.https://doi.org/10.2174/138920111794480633.

Chen, Q., Wang, Y., Sun, L., Zhang, S., Chai, W., Hong, Q., Long H, Wang L, Lyu Q,& Kuang, Y. (2017a). Controlled ovulation of the dominant follicle using progestin in minimal stimulation in poor responders. *Reproductive Biology and Endocrinology*, *15*, 1-9. https://doi.org/10.1186/s12958-017-0291-0.

Chen Q, Wang Y, Sun L, Zhang S, Chai W, Hong Q, Long H, Wang L, Lyu Q, Kuang Y. (2017b). Oral contraceptive pill, progestogen or oestrogen pretreatment for ovarian stimulation protocols for women undergoing assisted reproductive techniques. *The Cochrane database of systematic reviews*, *5*, Cd006109. https://doi.org/10.1002/14651858.CD006109.pub3.

Faulisi, S., Reschini, M., Borroni, R., Paffoni, A., Busnelli, A., & Somigliana, E. (2017). Clinical value of basal serum progesterone prior to initiate ovarian hyper-stimulation with GnRH antagonists: a retrospective cohort study. *Gynecologic and Obstetric Investigation*, *82*(2), 175-180.https://doi.org/10.1159/000446952.

Farquhar, C., Rombauts, L., Kremer, J. A., Lethaby, A., & Ayeleke, R. O. (2017). Oral contraceptive pill, progestogen or oestrogen pretreatment for ovarian stimulation protocols for women undergoing assisted reproductive techniques. *Cochrane Database of Systematic Reviews*, (5), 1-129. Feichtinger, W., & Kemeter, P. (1986). Transvaginal sector scan sonography for needle guided transvaginal follicle aspiration and other applications in gynecologic routine and research. *Fertility and sterility*, *45*(5), 722-725. https://doi.org/ 10.1016/s0015-0282(16)49349-0.

Ferraretti, A., La Marca, A., Fauser, B. C. J. M., Tarlatzis, B., Nargund, G., Gianaroli, L., & ESHRE working group on Poor Ovarian Response Definition. (2011). ESHRE consensus on the definition of 'poor response'to ovarian stimulation for in vitro fertilization: the Bologna criteria. *Human reproduction*, *26*(7), 1616-1624. https://doi.org/ 10.1093/humrep/der092.

Frydman, R., Parneix, I., Belaisch-Allart, J., Forman, R., Hazout, A., Fernandez, H., & Testart, J. (1988). LHRH agonists in IVF: different methods of utilization and comparison with previous ovulation stimulation treatments. *Human Reproduction*, *3*(4), 559-561. https://doi.org/ 10.1093/oxfordjournals.humrep.a136744.

Griesinger, G., Verweij, P. J., Gates, D., Devroey, P., Gordon, K., Stegmann, B. J., & Tarlatzis, B. C. (2016). Prediction of ovarian hyperstimulation syndrome in patients treated with corifollitropin alfa or rFSH in a GnRH antagonist protocol. *PloS one*, *11*(3), e0149615. https://doi.org/10.1371/journal.pone.0149615.

ESHRE Reproductive Endocrinology Guideline Group (2019). *Ovarian Stimulation for IVF/ICSI Guideline of the European Society of Human Reproduction and Embryology*. ESHRE. https://doi.org/10.1093/hropen/hoaa009.

Hamdi, K., Farzadi, L., Ghasemzadeh, A., Navali, N., Atashkhoei, S., Pia, H., Shahnazi, V., Fattahi, A., Bahrami-asl, Z., Sepasi, F., Faliz, M. D., Lahroudi, N.,& Hakimi, P. (2018). Comparison of medroxyprogesterone acetate with cetrotide for prevention of premature luteinizing hormone surges in women undergoing in vitro fertilization. *Int J Women Health Reprod Sci*, *6*, 187-191. https://doi.org/10.15296/ijwhr.2018.31

Hamdine, O., Macklon, N. S., Eijkemans, M. J., Laven, J. S., Cohlen, B. J., Verhoeff, A., van Dop PA, Bernardus RE, Lambalk CB, Oosterhuis GJ,Holleboom CA, van den Dool-Maasland GC, Verburg HJ, van der Heijden PF, Blankhart A, Fauser BC, Broekmans FJ & CETRO trial study group. (2014). Elevated early follicular progesterone levels and in vitro fertilization outcomes: a prospective intervention study and meta-analysis. *Fertility and sterility*, *102*(2), 448-454. https://doi.org/10.1016/j.fertnstert.2014.05.002

Kingsland, C., Tan, S. L., Bickerton, N., Mason, B., & Campbell, S. (1992). The routine use of gonadotropin-releasing hormone agonists for all patients undergoing in vitro fertilization. Is there any medical advantage? A prospective randomized study. *Fertility and sterility*, *57*(4), 804-809. https://doi.org/ 10.1016/ s0015-0282(16)54962-0.

Kolibianakis, E. M., Zikopoulos, K., Smitz, J., Camus, M., Tournaye, H., Van Steirteghem, A. C., & Devroey, P. (2004). Elevated progesterone at initiation of stimulation is associated with a lower ongoing pregnancy rate after IVF using GnRH antagonists. *Human reproduction*, *19*(7), 1525-1529. https://doi.org/10 .1093/humrep/deh272.

Kovacs, G., Rutherford, A., & Gardner, D. K. (Eds.). (2019). *How to Prepare the Egg and Embryo to Maximize IVF Success.* Cambridge Press .

Kuang Y, Chen Q, Fu Y, Wang Y, Hong Q, Lyu Q, Ai A, Shoham Z. (2015). Medroxyprogesterone acetate is an effective oral alternative for preventing premature luteinizing hormone surges in women undergoing controlled ovarian hyperstimulation for in vitro fertilization. *Fertility and sterility,* 104, 62-70.e63. https://doi.org/10.1016/j.fertnstert.2015.03.022.

Lambalk, C. B., Banga, F. R., Huirne, J. A., Toftager, M., Pinborg, A., Homburg, R., van der Veen F,& Van Wely, M. (2017). GnRH antagonist versus long agonist protocols in IVF: a systematic review and meta-analysis accounting for patient type. *Human reproduction update*, *23*(5), 560-579. https://doi.org/10.1093/ humupd/dmx017.

Lenz, S., & Lauritsen, J. G. (1982). Ultrasonically guided percutaneous aspiration of human follicles under local anesthesia: a new method of collecting oocytes for in vitro fertilization. *Fertility and sterility*, *38*(6), 673-677.https://doi.org/10 .1016/s0015-0282(16)46692-6.

Lewin, A., Laufer, N., Rabinowitz, R., & Schenker, J. G. (1986). Ultrasonically guided oocyte recovery for in vitro fertilization: An improved method. *Journal of in vitro fertilization and embryo transfer*, *3*, 370-373. 3: 370–3. https://doi.org /10.1007/BF01133250.

Lowe, B., Osborn, J. C., Fothergill, D. J., & Lieberman, B. A. (1988). Factors associated with accidental fractures of the zona pellucida and multipronuclear human oocytes following in-vitro fertilization. *Human Reproduction*, *3*(7), 901-904.

Rose, B. I. (2014). Follicle flushing for oocyte retrieval: Targeted analysis for patients with few follicles. *IVF Lite*, *1*(2), 75-80. https://doi.org/10.4103/2348-2907 .140119

Siristatidis, C. S., Gibreel, A., Basios, G., Maheshwari, A., & Bhattacharya, S. (2015). Gonadotrophin-releasing hormone agonist protocols for pituitary suppression in assisted reproduction. *Cochrane Database of Systematic Reviews*, (11), Cd006919. https://doi.org/10.1002/14651858.CD006919.pub4.

Stanger, J. D., & Yovich, J. L. (1985). Reduced in-vitro fertilization of human oocytes from patients with raised basal luteinizing hormone levels during the follicular phase. *BJOG: An International Journal of Obstetrics & Gynaecology*, *92*(4), 385-393.https://doi.org/10.1111/j.1471-0528.1985.tb01113.x

Sunkara, S. K., Rittenberg, V., Raine-Fenning, N., Bhattacharya, S., Zamora, J., & Coomarasamy, A. (2011). Association between the number of eggs and live birth in IVF treatment: an analysis of 400 135 treatment cycles. *Human reproduction*, *26*(7), 1768-1774. https://doi.org/10.1093/humrep/der106.

Urbancsek, J., & Witthaus, E. (1996). Midluteal buserelin is superior to early follicular phase buserelin in combined gonadotropin-releasing hormone analog and gonadotropin stimulation in in vitro fertilization. *Fertility and sterility*, *65*(5), 966-971.

Feichtinger, W. (1998). Follicle aspiration with interactive three-dimensional digital imaging (Voluson): a step toward real-time puncturing under three-dimensional ultrasound control. *Fertility and sterility*, *70*(2), 374-377.https://doi.org/10.1016 /s0015-0282(98)00131-9.

Feichtinger, W., & Kemeter, P. (1986). Transvaginal sector scan sonography for needle guided transvaginal follicle aspiration and other applications in gynecologic routine and research. *Fertility and sterility*, *45*(5), 722-725.

Zegers-Hochschild, F., Adamson, G. D., Dyer, S., Racowsky, C., De Mouzon, J., Sokol, R.,Rienzi L, Sunde A,Schmidt L, Cooke ID& Van Der Poel, S. (2017). The international glossary on infertility and fertility care, 2017. *Human reproduction*, *32*(9), 1786-1801.https://doi.org/10.1093/humrep/dex234

Chapter 10

Evaluation and Denudation of Oocytes

Elif Seda Özdemir, MD*
Department of Assisted Reproductive Technologies, Embryology, Ankara City Hospital, Ankara, Turkey

Abstract

Many factors can affect clinical outcomes in assisted reproductive therapies. One of these, perhaps the first step, is the quality of the gametes. It has been shown that not all collected oocytes are of the same quality, with only 5% resulting in live birth. For this reason, it is important to evaluate the morphology of the oocyte before the procedure and to complete its maturation. Cumulus corona cells around the oocyte are used to assess maturation. Incubation of oocytes with cumulus cells helps their maturation. However, an evaluation of nuclear maturation can only be done clearly when denudation has occurred. Enzymatic and mechanical methods are used to separate the oocyte from the cumulus cells. In this section, the evaluation of the oocyte together with the cumulus cells and the methods used in the application of denudation are compiled in terms of literature and practice.

Key Words: Cumulus oocyte complex, Oocyte denudation

Introduction

Oocyte maturation is a complex and dynamic process necessary for fertilization and early embryo development (Carvalho et al., 2020). Cumulus cells are the cells of the Graafian follicle that surround and nourish the oocyte during its

---

* Corresponding Author's E-mail: elifsedabilgic@gmail.com

In: Holistic Approach to Assisted Reproductive Technology
Editor: Kenan Demir and Rümeysa Yılmaz Göç
ISBN: 979-8-89113-017-3
© 2023 Nova Science Publishers, Inc.

development in the ovary. The corona radiata layer, which is the innermost layer of the cumulus cells, is adjacent to the zona pellucida. Corona radiata sustains its contact with the oocyte by crossing the zona pellucida with cytoplasmic extensions called transzonal projections. This organized structure is called the cumulus-oocyte complex (COC) (Albertini et al., 2001). Incubation of the oocyte with surrounding cumulus cells remains the most commonly used method to achieve the completion of cytoplasmic maturation (Carvalho et al., 2020).

During the oocyte collection process, the follicle fluid is brought to the embryology laboratory in a preheated sterile tube. The content of the tube is poured into a Petri dish heated to 37°C and examined first macroscopically and then microscopically. The oocyte should be taken to the incubator as soon as possible. Therefore, the communication between the laboratory and the operating room is important during the collection process. If the procedure takes a long time, the collected oocytes should be removed before the end of the procedure.

Since the follicle fluid contains free oxygen radicals, the cumulus-oocyte complex should be removed from the follicle fluid as soon as possible in the oocyte retrieval process (Wale & Gardner, 2016). For this, it is important to use buffered media such as HEPES and MOPS (Swain et al., 2016). COCs seen under the microscope are taken with the help of a suitable pipette. Center-well culture dishes are generally used for oocyte collection. COCs, which are prepared with buffered culture medium inside and outside, are washed on the outside, and purified from the follicle fluid are collected in the interior. MOPS and HEPES buffered media should be used at ~ 37°C due to their optimal buffering capacity. Temperature changes can cause pH instability in these culture media and therefore cause serious damage to cells (Swain & Wilding, 2012).

The collected cumulus-oocyte complexes are incubated for an appropriate time according to the procedure to be applied and the appearance of the cumulus. During the oocyte retrieval process, both the detection and evaluation of COCs are performed. It is more appropriate to perform a morphological evaluation, which is the main factor in determining the incubation period of the oocyte, during the collection process to reduce the exposure of the oocyte to external factors.

Evaluation of oocyte morphology

Although the cumulus cells surrounding the oocyte seem to be separated from the oocyte by the zona pellucida, they continue to communicate. Communication between oocyte and cumulus cells occurs through paracrine signaling or gap junctions in their transzonal projections passing through the zona pellucida. Thanks to this interaction, the oocyte maintains its nutrition and development until the diplotene stage of meiosis II (Alam & Miyano, 2020; Albertini et al., 2001; Dong et al., 1996). The cumulus-corona mass appears as an enlarged mucus-like layer in mature oocytes, as it actively secretes hyaluronic acid. This hyaluronic acid-rich mucus-like matrix normally connects the oocyte to the cumulus, allowing sperm penetration and fertilization (Salustri et al., 1996). Hyaluronic acid spreads among cells and separates them from each other. For this reason, the cumulus-corona layer gains an enlarged appearance. Cumulus enlargement is essential for in vivo oocyte development, and oocytes without cumulus enlargement have limited implantation potential (Veeck & Zaninovic, 2003). In unstimulated cycles, nuclear maturation of the oocyte is concurrent with the expansion and musification of the cumulus layer (Testart et al., 1983). However, this synchronization is impaired in stimulated cycles (Laufer et al., 1984). It is thought that this may be due to the fact that oocyte and cumulus cells do not show the same sensitivity to incoming stimuli (Bar-Ami et al., 1989; Laufer et al., 1984). On the other hand, current publications reveal that cumulus cells play an important role in cytoplasmic maturity, which is critically important for fertilization, pronucleus formation and afterwards (Das et al., 1991; Ng et al., 1999).

Only 5% of the oocytes obtained from stimulated cycles go to live birth, suggesting that not all oocytes have the same developmental characteristics (Lemmen et al., 2016). It is known that the quality of gametes is one of the effective factors in embryo development. Therefore, it is important to examine the morphological features of the oocyte after retrieval of the oocyte in the embryology laboratory. There is a consensus on the importance of oocyte morphology in cases of low fertilization rates or total fertilization failure, particularly in cases of ICSI and classical IVF (ESHRE, 2017).

The cumulus-corona-oocyte complexes collected after oocyte collection can be examined to determine the morphology and to get an idea of the quality and maturation of the oocytes (Figure 10.1 and Figure 10.2). Based on the

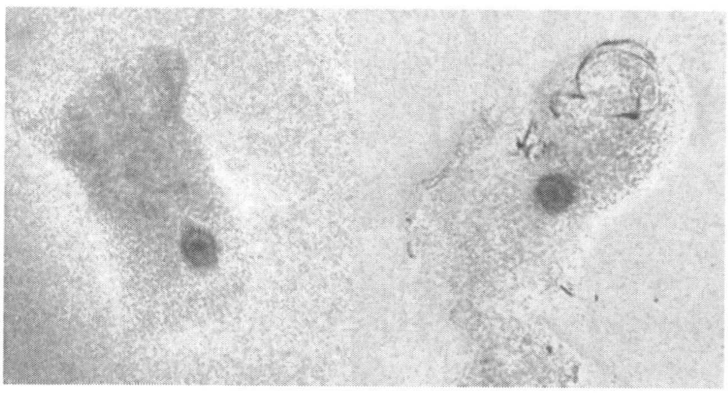

Figure 10.1 Appearances of mature COCs collected during OPU (Author's own archive).

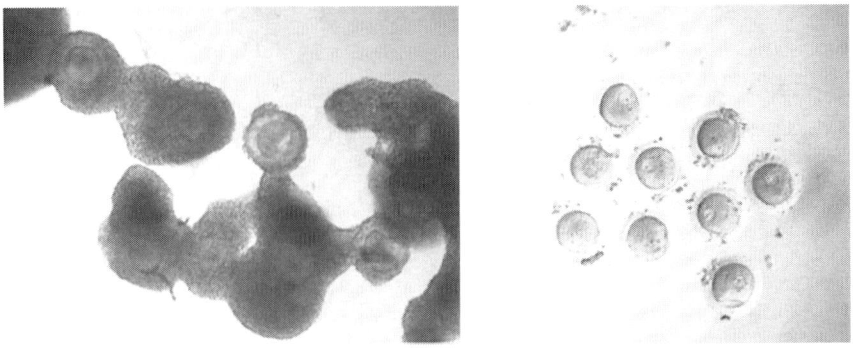

Figure 10.2 Appearances of immature COCs and their immature oocytes after denudation (Author's own archive).

Table 10.1 Grading system for cumulus oocyte complexes (Wolf, 1988)

Grade 1 (A)	Cumulus cells are absent or sparse, and corona cells are in 1-3 rows
Grade 2 (B)	Cumulus cells are dense, and corona cells are tightly packed.
Grade 3 (C)	Cumulus and corona cells are expanded and fluffy
Grade 4 (D)	Cumulus cells are common and scarce, and corona cells are scattered and may be partially lost.

morphological features of the cumulus-corona complex, Wolf et al. introduced a classification system (Wolf, 1988) (Table 10.1). A study in which the classification is made according to the cumulus-corona complex classification system revealed that grade 3 COCs have higher fertilization rates. Furthermore, it was pointed out that patients with a grade 3 COC proportion greater than 50% have higher pregnancy rates regardless of the parameters including age and count of grade 3 COC (Ng et al., 1999). In the following years, a classification system based on the evaluation of the oocyte with surrounding cells has been presented for the maturation of oocytes (Lin et al., 2003) (Table 10.2). These classifications based on the cumulus-corona-oocyte complex morphologies are highly dependent on the embryologist's experience. Therefore, it was thought that they may be insufficient for evaluating oocyte morphology (Hammitt et al., 1992; Hammitt et al., 1993). Despite the research showing that COC morphology cannot provide sufficient information, there are also studies indicating that it can be correlated with fertilization, blastocyst development, and pregnancy rates (Lin et al., 2003; Ng et al., 1999).

Although a discrepancy between was reported, the morphology of the cumulus-corona cell is still used to determine approximately oocyte maturation due to its ease of applicability and the desire to preserve the cumulus

Table 10.2 Oocyte maturity grading system (Lin et al., 2003)

Grade 1	Expanded cumulus, distinct zona pellucida, very radiant corona, clear cytoplasm, well aggregated expanded granulosa cells (mature – preovulatory)
Grade 2	Expanded cumulus cells, slightly compact corona radiata, expanded well aggregated granulosa cells (approximately mature- M1)
Grade 3	Compact dense cumulus if present, compact very adherent layer of corona cells, germinal vesicle in the cytoplasm if visible, compact and non- aggregated membrana granulosa cells (immature –GV
Grade 4	Much expanded cumulus mass with clumps, irregularly radiant or clumped corona radiata, prominent zona, slightly granular or dark ooplasm, small and relatively unaggregated granulosa cells (postmature)
Grade 5	Rarely with associated cumulus cells, clumped and very irregular corona radiata if present, very prominent zona, dark and frequently misshapen ooplasm, membrana granulosa cells in very small clusters (atretic)

for sperm activation. Evaluation of oocyte maturation is considered a prudent approach in determining the incubation period with sperm in conventional IVF cycles (Trounson et al., 1982; Veeck, 1986).

There are studies reporting that there is no relationship between predenudation COC morphology and nuclear maturity, fertilization rate, and cleavage rates in oocytes planned for insemination with ICSI. However, these studies have shown that the density of the corona radiate layer is associated with a decrease in oocyte maturity (Ebner et al., 2008; Rattanachaiyanont et al., 1999). In addition, the presence of blood clots in COC has been noted to be associated with dense central granulation in the oocyte and has a negative effect on fertilization and blastocyst development rates (Ebner et al., 2008). It has been shown that COC classification is associated with fertilization and pregnancy rates, and blastocyst quality and development (Lin et al., 2003; Ng et al., 1999).

The 2017 Vienna consensus of the European Society for Human Reproduction and Embryology (ESHRE) found that the ratio of the cumulus-oocyte complex with the enlarged cumulus during oocyte retrieval is a potential indicator of oocyte classification. Since ovulation triggers cumulus expansion by providing a stable structure of the cellular matrix together with hyaluronic acid synthesis (Russell & Salustri, 2006), it has been observed that this indicator – the ratio of COCs with enlarged cumulus – can provide an assessment of the quality of communication between oocytes and cumulus cells. Concerns about the applicability of this indicator in the laboratory, the lack of objective criteria to make the assessment, and the fact that cumulus cell growth and nuclear maturation do not always correlate well have been cited as potential problems (Balaban & Urman, 2006; ESHRE, 2017).

It is possible to clearly evaluate the maturity and morphology of the oocyte by separating the oocyte from the cumulus and corona cells. If conventional IVF is planned, maturation evaluation is made according to COC morphology, and oocyte denudation is not applied (Veeck, 1986). In vitrified oocytes, vitrification, together with surrounding cumulus cells, can cause damage to the oocyte and decrease the effect of cryoprotectant on the oocyte. Therefore, as a step to improve oocyte viability after thawing, vitrified oocytes should be denuded prior to procedure (Iussig et al., 2019; Kuwayama et al., 2005; Minasi et al., 2012).

Denudation

Oocytes incubated at 37°C after OPU are separated from the cumulus layer by enzymatic and mechanical steps under a stereo microscope. Although the information on how much time to incubate should pass between oocyte retrieval and denudation is still unclear, each laboratory has determined the appropriate protocols. Although denudation varies according to the routine procedure of laboratories, it consists of an enzyme solution prepared in Petri dishes or culture plates with 4-5 wells followed by MOPS or HEPES buffered solutions. Oocyte denudation occurs in two stages, enzymatic and mechanical denudation.

Enzymatic Denudation

Hyaluronic acid forms the main component of the cumulus surrounding the mature oocyte. Therefore, in the first step of denudation, hyaluronidase is used to enzymatically remove cumulus cells. Physiological medium containing this enzyme is often used in ready-to-use form at a concentration of 80 IU/ml or by diluting the stock solution with MOPS or HEPES buffered solutions. Although it is often used at this concentration, there are also studies showing that effective denudation is provided at lower concentrations (Van de Velde et al., 1997).

COC is taken into hyaluronidase with a sterile glass pasteur pipette and repeatedly aspirated for a period not exceeding one minute to try to separate it from the oocyte cumulus. The ideal enzymatic concentration and duration to which COCs are exposed for denudation are uncertain. Therefore, attention should be paid to exposure to hyaluronidase, and enzymatic denudation should be terminated in a minimum time. The centers optimize this time themselves according to the workload and/or protocols of the laboratories.

Enzyme Concentration

Information about the ideal concentration of hyaluronidase is not certain. However, a similar cumulus removal efficiency was found when used at a concentration of 80 IU/ml and 20 IU/ml. Additionally, there are studies that detect better fertilization and embryo development at concentrations of 20 IU/ml and 8 IU / ml (de Moura et al., 2017; Taylor et al., 2006). In the study carried out at a concentration of 10 IU/ml, fertilization, embryo development, and pregnancy rates were found similar to 80 IU/ml (Van de Velde et al., 1997).

Duration of Enzyme Exposure

On the basis of animal studies, the harmful effects of long-term exposure to hyaluronidase have been demonstrated. Exposure to hyaluronidase for more than 5 minutes in mice has been associated with a reduced rate of fertilization and cleavage (Ishizuka et al., 2014). A decrease in embryo development rates was detected in pig oocytes exposed to hyaluronidase for more than 20 minutes (Lee et al., 2021). Considering human studies published to date, it seems that keeping human oocytes under the effect of hyaluronidase for less than 1 minute can preserve oocyte quality (Rosas et al., 2022).

Mechanical Denudation

At the second stage of denudation, glass pasteur pipettes and stripper pipettes of different calibers are used. Buffered medium droplets are prepared following hyaluronidase. The cumulus-oocyte complex transferred from hyaluronidase to the buffered medium without the enzyme in the shortest time and in the smallest volume possible. Cumulus cells are mechanically stripped by passing through pipettes with gradually decreasing inner diameter (from 180/150 μm to 135-130 μm) and washed by passing through medium to completely eliminate the effect of hyaluronidase. The stripping process requires considerable caution and experience not to harm the oocyte (Rosas et al., 2022).

Denudation Pipettes

The minimum inner diameter of the pipettes for oocyte denudation is unclear. Pipettes with small inner diameter have been shown to harm the oocyte cell skeleton by compressing and also increase oocyte degeneration rates after ICSI (Nagy et al., 1995). The use of pipettes with inner diameter 130-150 μm has not been found to be associated with increased oocyte lysis (de Moura et al., 2017; Rosen et al., 2006; Taylor et al., 2006) and no important change in the original location of the spindle and polar bodies has been detected in these diameters

(Van de Velde et al., 1997). The importance of the location of the meiotic spindle and polar body for the application and success of ICSI has been emphasized (Rienzi et al., 2003).

Denudation with Automated Systems

Based on the idea that manual denudation varies among practitioners and that oocytes are exposed to mechanical stress during pipetting, the search for new methods has emerged. The fact that denudation is not a standard procedure and the effects of enzymatic denudation are still not fully clarified have also supported this search. Although pipettes with an inner diameter greater than the diameter of the oocyte are used for safe manual denudation, denudation should be completed with a minimal number of aspirations to avoid disruption of the meiotic spindle (Luo et al., 2015). These searches have led to a rise in research on the use of microfluidics in denudation, with the idea that this step can also benefit from the use of microfluidics, which has recently been on the agenda in assisted reproductive procedures. Successful denudation of the oocyte has been demonstrated using microfluidic channel systems that apply laminar flow (Beebe et al., 2002; Weng et al., 2018; Zeringue & Beebe, 2004). In addition, ideas such as providing denudation with ultrasound without contacting the oocyte have emerged (Mokhtare et al., 2022).

Conclusion

Assessing COC morphology after oocyte retrieval is an important guide in conventional IVF. The preprocedure incubation time may be planned according to the grade of the oocytes determined by the COC morphology. However, the nuclear maturation of the oocyte becomes apparent after the denudation. The procedure of denudation of oocytes has not been standardized yet. There should be more data to determine the diameters of pipettes, optimal enzyme concentration, and exposure time. Every laboratory is still applying its own procedure. The new automated systems to provide standardization have still limited data. It is important to do research to constitute standard procedures. The emergence of many new ideas on this topic may herald the technological developments that we will see in the near future.

References

Alam, M. H., & Miyano, T. (2020). Interaction between growing oocytes and granulosa cells in vitro. *Reproductive medicine and biology*, *19*(1), 13-23. https://doi.org/ https://doi.org/10.1002/rmb2.12292

Albertini, D. F., Combelles, C., Benecchi, E., & Carabatsos, M. J. (2001). Cellular basis for paracrine regulation of ovarian follicle development. *Reproduction*, *121*(5), 647-653. https://doi.org/https://doi.org/10.1530/rep.0.1210647

Balaban, B., & Urman, B. (2006). Effect of oocyte morphology on embryo development and implantation. *Reproductive biomedicine online*, *12*(5), 608-615. https://doi.org/https://doi.org/10.1016/S1472-6483(10)61187-X

Bar-Ami, S., Gitay-Goren, H., & Brandes, J. M. (1989). Different morphological and steroidogenic patterns in oocyte/cumulus-corona cell complexes aspirated at in vitro fertilization. *Biology of reproduction*, *41*(4), 761-770. https://doi.org/https://doi.org/10.1095/biolreprod41.4.761

Beebe, D., Wheeler, M., Zeringue, H., Walters, E., & Raty, S. (2002). Microfluidic technology for assisted reproduction. *Theriogenology*, *57*(1), 125-135. https://doi.org/https://doi.org/10.1016/S0093-691X(01)00662-8

Carvalho, M., Leal, F., Mota, S., Aguiar, A., Sousa, S., Nunes, J., & Calhaz-Jorge, C. (2020). The effect of denudation and injection timing in the reproductive outcomes of ICSI cycles: new insights into the risk of in vitro oocyte ageing. *Human reproduction*, *35*(10), 2226-2236. https://doi.org/https://doi.org/10.1093/humrep/deaa211

Das, K., Stout, L. E., Hensleigh, H. C., Tagatz, G. E., Phipps, W. R., & Leung, B. S. (1991). Direct positive effect of epidermal growth factor on the cytoplasmic maturation of mouse and human oocytes. *Fertility and sterility*, *55*(5), 1000-1004. https://doi.org/https://doi.org/10.1016/S0015-0282(16)54313-1

de Moura, B. R., Gurgel, M. C., Machado, S. P., Marques, P. A., Rolim, J. R., de Lima, M. C., & Salgueiro, L. L. (2017). Low concentration of hyaluronidase for oocyte denudation can improve fertilization rates and embryo quality. *JBRA Assisted Reproduction*, *21*(1), 27. https://doi.org/https://doi.org/10.5935/1518-0557.20170008

Dong, J., Albertini, D. F., Nishimori, K., Kumar, T. R., Lu, N., & Matzuk, M. M. (1996). Growth differentiation factor-9 is required during early ovarian folliculogenesis. *Nature*, *383*(6600), 531-535. https://doi.org/https://doi.org/10.1038/383531a0

Ebner, T., Moser, M., Shebl, O., Sommergruber, M., Yaman, C., & Tews, G. (2008). Blood clots in the cumulus–oocyte complex predict poor oocyte quality and post-fertilization development. *Reproductive biomedicine online*, *16*(6), 801-807. https://doi.org/https://doi.org/10.1016/S1472-6483(10)60145-9

ESHRE (2017). The Vienna consensus: report of an expert meeting on the development of art laboratory performance indicators. *Human Reproduction Open*, *2017*(2), hox011. https://doi.org/https://doi.org/10.1016/j.rbmo.2017.06.015

Hammitt, D., Syrop, C., Van Voorhis, B., Walker, D., Miller, T., Barud, K., & Hood, C. (1992). Prediction of nuclear maturity from cumulus-coronal morphology: influence of embryologist experience. *Journal of assisted reproduction and genetics*, *9*(5), 439-446. https://doi.org/https://doi.org/10.1007/BF01204049

Hammitt, D. G., Syrop, C. H., Van Voorhis, B. J., Walker, D. L., Miller, T. M., & Barud, K. M. (1993). Maturational asynchrony between oocyte cumulus-coronal morphology and nuclear maturity in gonadotropin-releasing hormone agonist stimulations. *Fertility and sterility*, *59*(2), 375-381. https://doi.org/https://doi.org/10.1016/S0015-0282(16)55680-5

Ishizuka, Y., Takeo, T., Nakao, S., Yoshimoto, H., Hirose, Y., Sakai, Y., Horikoshi, Y., Takeuji, S., Tsuchiyama, S., & Nakagata, N. (2014). Prolonged exposure to hyaluronidase decreases the fertilization and development rates of fresh and cryopreserved mouse oocytes. *Journal of Reproduction and Development*. https://doi.org/https://doi.org/10.1262/jrd.2014-045

Iussig, B., Maggiulli, R., Fabozzi, G., Bertelle, S., Vaiarelli, A., Cimadomo, D., Ubaldi, F. M., & Rienzi, L. (2019). A brief history of oocyte cryopreservation: Arguments and facts. *Acta obstetricia et gynecologica Scandinavica*, *98*(5), 550-558. https://doi.org/https://doi.org/10.1111/aogs.13569

Kuwayama, M., Vajta, G., Kato, O., & Leibo, S. P. (2005). Highly efficient vitrification method for cryopreservation of human oocytes. *Reproductive biomedicine online*, *11*(3), 300-308. https://doi.org/https://doi.org/10.1016/S1472-6483(10)60837-1

Laufer, N., Tarlatzis, B. C., DeCherney, A. H., Masters, J. T., Haseltine, F. P., MacLusky, N., & Naftolin, F. (1984). Asynchrony between human cumulus-corona cell complex and oocyte maturation after human menopausal gonadotropin treatment for in vitro fertilization. *Fertility and sterility*, *42*(3), 366-372. https://doi.org/https://doi.org/10.1016/S0015-0282(16)48074-X

Lee, J. H., Yoo, M., Lee, S. M., Park, S.-J., Kil, T. Y., & Kim, M. K. (2021). Toxicity of the recombinant human hyaluronidase ALT-BC4 on embryonic development. *Journal of Animal Science and Technology*, *63*(2), 272. https://doi.org/https://doi.org/10.5187/jast.2021.e34

Lemmen, J., Rodriguez, N., Andreasen, L., Loft, A., & Ziebe, S. (2016). The total pregnancy potential per oocyte aspiration after assisted reproduction—in how many cycles are biologically competent oocytes available? *Journal of assisted reproduction and genetics*, *33*(7), 849-854. https://doi.org/https://doi.org/10.1007/s10815-016-0707-3

Lin, Y.-C., Chang, S.-Y., Lan, K.-C., Huang, H.-W., Chang, C.-Y., Tsai, M.-Y., Kung, F.-T., & Huang, F.-J. (2003). Human oocyte maturity in vivo determines the outcome of blastocyst development in vitro. *Journal of assisted reproduction and genetics*, *20*(12), 506-512. https://doi.org/https://doi.org/10.1023/B:JARG.0000013651.37866.0c

Luo, Z., Güven, S., Gozen, I., Chen, P., Tasoglu, S., Anchan, R. M., Bai, B., & Demirci, U. (2015). Deformation of a single mouse oocyte in a constricted microfluidic channel. *Microfluidics and nanofluidics*, *19*(4), 883-890. https://doi.org/https://doi.org/10.1007/s10404-015-1614-0

Minasi, M. G., Fabozzi, G., Casciani, V., Ferrero, S., Litwicka, K., & Greco, E. (2012). Efficiency of slush nitrogen vitrification of human oocytes vitrified with or without cumulus cells in relation to survival rate and meiotic spindle competence. *Fertility and sterility*, *97*(5), 1220-1225. https://doi.org/https://doi.org/10.1016/j.fertnstert.2012.02.022

Mokhtare, A., Davaji, B., Xie, P., Yaghoobi, M., Rosenwaks, Z., Lal, A., Palermo, G., & Abbaspourrad, A. (2022). Non-contact ultrasound oocyte denudation. *Lab on a Chip*, *22*(4), 777-792. https://doi.org/https://doi.org/10.1039/D1LC00715G

Nagy, Z., Liu, J., Joris, G., Bocken, G., Desmet, B., Van Ranst, A., Vankelecom, A., Devroey, P., & Van Steirteghem, A. (1995). The influence of the site of sperm deposition and mode of oolemma breakage at intracytoplasmic sperm injection on fertilization and embryo development rates. *Human reproduction, 10*(12), 3171-3177. https://doi.org/https://doi.org/10.1093/oxfordjournals.humrep.a135881

Ng, S. T., Chang, T.-H., & Wu, T. J. (1999). Prediction of the rates of fertilization, cleavage, and pregnancy success by cumulus-coronal morphology in an in vitro fertilization program. *Fertility and sterility, 72*(3), 412-417. https://doi.org/https://doi.org/10.1016/S0015-0282(99)00290-3

Rattanachaiyanont, M., Leader, A., & Léveillé, M.-C. (1999). Lack of correlation between oocyte-corona-cumulus complex morphology and nuclear maturity of oocytes collected in stimulated cycles for intracytoplasmic sperm injection. *Fertility and sterility, 71*(5), 937-940. https://doi.org/https://doi.org/10.1016/S0015-0282(99)00100-4

Rienzi, L., Ubaldi, F., Martinez, F., Iacobelli, M., Minasi, M., Ferrero, S., Tesarik, J., & Greco, E. (2003). Relationship between meiotic spindle location with regard to the polar body position and oocyte developmental potential after ICSI. *Human reproduction, 18*(6), 1289-1293. https://doi.org/https://doi.org/10.1093/humrep/deg274

Rosas, I. M., Anagnostopoulou, C., Singh, N., Gugnani, N., Singh, K., Desai, D., Darbandi, M., Manoharan, M., Darbandi, S., & Chockalingam, A. (2022). Optimizing embryological aspects of oocyte retrieval, oocyte denudation, and embryo loading for transfer: a state of the art review. *Panminerva Medica*. https://doi.org/https://doi.org/10.23736/s0031-0808.22.04675-4

Rosen, M. P., Shen, S., Dobson, A. T., Fujimoto, V. Y., McCulloch, C. E., & Cedars, M. I. (2006). Oocyte degeneration after intracytoplasmic sperm injection: a multivariate analysis to assess its importance as a laboratory or clinical marker. *Fertility and sterility, 85*(6), 1736-1743. https://doi.org/https://doi.org/10.1016/j.fertnstert.2005.12.017

Russell, D. L., & Salustri, A. (2006). Extracellular matrix of the cumulus-oocyte complex. Seminars in reproductive medicine,

Salustri, A., Camaioni, A., & D'Alessandris, C. (1996). Endocrine and paracrine regulation of cumulus expansion. *Zygote, 4*(4), 313-315. https://doi.org/https://doi.org/10.1017/S0967199400003312

Swain, J. E., Carrell, D., Cobo, A., Meseguer, M., Rubio, C., & Smith, G. D. (2016). Optimizing the culture environment and embryo manipulation to help maintain embryo developmental potential. *Fertility and sterility, 105*(3), 571-587. https://doi.org/https://doi.org/10.1016/j.fertnstert.2016.01.035

Swain, J. E., & Wilding, M. (2012). Practical pH for the IVF Laboratory. *Journal of Reproductive and Stem Cell Biotechnology, 3*(2), 62-76. https://doi.org/https://doi.org/10.1177/205891581200300205.

Taylor, T. H., Elliott, T., Colturato, L. F., Straub, R. J., Mitchell-Leef, D., & Nagy, Z. P. (2006). Comparison of bovine-and recombinant human-derived hyaluronidase with regard to fertilization rates and embryo morphology in a sibling oocyte model: a prospective, blinded, randomized study. *Fertility and sterility, 85*(5), 1544-1546. https://doi.org/https://doi.org/10.1016/j.fertnstert.2005.10.053

Testart, J., Frydman, R., De Mouzon, J., Lassalle, B., & Belaisch, J. (1983). A study of factors affecting the success of human fertilization in vitro. I. Influence of ovarian stimulation upon the number and condition of oocytes collected.

Biology of reproduction, *28*(2), 415-424. https://doi.org/https://doi.org/10.1095/biolreprod28.2.415

Trounson, A., Mohr, L. R., Wood, C., & Leeton, J. (1982). Effect of delayed insemination on in-vitro fertilization, culture and transfer of human embryos. *Reproduction*, *64*(2), 285-294. https://doi.org/https://doi.org/10.1530/jrf.0.0640285

Van de Velde, H., Nagy, Z., Joris, H., De Vos, A., & Van Steirteghem, A. (1997). Effects of different hyaluronidase concentrations and mechanical procedures for cumulus cell removal on the outcome of intracytoplasmic sperm injection. *Human reproduction (Oxford, England)*, *12*(10), 2246-2250. https://doi.org/https://doi.org/10.1093/humrep/12.10.2246

Veeck, L. (1986). Morphological estimation of mature oocytes and their preparation for insemination. *In vitro fertilization, Norfolk. Baltimore: Williams and Wilkins*, 81-93.

Veeck, L. L., & Zaninovic, N. (2003). *An atlas of human blastocysts*. CRC Press.

Wale, P. L., & Gardner, D. K. (2016). The effects of chemical and physical factors on mammalian embryo culture and their importance for the practice of assisted human reproduction. *Human reproduction update*, *22*(1), 2-22. https://doi.org/https://doi.org/10.1093/humupd/dmv034

Weng, L., Lee, G. Y., Liu, J., Kapur, R., Toth, T. L., & Toner, M. (2018). On-chip oocyte denudation from cumulus–oocyte complexes for assisted reproductive therapy. *Lab on a Chip*, *18*(24), 3892-3902. https://doi.org/https://doi.org/10.1039/C8LC01075G

Wolf, D. (1988). Oocyte quality and fertilization. *Invitro fertilization and Embryo Transfer, Plenum Pres, NY*, 129-138.

Zeringue, H. C., & Beebe, D. J. (2004). Microfluidic removal of cumulus cells from Mammalian zygotes. In *Germ Cell Protocols* (pp. 365-373). Springer. https://doi.org/https://doi.org/10.1385/1-59259-741-6:365

Chapter 11

Sperm Preparation for IVF and ICSI

Özge Kendirlinan, MD*

Fertility Center, Antalya Education and Research Hospital, Antalya, Turkiye

Abstract

To maximize the chance of successful reproduction, in vivo, the sperm selection process occurs in the female reproductive tract. This specialized sperm transport mechanism supports the selection of sperm with normal morphology and enhanced fertilization ability. These natural barriers encountered by spermatozoa in vivo are partially or completely absent when assisted reproductive techniques (ART) are applied. The success of ART depends mainly on the quality of gamete cells. Therefore, semen samples is a mixture and the content varies from one to another, and several separation techniques have been developed to maximize the chance of successful reproduction.

Key Words: Spermatozoa, Simple wash, Swim up, Gradient, HAB, Zeta potential, MSOME, MACS, Microfluidic systems

Introduction

In the 2018 speech by Dr. David Adamson at the International Committee for Monitoring Assisted Reproductive Technologies (ICMART) it was stated that there have been approximately 8 million childbirths from IVF since 1978 (European Society for Human Reproduction and Embryology, 2018). After

* Corresponding Author's E-mail: ozgekendirlinan@yahoo.com

In: Holistic Approach to Assisted Reproductive Technology
Editor: Kenan Demir and Rümeysa Yılmaz Göç
ISBN: 979-8-89113-017-3
© 2023 Nova Science Publishers, Inc.

maturation in the epididymis, mature spermatozoa are activated and acquire the ability to fertilize the oocyte within the female reproductive tract called capacitation. With capacitation, spermatozoa undergo membrane remodeling, intracellular signal pathway activation, and intracellular level of Ca and H change thus obtaining the correct interaction with the oocyte and preparing for the acrosome reaction. In in vivo conditions this process takes place in the genital tract, but in vitro procedures in ART it is necessary to eliminate seminal plasma proteins to remove the negative effect of seminal plasma proteins on sperm functions. In the first trials, semen was inseminated into the uterus without any preparation; uterine spasm was observed and it was predicted that it could cause infection. The aforementioned reasons have led to the development of various preparation methods. Initially in preparation methods, ejaculate was washed with Bavister's medium and then suspension was made with the same medium (Edwards et al., 1969) and allowed spermatoza to swim into columns of diluent (Lopata et al., 1976) and later more complicated techniques were developed.

The ideal sperm preparation method aims to

- be quick, easy, and cost-effective
- not causing damage to spermatozoa or nonphysiological alterations
- remove seminal plasma, decapacitant factors, dead spermatozoa, infectious agents, and leukocytes
- gain a motile, functional, and morphologically competent spermatozoa population

The feature of the sample is important in the selection of the method. If the number of semen motility morphology is within normal limits, dilution and centrifugation or swimming can be applied, whereas in low number, motility and morphology density gradient centrifugation is usually preferred. For example, the direct swim-up technique can be used to select motile sperm, as it reflects the capacity of sperm to swim into the culture medium. The purpose of use also determines the choice of method. When normozoospermic specimens prepararing for IUI diluting semen with culture medium and centrifuging have been recommended (World Health Organization, 2021).

In general, the first step in semen processing for ART is conventional sperm preparation techniques named, simple wash, swim up, density gradient, and glass wool filtration and can be used together or separately. Although these methods are mainly based on motility, adhesion, and filtration processes; afterward the aim shifted to the selection of functional sperm and advanced sperm selection techniques were developed.

Simple Wash

Simple washing procedure preferred if the semen sample is within normal limits and gives good yields in these examples.

The sample is placed in a conic sterile tube to collect sperm in the smallest volume, then the entire semen sample is diluted with the same volume of medium (1 / 2) for removing seminal plasma. The total mixture is shared in a maximum of 3 ml per tube to multiple tubes. Centrifugation is done at 300-500 g for 5-10 minutes, then the supernatants are discarded. Sperm pellets are combined and 1 ml of medium is added and pipetted. Centrifugation is carried out at 300–500 g for 3-5 minutes, then the supernatants are discarded. Upon the treatment protocol, for example, insemination, the final volume of medium is added to the pellet and pipetted (WHO, 2021).

If it is wanted to reduce the number of washes, the number of tubes can be decreased and the volume per tube can be increased. In this case, centrifugation time and force should be increased to allow the sperm to form pellets (WHO, 2021).

Simple washing of semen essentially removes the seminal plasma without any significant decrease in total sperm count. This method has the advantages of being inexpensive and easy to use, but has the disadvantages of containing other cell types and the potential harm of centrifugation. Reactive oxygen species (ROS) homeostasis is essential for male reproductive potential; at physiological levels, ROS plays a role in capacitation and fertilization, while surplus levels cause membrane protein and lipid oxidation and DNA damage, and thus fertility could be altered (Martin-Hidalgo et al., 2019). Seminal plasma contains different types of cells; but within these cell types, seminal leukocytes and immature spermatozoa are the main origin of ROS production (Garrido et al., 2004). The NADPH oxidase system and the NADPH-dependent oxidoreductase system in abnormal spermatozoa produce ROS, oxidative stress affects the plasma membrane and mitochondrion (Gavella and Lipovac, 1992). In addition, DNA damage, decreased motility, and increased apoptosis are seen in increased ROS levels. Therefore, capacitation can be inhibited by the numerous nonviable sperm in the prepared sample. (Makker et al., 2009). Centrifugation is generally used in preparation methods and is associated with ROS formation. But it is concluded that there will be no problem until 800x force is applied (Jeulin et al., 1982) and if the duration is kept short also in some sperm specimens it can ameliorate the quality (Shekarriz et al., 1995).

Swim Up (SU)

The method is based on the motility of the spermatozoa. It is not effective under the circumstances if the total motile sperm count is low or the morphology is below %5 (Delilbaşı, 2008). However, for the samples that are oligoteratozoospermia, culture medium can be lessened and the incubation period can be prolonged. Sperm obtained can be used in IUI or ICSI.

If culture media are put at the bottom and downward floating is done, the method is called *swim down.*

Direct swim up from semen: Under the culture medium, liquefied semen is placed, then the tube is placed at a 45-degree angle to widen the surface area interface between semen and the culture medium and kept at 37° C for 45-60 minutes to allow sperm to swim and obtain a highly motile sperm population. To increase the recovery of motile spermatozoa, the number of tubes can be increased depending on the volume of the ejaculate, the concentration of the sperm and the motility of the sperm. Then the upper layer of each tube is collected on a new tube (Gardner, 2007).

Swim up from washed pellet: After the washing procedure, the appropriate amount of medium (depending on the characteristics of the sample and the size of the pellet from 0.5 ml to 1.5 ml) is slowly added from the side of the tube over the pellet. The tube is then kept at 37° C, at an angle of 45°, depending on the nature of the sample, for on average 45 minutes. In this process, progressive spermatozoa migrate from the pellet to the upper part of the medium.

The procedure is easy to perform and allows the recovery of a good number of progressive spermatozoa in normozoospermic cases.

Although the advantages of washed pellet usage are obtaining a higher percentage of motile sperm and preventing contamination with debris and other cells, the disadvantages of this method are obtaining less motile spermatozoa and failure of bottom spermatozoa reaching culture media.

Migration Sedimentation: Tea et al. (1984) discarded centrifugation and combined migration with a sedimentation step. The selection process takes place in two homocentric tubes consisting of an outer chamber in which the medium over semen is placed and the spermatozoa swim to the medium and an inner chamber where progressive spermatozoa are sedimented by the effect of gravity and collected. Oxidative stress is reduced because centrifugation is not applied, as a result spermatozoa damage is kept minimum. The spermatoza population is obtained without unwanted components. However, a lower yield is a major disadvantage and restricts usage in in vitro fertilization and intrauterine insemination (Friedler, 2012).

Density gradient centrifugation (DGC)

Abnormal spermatozoa are reported to have a density between 1.06 and 1.09 g/ml and normal spermatozoa have a density greater than 1.10 g/ml. Because normal, abnormal spermatozoa and other cells have different densities, they accumulate at equilibration points identical to their own densities in the density gradient column after centrifugation. As a result, other cells and abnormal spermatozoa stay upside, while highly motile and morphologically normal spermatozoa pelleted bottom (Malvezzi et al., 2014).

In the mid to late 1980s a colloidal suspension of polyvinylpyrrolidone (PVP) coated silica particles Percoll® gained widespread acceptance as the product of choice for use in density gradient separation of spermatozoa. Afterward, due to concerns about the high content of endotoxins, it was withdrawn from usage. Subsequently, silane-coated silica particles, Ficoll and iodixanol mixture or highly purified arabinogalactan were used for this purpose.

The density gradient centrifugation can be done with either one layer (continuous) or multiple layers (discontinuous gradients). With continuous gradients, one layer is used whereas in discontinuous gradients multiple layers lay with clear borders between each other. The ejaculate is placed on top of the density media and then centrifuged. In studies in which %72 and %95 concentrations were tested, %80 was accepted as the threshold value at the bottom (Delilbaşı, 2008). The most preferred discontinuous density gradient is formed by a high density (80%–90%) on the bottom, a low density (40%–45%) over and the sample put on top. For oligospermia, discontinuous density gradient centrifugation can be a method for sample preparation. However, the yield obtained in standard method may be low to ameliorate sperm recovery from oligospermia samples, mini-gradient in which 0.5 ml of gradients are used or single-layer centrifugation (90% or 45% density) can be used.

The method has been shown to be effective in eliminating aneuploid and diploid spermatozoa (Brahem et al., 2013). There have been many studies investigating which method is better in sperm preparation, unfortunately the results have been contradictory. DNA integrity in processed spermatozoa was shown to be higher in swim-up than density gradient centrifugation (Zini et al., 2000) while Viswambharan and Murugan concluded the opposite (Viswambharan and Murugan, 2021). Combining DGC and SU was shown to be better in separating sperm cells with damaged DNA (Ghumman et al., 2011) and decreased the number of sperm with head and tail ultrastructural abnormalities (Yamanaka et al., 2016). Furthermore, Hernández-Silva concluded that indicators showing capacitation are higher in spermatozoa with DGC than in SU. Therefore, choosing DGC could be more appropriate for intracytoplasmic sperm injection, while SU can be suitable for procedures such as intrauterine insemination in which capacitation takes place in the female genital tract or in vitro fertilization in which incubation with cumulus oocyte complex is performed (Hernández-Silva et al., 2021).

Glass Wool Filtration (GWF)

In 1977 Paulson and Polakoski added ejaculate in glass pasteur pipette filled with loosely packed glass wool and showed that agglutinated and dead spermatozoa adhered to glass fibers. With the hypothesis that if the fibers are too loosely compressed, some of the dead sperm and debris in the semen may pass through, in 1986 Jeyendran added 30 mg glass wool in 3 ml syringe into depth of 3mm and put it vertically and to get rid of loose particles rinsed afterward 0.3-0.5 ml concentrated spermatozoa put over wet glass wool and filtered by gravity (Jeyendran et al., 1986). The filtered sample is then rinsed with media to clean the wool fibers. Motile spermatozoa are dispersed from immotile spermatozoa, leukocytes, and seminal fluid. Since higher yield is obtained with the use of full semen, oligozoospermia and asthenozoospermia and retrograde ejaculation can be used. In addition, it was concluded in the study that glass wool filtration is better in oocyte fertilization in IVF than the swim up procedure (Jeyendran et al., 1987). In a study investigating whether annexin V can be combined with GWF compared: (i) raw glass wool, (ii) commercial SpermFertil® columns, (iii) annexin V-GW (iv) MACS separation and showed that the effect of conventional GWF can be ameliorated by combining with annexin V. Thus, gained spermatozoa population without apoptotic markers improved to grade of annexin V magnetic separation (Grunewald et al., 2007).

Hyaluronic Acid Binding

The extracellular compartment of the cumulus oophorus complex contains hyaluronic acid (HA). In normal sperm maturation, zona pellucida and HA binding regions are created with plasma membrane remodeling (Parmegiani et al., 2012). Spermatozoa with HA binding sites can bind and digest HA, while immature spermatozoa have less affinity for HA and a high risk of aneuploidy and DNA fragmentation (Moretti et al., 1997; Prinosilova et al., 2009; Sati et al., 2008). Because of this arrangement in the maturation process, commercial products are based on HA binding. For this purpose, physiological intracytoplasmic sperm injection (PICSI) or hyaluronan (or hyaluronic acid) rich medium can be used. In PICSI (PICSI; Origio, Måløv, Denmark) petri with microdots of hyaluronan is used and spermatozoa are added to microdot, after waiting for binding bonded spermatozoa are selected for ICSI. In a hyaluronan-rich medium procedure (Spermslow®, Cooper Surgical) bridge is made between sperm droplet and SpermSlow droplet and spermatozoa that bind to hyaluronic acid slow and are selected.

In a prospective randomized trial comparing PICSI and Sperm Slow, no statistically significant differences in good quality embryo, fertilization ratio, and clinical pregnancy were found (Parmegiani et al., 2012). Furthermore, in the Cochrane 2019 review evaluating two randomized controlled trials (RCTs) comparing live birth and four RCTs comparing clinical pregnancy in the HAICSI and ICSI groups with the low quality of evidence, it concluded that little or no difference was found between groups. Also, it was concluded that miscarriage rates decreased compared to ICSI (Lepine et al., 2019).

Zeta Potential

The electrokinetic potential between the sperm membrane and its environment defined as the sperm zeta potential (Lepine et al., 2019) that is gained by epididymal maturation and spermatogenesis is around -16 to -20 mV (Kirchhoff and Hale, 1996) and decreases with capacitation, which is due to the release of the gp20-CD52 low charge form (Giovampaola et al., 2001). Since the zeta potential decreases with capacitation, the method should be applied immediately after liquefaction.

Briefly, to obtain a positively charged tube, centrifugation tubes (preferably glass tubes) are rotated two to three times in a latex glove and quickly drawn out, then the tube is kept 1 minute at room temperature to allow charged sperm to stick to the wall and then centrifugated and then inverted to remove non-adherent spermatozoa. Adherent spermatozoa are collected by draining serum supplemented medium from the wall of the tube to neutralize the charge (Chan et al., 2006). The main advantages are simplicity and low cost. Disadvantages include limited use in oligozoospermia or testicular spermatozoa due to low recovery of processed sperm, potential biases in choosing X-bearing sperm, since there is no correlation between zeta potential and motility, it is recommended to apply the method to selected sperm.

Esfahani investigated 102 women in the DGC-selective sperm group and 101 in the DGC+ Zeta group and reported improvement of the embryo and pregnancy rate of the highest quality in the DGC + Zeta group (Esfahani et al., 2016). However, in a comparative review Lepine concluded that the quality of evidence was very low and that the effect of Zeta sperm selection on live birth, clinical pregnancy, nor miscarriage per woman or per clinical pregnancy is uncertain (Lepine et al., 2019).

Motile Sperm Organelle Morphology Examination (MSOME)

In ICSI sperm selection is made with morphological evaluation under 400x, Bartoov used an inverted light microscope equipped with high-power Nomarski optics enhanced by digital imaging to achieve a magnification of 6300x to evaluate ultrastructure (Bartoov et al., 2002). Incorporation of this technique together with a micromanipulation system is called intracytoplasmic morphologically selected sperm injection (IMSI). Through it the acrosome, postacrosome lamina, nucleus, mitochondria, neck, tail, and vacuoles are examined.

In this process, motile sperm is obtained by routine sperm preparation methods, and microdroplet is prepared from this suspension then evaluation is done under immersion oil.

The selection of sperm with IMSI is a time-consuming and complex process and requires a skilled embryologist beyond that guidelines and standardization are insufficient. In addition, IMSI is expensive as it is performed on a conventional inverted microscope attached with certain accessories.

It was shown that in severe cases (oligoastenotheratozoospermia and teratozoospermia) could benefit (Mangoli and Khalili, 2020). Also, it was shown that the miscarriage rate is decreased, the number of good quality embryos, and pregnancy rates can be ameliorated when IMSI is applied to repeated ICSI failures (Delaroche et al., 2013).

The ICSI IMSI comparison remains conflicting. Compared to IMSI with ICSI, Duran-Retamal has not found any difference in miscarriage rate and live birth rate in meta-analysis of randomized studies, has observed an increase in live birth rate and a decrease in miscarriage rate with IMSI in meta-analysis of observational studies (Duran-Retamal et al., 2020). In the meta-analysis of He on male factor infertility, IMSI is associated with a higher clinical pregnancy rate than ICSI with low evidence quality (He et al., 2018). In addition, these authors do not support the routine use of IMSI (Duran-Retamal et al., 2020; He et al., 2018). In a meta-analysis, Setti was concluded that with IMSI not only pregnancy rates, implantation, and top quality embryos increased significantly, but also miscarriage rates were significantly reduced from ICSI (Setti et al., 2010). In a review comparing IMSI with ICSI Teixitera concluded that the chances of having a live birth and the risk of having a miscarriage are uncertain, very low quality evidence found that IMSI increases clinical pregnancy, which means that it is still very uncertain about any real difference (Teixeira et al., 2020).

Magnetic Activated Cell Sorting (MACS)

The most common features seen in apoptotic spermatozoa are i) movement of phosphatidylserine to the outer leaflet of the plasma membrane; ii) activation of caspase; iii) fragmentation of DNA; iv) alterations in the mitochondrial membrane potential (Agarwal et al., 2016). Phosphatidylserine is normally an inner membrane phospholipid; its movement to the outer membrane is an early reversible change, but with massive DNA damage, becomes irreversible (Oosterhuis et al., 2000). Since Annexin V has high affinity to phosphatidylserine, annexin V conjugated paramagnetic beads bind to externalized phosphatidylserine, thus sperm population with externalized phosphatidylserine can be separated using a magnetic activated cell sorting system (MACS, Miltenyi Biotec GmbH, Bergisch Gladbach, Germany) (Grunewald et al., 2001). This suspension is placed inside a MACS column that produces an external magnetic field, trapping the apoptotic spermatozoa that are bound to the Annexin-V-coated magnetic beads, while the nonapoptotic spermatozoa pass through and are collected (Said and Land, 2011). With rinsing, the nonapoptotic unlabeled spermatozoa will be washed out and could be used for procedures.

Although there are variabilities between laboratories, the procedure can be done by Ziarati et al. prescribed before: twice 1x buffer washing of semen samples, usage of 100 μl of microbead solution per 10 million / ml spermatozoa, (Milteny Biotec, Bergisch Gladbach, Germany) and incubation at room temperature for 15 minutes after loading into the MACS column (Miltenyi Biotec, Bergisch Gladbach, Germany). As apoptotic spermatozoa were retained in the column applying the DGC procedure to unlabeled spermatozoa (Ziarati et al., 2018). It should be taken into account that MACS microbeads may be fragmented or magnetic micromolecules may be present in the solution of nonapoptotic spermatozoa, thus affecting viability; to avoid this an alternative to the magnetic beads, Annexin V coated glass wool can be used. Since the purpose of removing debris and infectants by sperm processing cannot be achieved with MACS, additional methods such as density gradient centrifugation could be applied. PS is externalized not only in apoptosis but also in capacitation. For this purpose, Berteli applied density gradient centrifugation (DGC) before and after MACS and showed in his study that the efficiency was higher in the application of DGC after MACS than before the application (Berteli et al., 2017).

In a study investigating whether MACS could be effective in detecting viable spermatozoa from the asthenozoospermic sample, spermatozoa population gained with the combination of DGC and MACS had a lower DNA fragmentation from the single DGC and MACS procedure and a higher morphology than the single DGC (Zhang et al., 2018).

Also in another study it was shown that cryosurvival rates and motility were higher when MACS was applied before cryopreservation (Said et al., 2005).

But the literature on clinical outcomes remains incomplete. The effects of MACS in oocyte donated couples ICSI application was examined by means of fertilization rates, percentage of good-quality embryos, implantation ratios, positive beta-hCG tests and live birth rates; it was showed no statistically significant difference with control group (swim-up) (Romany et al., 2014). Dirican et al. evaluated the outcome of male fertility treatment for this purpose and selected MACS and DGS selected sperm were used in ICSI and higher cleavage and pregnancy rates were found in MACS (Dirican et al., 2008). In 2019 the systematic review of the comparison between MACS with ICSI; live birth, clinical pregnancy, miscarriage per pregnancy were uncertain (Lepine et al., 2019).

Microfluidic Systems

In the development of this method, the natural environment was inspired in this manner intrauterine, cervical, and vaginal canal microenvironment-like microchannels were developed. Present microfluidic devices for sperm sorting are passively, chemoattractant-mediated, flow-mediated, thermotaxis-mediated, or combination forms.

In the passively driven model, raw semen or sperm solution injected from the inlet immotile or low motile sperm stayed in the microchannels while higher motile ones were collected from the outlet.

In flow driven models, either pumping or gravity mediated flow (Cho et al., 2003) or hydrostatic pressure difference mediated flow (Seo et al., 2007) is used to separate motile sperm with the ability to get away from stream from debris and immotile sperm.

In in vivo conditions, sperm swim to the oocyte for many reasons, one of which is oocyte-derived substances. On the basis of this, chemoattractant-driven sperm sorting allows collection of spermatozoa to chemoattractivity in optimal time. Atrial natriuretic peptide, bourgeonal, peptides, progesterone, and RANTES are confirmed as chemoattractants (Eisenbach and Giojalas, 2006).

Thermotaxis-driven driven system uses the temperature gradient system to produce a thermal gradient. Thermal-responsive spermatozoa aggregate at higher temperatures, while non-responsive ones accumulated both lower and higher temperatures (Li et al., 2014).

The microfluidic device designed by Ko and colleagues designed a microfluidic device that used acetylcholine as a chemoattractant and a microheater and microsensor for the temperature gradient was experimented in mice and showed that the use of both thermotaxis and chemotaxis was more effective than single ones (Ko et al., 2018)

As most microchannel systems use raw samples, damage due to centrifugation is avoided, and short preparation time and automation are other advantages of this method. Unfortunately, expensive instruments and low volume yield are disadvantages of the method.

In a study comparing centrifugation and swim up with two gravity-driven laminar flow used microfluidic sperm sorter about DNA damage, it is concluded that the DNA fragmentation rate is ameliorated (Shirota et al., 2016). Since microfluidic chips are in the development phase, concerns about clinical outcomes remain unclear. A study in comparison of density gradient centrifugation with microfluidic chips in male factor infertility, an improvement was reported in the clinical pregnancy group using microfluidic chips (Ozcan et al., 2019). Yildiz and Yuksel used density gradient centrifugation and a microfluidic chip (Fertile Plus®) in unsuccessful recurrent IVF treatments and unexplained infertility and compared fertilization and pregnancy rates. In first-time IVF treatment patients, no statistically significant differences were found between fertilization and pregnancy rates compared to study groups. However, in recurrent IVF failure, there was a significant difference in fertilization rates but no statistically significant differences were found in pregnancy rates. In addition, the microfluidic chip method was found to significantly decrease the sperm DNA fragmentation index according to the density gradient method (Yildiz and Yuksel, 2019).

Case-Specific Recommendations

Selection Methods for Reduced Motility

Hypo-osmotic swelling test

The HOST has already been used as a diagnostic test to determine if the sperm membrane is intact. Due to the flow of water, intact membranes (live cells) swell and bend in the hypoosmotic environment. In this method, spermatozoa are incubated in a hypo-osmotic solution and spermatozoa with coiled tails are selected and washed prior to conventional ICSI. It has been suggested that different HOST class was associated with different nuclear maturity (Bloch et al., 2021). It was shown that if HOST sperm selection was performed in patients with only nonmotile spermatozoa, without statistical significance, a higher rate of pregnancy and implantation is obtained (El-Nour et al., 2001). But there are insufficient or inconclusive data on the results of ART.

Laser-assisted immotile sperm selection (LAISS)

Lasers have been used in ART for spermatozoa immobilization, assisted hatching, and biopsy. In typical, sperm are selected for ICSI according to motility which evinces vitality; however, it is hard to estimate vitality for asthenozoospermia. To detect viable in immotile spermatozoa, a single laser shot is utilized at the tail of the sperm and tail curling is observed solely in viable (Aktan et al., 2004). The use of laser for this purpose has also given rise to concerns like excess ROS formation and due to Ca^{+2}-ATPase calcium channel hyperactivity, excess energy consumption, and plasma membrane injury. In a study aimed at determining effects on TESA patients divided into routine ICSI (control) and laser applied (test) groups, there was no statistically differance in embriyo development, no negative effects on obstetric and neonatal outcomes (Chen et al., 2021).

Polarization microscopy

Birefringence is observed when a light beam passes an anisotropic object. Hence the method is based on longitudinal nucleoprotein filaments reasoned anisotropy of sperm cells (Gianaroli et al., 2008). The polarization microscope allows evaluation of the nuclear structural organization and the state of the acrosome reaction. If an acrosomal reaction has occurred in sperm, birefringence is seen in the postacrosomal region, while uniform birefringence is seen at the head when the acrosome is intact. In a study verifying whether the acrosome reaction affected clinical outcome, fertilizing capacity, initial cleavage divisions, embryo quality was found similar, whereas the implantation rate was higher in ICSI is done with reacted spermatozoa (Gianaroli et al., 2010). Besides advantages, further studies are needed to be done also birefringence pattern determination required a skilled embryologist and polarized light equipment is expensive.

Preparation of epididymal and testicular samples

Obstructive azoospermia is the most common cause of epididymal aspiration, in which enough spermatozoa are generally obtained, then DGC can be used; in contrast, if spermatozoa number is inadequate, a simple wash can be performed.

Because testicular specimens contain many erythrocytes and non-germ cells, enzymatic or mechanical methods are needed to get away from those. Since the sperm count will be low, ICSI preparation will be done (World Health Organization, 2021).

Crabbé et al. reported the use of enzymatic treatment with collagenase type IV and DNAse as a safe procedure in patients for whom no spermatozoa was found after mechanical mincing, with an acceptable fertilization rate

(Crabbé et al., 1998). Mechanically, testicular tissue can be shredded in culture medium with glass coverslips or seminiferous tubules can be removed by fine needles (World Health Organization, 2021).

Preparation of retrograde ejaculation samples

For sperm to be obtained from the postejaculatory urine sample, the urine should be alkalized by sodium bicarbonate to avoid losing sperm motility. For this, the patient can drink water with sodium chloride or sodium bicarbonate or urinate in a container with culture medium. According to the WHO guideline, the concentrated retrograde and anterograde specimen can be processed by the density gradient preparation method.

Preparing HIV-infected semen samples

If the human immunodeficiency virus (HIV) is present in semen, viral ribonucleic acid (RNA) and proviral DNA can be found free in seminal plasma and nonsperm cells. In a systematic review and meta-analysis it was shown that without viral suppression, HIV transmission was prevented by washing 56.3% clinical pregnancy (Zafer et al., 2016). Also, it was recommended to use DGC for the separation of spermatozoa because only non-sperm cells express HIV receptors plus swim up to obtain motile spermatozoa (Gilling-Smith et al., 2006; Savasi et al., 2007). It is worth mentioning that in a systematic review it was shown that when antiretroviral treatment is used and viral load is suppressed there is negligible risk of transmission (LeMessurier et al., 2018).

Conclusion

It is difficult to compare studies and results, as it is difficult to standardize protocols and laboratories. Although promising results have been obtained from a large number of methods so far, there have not been enough randomized controlled studies that give data to establish any method as the gold standard. Furthermore, the effectiveness of the method should be determined by making long-term follow-up of the children born. When choosing a method, the advantages and disadvantages of each method should be considered.

References

Agarwal, A., Borges Jr, A., & Setti, A. (2016). *Non-invasive sperm selection for in vitro fertilization*. Springer-Verlag New York.

Aktan, T. M., Montag, M., Duman, S., Gorkemli, H., Rink, K., & Yurdakul, T. (2004). Use of a laser to detect viable but immotile spermatozoa. *Andrologia*, *36*(6), 366-369. https://doi.org/10.1111/j.1439-0272.2004.00636.x

Bartoov, B., Berkovitz, A., Eltes, F., Kogosowski, A., Menezo, Y., & Barak, Y. (2002). Real-time fine morphology of motile human sperm cells is associated with IVF-ICSI outcome. *Journal of andrology*, 23(1), 1-8. https://doi.org/10.1002/j.1939-4640.2002.tb02595.x

Berteli, T.S., Da Broi, M.G., Martins, W.P., Ferriani, R.A., & Navarro, P.A. (2017). Magnetic activated cell sorting before double gradient centrifugation improves recovery of high quality spermatozoa. *Andrology*, 5, 776–782. https://doi.org/10.1111/andr.12372

Bloch, A., Rogers, E. J., Nicolas, C., Martin-Denavit, T., Monteiro, M., Thomas, D., Morel, H., Levy, R., Siffroi, J., Dupont, C., Rouen, A. (2021). Detailed cell-level analysis of sperm nuclear quality among the different hypo-osmotic swelling test (HOST) classes. *Journal of Assisted Reproduction and Genetics*, *38*(9), 2491-2499. https://doi.org/10.1007/s10815-021-02232-y

Brahem, S., Letaief, K., Ben Ali, H., Saad, A., & Mehdi, M. (2013). Efficacy of the density gradient centrifugation method in eliminating sperm with aneuploidy. *Andrologia*, 45(3), 158-162. https://doi.org/10.1111/j.1439-0272.2012.01327.x

Chan, P. J., Jacobson, J. D., Corselli, J. U., & Patton, W. C. (2006). A simple zeta method for sperm selection based on membrane charge. *Fertility and sterility*, 85(2), 481-486. https://doi.org/10.1016/j.fertnstert.2005.07.1302

Chen, H., Wang, C., Zhou, H., Shu, J., Gan, X., Xu, K., Wu, S., DEng, X., Huang, G., & Lin, R. (2021). Laser-assisted selection of immotile spermatozoa has no effect on obstetric and neonatal outcomes of TESA-ICSI pregnancies. *Reproductive Biology and Endocrinology*, *19*, 1-9. https://doi.org/10.1186/s12958-021-00835-9

Cho, B. S., Schuster, T. G., Zhu, X., Chang, D., Smith, G. D., & Takayama, S. (2003). Passively driven integrated microfluidic system for separation of motile sperm. *Analytical chemistry*, 75(7), 1671-1675. https://doi.org/10.1021/ac020579e

Crabbé, E., Verheyen, G., Silber, S., Tournaye, H., Van de Velde, H., Goossens, A., & Van Steirteghem, A. (1998). Enzymatic digestion of testicular tissue may rescue the intracytoplasmic sperm injection cycle in some patients with non-obstructive azoospermia. *Human Reproduction* (Oxford, England), 13(10), 2791-2796 https://doi.org/10.1093/humrep/13.10.2791

Delaroche, L., Yazbeck, C., Gout, C., Kahn, V., Oger, P., & Rougier, N. (2013). Intracytoplasmic morphologically selected sperm injection (IMSI) after repeated IVF or ICSI failures: a prospective comparative study. *European Journal of Obstetrics & Gynecology and Reproductive Biology*, 167(1), 76-80. https://doi.org/10.1016/j.ejogrb.2012.11.011

Delilbaşı, L. (2008). İn vitro fertilizasyon (IVF) laboratuvar yöntemleri [In vitro fertilization (IVF) laboratory methods]. Ankara: Öncü Publishing.

Dirican, E. K., Özgün, O. D., Akarsu, S., Akın, K. O., Ercan, Ö., Uğurlu, M., Çamsarı, Ç., Kanyılmaz, O., Kaya, A., Ünsal, A. (2008). Clinical outcome of magnetic activated cell sorting of non-apoptotic spermatozoa before density gradient centrifugation for assisted reproduction. *Journal of assisted reproduction and genetics*, 25(8), 375-381. https://doi.org/10.1007/s10815-008-9250-1

Duran-Retamal, M., Morris, G., Achilli, C., Gaunt, M., Theodorou, E., Saab, W., Serhal, P., & Seshadri, S. (2020). Live birth and miscarriage rate following intracytoplasmic morphologically selected sperm injection vs intracytoplasmic sperm injection: an updated systematic review and meta-analysis. *Acta Obstetricia et Gynecologica Scandinavica,* 99(1), 24-33. https://doi.org/10.1111/aogs.13703

Edwards RG, Bavister BD, Steptoe PC (1969). Early stages of fertilization in vitro of human oocytes matured in vitro. *Nature.*, 221, 632–635. https://doi.org/10.1038/221632a0

Eisenbach, M., & Giojalas, L. C. (2006). Sperm guidance in mammals—an unpaved road to the egg. *Nature reviews Molecular cell biology*, *7*(4), 276-285. https://doi.org/10.1038/nrm1893

El-Nour, A. M., Al Mayman, H. A., Jaroudi, K. A., & Coskun, S. (2001). Effects of the hypo-osmotic swelling test on the outcome of intracytoplasmic sperm injection for patients with only nonmotile spermatozoa available for injection: a prospective randomized trial. *Fertility and sterility*, *75*(3), 480-484. https://doi.org/10.1016/S0015-0282(00)01762-3

Esfahani, M. H. N., Deemeh, M. R., Tavalaee, M., Sekhavati, M. H., & Gourabi, H. (2016). Zeta sperm selection improves pregnancy rate and alters sex ratio in male factor infertility patients: a double-blind, randomized clinical trial. *International Journal of Fertility & Sterility*, 10(2), 253. https://doi.org/10.22074/ijfs.2016.4917

European Society for Human Reproduction and Embryology. (2018). More than 8 million babies born from IVF since the world's first in 1978: European IVF pregnancy rates now steady at around 36 percent, according to ESHRE monitoring. *ScienceDaily*. Retrieved March 12, 2023 from www.sciencedaily.com/releases/2018/07/180703084127.htm

Friedler, S. (Ed.). (2012). In Vitro Fertilization: Innovative Clinical and Laboratory Aspects. BoD–Books on Demand.

Gardner, D. K. (2007). İn vitro fertilization a clinical approach. CRC press.

Garrido, N., Meseguer, M., Simon, C., Pellicer, A., & Remohi, J. (2004). Pro-oxidative and anti-oxidative imbalance in human semen and its relation with male fertility. *Asian journal of andrology*, 6(1), 59-66. Http://www.asiaandro.com/archive/1008-682X/6/59.htm

Gavella, M., & Lipovac, V. (1992). NADH-dependent oxidoreductase (diaphorase) activity and isozyme pattern of sperm in infertile men. *Archives of andrology*, 28(2), 135-141. https://doi.org/10.3109/01485019208987691

Ghumman, S., Adiga, S. K., Upadhya, D., Kalthur, G., Jayaraman, V., Rao, S. B., & Kumar, P. (2011). Combination of swim-up and density gradient separation methods effectively eliminate DNA damaged sperm. *Journal of the Turkish German Gynecological Association*, 12(3), 148. https://doi.org/10.5152/jtgga.2011.35

Gianaroli, L., Magli, M. C., Collodel, G., Moretti, E., Ferraretti, A. P., & Baccetti, B. (2008). Sperm head's birefringence: a new criterion for sperm selection. *Fertility and sterility*, *90*(1), 104-112. https://doi.org/10.1016/j.fertnstert.2007.05.078

Gianaroli, L., Magli, M. C., Ferraretti, A. P., Crippa, A., Lappi, M., Capitani, S., & Baccetti, B. (2010). Birefringence characteristics in sperm heads allow for the selection of reacted spermatozoa for intracytoplasmic sperm injection. *Fertility and sterility*, *93*(3), 807-813. https://doi.org/10.1016/j.fertnstert.2008.10.024

Gilling-Smith, C., Nicopoullos, J. D. M., Semprini, A. E., & Frodsham, L. C. G. (2006). HIV and reproductive care—a review of current practice. *BJOG: An International Journal of Obstetrics & Gynaecology*, 113(8), 869-878. https://doi .org/10.1111/j.1471-0528.2006.00960.x

Giovampaola, C. D., Flori, F., Sabatini, L., Incerti, L., La Sala, G. B., Rosati, F., & Focarelli, R. (2001). Surface of human sperm bears three differently charged CD52 forms, two of which remain stably bound to sperm after capacitation. *Molecular Reproduction and Development: Incorporating Gamete Research*, 60(1), 89-96. https://doi.org/10.1002/mrd.1065

Grunewald, S., Miska, W., Miska, G., Rasch, M., Reinhardt, M., Glander, H. J., & Paasch, U. (2007). Molecular glass wool filtration as a new tool for sperm preparation. *Human Reproduction*, 22(5), 1405-1412. https://doi.org/10.1093/humrep/dem015

Grunewald, S., Paasch, U., & Glander, H. J. (2001). Enrichment of non–apoptotic human spermatozoa after cryopreservation by immunomagnetic cell sorting. *Cell and tissue banking*, 2(3), 127-133. https://doi.org/10.1023/A:1020188913551

He, F., Wang, M. J., Li, S. L., Zhang, C. Y., & Hu, L. N. (2018). IMSI versus ICSI for male factor infertility: A meta-analysis. *Zhonghua nan ke xue= National Journal of Andrology*, 24(3), 254-262.

Hernández-Silva, G., López-Torres, A. S., Maldonado-Rosas, I., Mata-Martínez, E., Larrea, F., Torres-Flores, V., Treviño, C. L., & Chirinos, M. (2021). Effects of semen processing on sperm function: differences between swim-up and density gradient centrifugation. *The world journal of men's health*, 39(4), 740. https://doi.org/10.5534/wjmh.200115

Jeulin, C., Serres, C., & Jouannet, P. (1982). The effects of centrifugation, various synthetic media and temperature on the motility and vitality of human spermatozoa. *Reproduction Nutrition Développement,* 22(1A), 81-91.

Jeyendran, R. S., Perez-Pelaez, M., & Crabo, B. G. (1986). Concentration of viable spermatozoa for artificial insemination. *Fertility and sterility*, *45*(1), 132-134. https://doi.org/10.1016/S0015-0282(16)49111-9

Jeyendran, R. S., Van der Ven, H. H., Perez-Pelaez, M., Al-Hasani, S., & Diedrich, K. (1987). Separation of viable spermatozoa by standardized glass wool column. In: *Vitro Fertilisation.* Carnforth, UK: Parthenon Publishing.

Kirchhoff, C., & Hale, G. (1996). Cell-to-cell transfer of glycosylphosphatidylinositol-anchored membrane proteins during sperm maturation. *MHR: Basic science of reproductive medicine*, 2(3), 177-184. https://doi.org/10.1093/molehr/2.3.177

Ko, Y. J., Maeng, J. H., Hwang, S. Y., & Ahn, Y. (2018). Design, fabrication, and testing of a microfluidic device for thermotaxis and chemotaxis assays of sperm. *SLAS TECHNOLOGY: Translating Life Sciences Innovation*, *23*(6), 507-515.

LeMessurier, J., Traversy, G., Varsaneux, O., Weekes, M., Avey, M. T., Niragira, O., Gervais, R., Guyatt, G.,& Rodin, R. (2018). Risk of sexual transmission of human immunodeficiency virus with antiretroviral therapy, suppressed viral load and condom use: a systematic review. *Cmaj*, *190*(46), E1350-E1360.

Lepine, S., McDowell, S., Searle, L. M., Kroon, B., Glujovsky, D., & Yazdani, A. (2019). Advanced sperm selection techniques for assisted reproduction.

Cochrane Database of Systematic Reviews, (7), 1-12. https://doi.org/10.1002/14651858.CD010461

Li, Z., Liu, W., Qiu, T., Xie, L., Chen, W., Liu, R., Lu, Y., Mitchelson, K., Wang, J., Qiao, J., & Cheng, J. (2014). The construction of an interfacial valve-based microfluidic chip for thermotaxis evaluation of human sperm. *Biomicrofluidics*, *8*(2), 024102. https://doi.org/10.1063/1.4866851

Lopata, A., Patullo, M. J., Chang, A., & James, B. (1976). A method for collecting motile spermatozoa from human semen. *Fertility and Sterility*, 27(6), 677-684. https://doi.org/10.1016/S0015-0282(16)41899-6

Makker, K., Agarwal, A., & Sharma, R. (2009). Oxidative stress & male infertility. *Indian Journal of Medical Research,* 129(4), 357.

Malvezzi, H., Sharma, R., Agarwal, A., Abuzenadah, A. M., & Abu-Elmagd, M. (2014). Sperm quality after density gradient centrifugation with three commercially available media: a controlled trial. *Reproductive Biology and Endocrinology*, 12(1), 1-7.

Mangoli, E., & Khalili, M. A. (2020). The Beneficial role of intra cytoplasmic morphologically selected sperm injection (IMSI) in assisted reproduction. *Journal of reproduction & infertility*, 21(1), 3.

Martin-Hidalgo, D., Bragado, M. J., Batista, A. R., Oliveira, P. F., & Alves, M. G. (2019). Antioxidants and male fertility: from molecular studies to clinical evidence. *Antioxidants*, 8(4), 89.

Moretti, E., Gergely, A., Zeyneloglu, H. B., Ward, P., Ward, D., Baccetti, B., & Huszar, G. (1997). Relationship among head size, morphology and chromosome structure in human spermatozoa. *Fertility and Sterility*, 1001(1997), S158.

Oosterhuis, G. J. E., Mulder, A. B., Kalsbeek-Batenburg, E., Lambalk, C. B., Schoemaker, J., & Vermes, I. (2000). Measuring apoptosis in human spermatozoa: a biological assay for semen quality?. *Fertility and sterility,* 74(2), 245-250.

Ozcan, P., Takmaz, T., Yazici, M. G. K., Alagoz, O. A., Yesiladali, M., Fıçıcıoğlu, C. N., & Sevket, O. (2019). Does the use of microfluidic sperm sorting for the sperm selection improve IVF success rates in male factor infertility?. *Fertility and Sterility, 112*(3), e282-e283.

Parmegiani, L., Cognigni, G. E., Bernardi, S., Troilo, E., Taraborrelli, S., Arnone, A., Maccarini, A. M., & Filicori, M. (2012). Comparison of two ready-to-use systems designed for sperm–hyaluronic acid binding selection before intracytoplasmic sperm injection: PICSI vs. Sperm Slow: a prospective, randomized trial. *Fertility and sterility*, 98(3), 632-637. https://doi.org/10.1016/j.fertnstert.2012.05.043

Paulson, J. D., & Polakoski, K. L. (1977). A glass wool column procedure for removing extraneous material from the human ejaculate. *Fertility and Sterility*, *28*(2), 178-181. https://doi.org/10.1016/S0015-0282(16)42379-4

Prinosilova, P., Kruger, T., Sati, L., Ozkavukcu, S., Vigue, L., Kovanci, E., & Huszar, G. (2009). Selectivity of hyaluronic acid binding for spermatozoa with normal Tygerberg strict morphology. *Reproductive biomedicine online*, 18(2), 177-183.

Romany, L., Garrido, N., Motato, Y., Aparicio, B., Remohi, J., & Meseguer, M. (2014). Removal of annexin V-positive sperm cells for intracytoplasmic sperm injection in ovum donation cycles does not improve reproductive outcome: A controlled and randomized trial in unselected males. *Fertility and Sterility*, 102(6), 1567–1575.e1. https://doi.org/10.1016/j.fertnstert.2014.09.001

Ross, M. H. and Pawlina W. (2011). Histology: a text and atlas: with correlated cell and molecular biology Histology (p 840).6th edition. China; Lippincott Williams & Wilkins.

Said, T. M., Grunewald, S., Paasch, U., Rasch, M., Agarwal, A., & Glander, H. J. (2005). Effects of magnetic-activated cell sorting on sperm motility and cryosurvival rates. *Fertility and sterility*, 83(5), 1442-1446.

Said, T. M., & Land, J. A. (2011). Effects of advanced selection methods on sperm quality and ART outcome: A systematic review. *Human Reproduction Update,* 17(6), 719–733. https://doi.org/10.1093/ humupd/dmr032

Sati, L., Ovari, L., Bennett, D., Simon, S. D., Demir, R., & Huszar, G. (2008). Double probing of human spermatozoa for persistent histones, surplus cytoplasm, apoptosis and DNA fragmentation. *Reproductive biomedicine online*, 16(4), 570-579.

Savasi, V., Ferrazzi, E., Lanzani, C., Oneta, M., Parrilla, B., & Persico, T. (2007). Safety of sperm washing and ART outcome in 741 HIV-1-serodiscordant couples. *Human reproduction*, 22(3), 772-777.

Seo, D. B., Agca, Y., Feng, Z. C., & Critser, J. K. (2007). Development of sorting, aligning, and orienting motile sperm using microfluidic device operated by hydrostatic pressure. *Microfluidics and Nanofluidics*, *3*, 561-570.

Setti, A. S., Ferreira, R. C., Braga, D. P. D. A. F., Figueira, R. D. C. S., Iaconelli Jr, A., & Borges Jr, E. (2010). Intracytoplasmic sperm injection outcome versus intracytoplasmic morphologically selected sperm injection outcome: a meta-analysis. *Reproductive biomedicine online*, 21(4), 450-455.

Shekarriz, M., DeWire, D. M., Thomas Jr, A. J., & Agarwal, A. (1995). A method of human semen centrifugation to minimize the iatrogenic sperm injuries caused by reactive oxygen species. *European urology*, 28, 31-31.

Shirota, K., Yotsumoto, F., Itoh, H., Obama, H., Hidaka, N., Nakajima, K., & Miyamoto, S. (2016). Separation efficiency of a microfluidic sperm sorter to minimize sperm DNA damage. *Fertility and sterility*, 105(2), 315-321.

Tea, N. T., Jondet, M., & Scholler, R. (1984). A 'migration-gravity sedimentation'method for collecting motile spermatozoa from human semen. *In Vitro Fertilizàtion, Embryo Transfer and Early Pregnancy* (pp. 117-120). Springer, Dordrecht.

Teixeira, D. M., Miyague, A. H., Barbosa, M. A., Navarro, P. A., Raine-Fenning, N., Nastri, C. O., & Martins, W. P. (2020). Regular (ICSI) versus ultra-high magnification (IMSI) sperm selection for assisted reproduction. *Cochrane Database of Systematic Reviews*, (2), 1-46. https://doi.org/10.1002/14651858 .CD010167.pub3

Viswambharan, N., & Murugan, M. (2021). Effect of wash and swim-up and density gradient sperm preparation on sperm DNA fragmentation. *Materials Today: Proceedings*, 45, 2002-2005. https://www.sciencedirect.com/science/article/pii /S221478532037139X#!

World Health Organization. (2021). *WHO laboratory manual for the examination and processing of human semen (6th edition).* World Health Organization. https:// www.who.int/publications/i/item/9789240030787

Yamanaka, M., Tomita, K., Hashimoto, S., Matsumoto, H., Satoh, M., Kato, H., Hosoi, Y., Inoue, M., Nakaoka, Y., & Morimoto, Y. (2016). Combination of density gradient centrifugation and swim-up methods effectively decreases morphologically abnormal sperms. *Journal of Reproduction and Development, 62*(2), 599-606. https://doi.org/10.1262/jrd.2016-112

Yildiz, K., & Yuksel, S. (2019). Use of microfluidic sperm extraction chips as an alternative method in patients with recurrent in vitro fertilisation failure. *Journal of Assisted Reproduction and Genetics*, 36(7), 1423-1429.

Zafer, M., Horvath, H., Mmeje, O., van der Poel, S., Semprini, A. E., Rutherford, G., & Brown, J. (2016). Effectiveness of semen washing to prevent human immunodeficiency virus (HIV) transmission and assist pregnancy in HIV-discordant couples: a systematic review and meta-analysis. *Fertility and sterility*, 105(3), 645-655.

Zhang, H., Xuan, X., Yang, S., Li, X., Xu, C., & Gao, X. (2018). Selection of viable human spermatozoa with low levels of DNA fragmentation from an immotile population using density gradient centrifugation and magnetic-activated cell sorting. *Andrologia*, 50(1), e12821. https://doi.org/10.1111/and.12821

Ziarati, N., Tavalaee, M., Bahadorani, M., & Esfahani, M. H. N. (2018). Clinical outcomes of magnetic activated sperm sorting in infertile men candidate for ICSI. *Human Fertility,* 22(2), 118-125. https://doi.org/10.1080/14647273.2018.1424354

Zini, A., Finelli, A., Phang, D., & Jarvi, K. (2000). Influence of semen processing technique on human sperm DNA integrity. *Urology*, 56(6), 1081-1084. https://doi.org/10.1016/S0090-4295(00)00770-6

Chapter 12

Assisted Fertilization

Aynura Aghayeva[1], MD* and Tunahan Yapıcı[2], MD

[1]Department of Histology and Embryology, Uludağ University, Bursa, Turkiye

[2]Department of Histology and Embryology, Manisa Celal Bayar University, Manisa, Turkiye

Abstract

Assisted reproduction has recently entered the field of interest of researchers and physicians and has become an open topic of research. Considering the 1.5 million babies born with assisted reproductive techniques today, we can also understand why this topic has become so popular. By 1978, 112 embryo transfers had been performed. The last transfer, which was made in July 1978, resulted in pregnancy and the first IVF baby was born in the history of ECO.By the end of the 1980s, a series of methods had been developed, the most famous of which were partial zone dissection (PZD) and subzonal sperm insemination (SUZI). A technical accident in 1992 led to the achievement of clinical success by microinjecting one sperm directly into the ooplasm of the oocyte, and thus to the discovery that successful in vitro fertilization can be achieved. The concept of assisted reproductive techniques refers to the whole process, including in vitro interventions of human oocytes, sperm, and embryos for reproductive purposes. These interventions include classical in vitro fertilization (IVF), intracytoplasmic sperm injection (ICSI), and intrauterine insemination (IUI) (de Geyter, 2019). In this section, the medical indications of these applications will be explained. In vitro fertilization is a set of procedures that involve extracorporeal fertilization of gametes. It includes traditional in vitro insemination and ICSI. The in vitro fertilization method was first used in infertile individuals with tuba uterine dysfunction. With the change and development of assisted reproductive techniques over time, IVF has begun to be used for a wide variety of indications.

---

* Corresponding Author's E-mail: dr.a.agayeva@gmail.com

In: Holistic Approach to Assisted Reproductive Technology
Editor: Kenan Demir and Rümeysa Yılmaz Göç
ISBN: 979-8-89113-017-3
© 2023 Nova Science Publishers, Inc.

Key Words: Assisted fertilization, IVF, Infertility, PZD, SUZI, ICSI

Introduction

History of assisted fertilization

Assisted reproduction has recently entered the field of interest of researchers and physicians and has become an open topic of research. Considering the 1.5 million babies born with assisted reproductive techniques today, we can also understand why this topic has become so popular. For the first time, information about assisted reproduction was presented in 1970 and has not lost its importance.

Embryologist Gregory Pinkus, one of the first researchers, was the first to demonstrate the in vitro maturation processes of oocytes aspirated from the follicles, the expulsion of the first polar body, in his work on the in vitro maturation of mammalian oocytes. In addition, by examining the oocytes removed from human ovaries, he identified the chromosome numbers and showed this as a marker for the completion of in vitro maturation (Pinkus et al., 1956).

In the late 1960s, Austin and Chang noted that spermatozoa remain in the female reproductive system for a certain time before fermenting the oocyte, in other words, they spend a period for capacitation (Toyoda et al., 1974).

In immature female rats in estrus Allen and Gates work, the researcher to induce ovulation, follicle-stimulating hormone (FSH) - rich serum from pregnant horses (PMS) and luteinizing hormone (LH) activity of human chorionic gonadotropin (hCG) was used (Gates & Bozarth, 1978).

Later, in their work with Mervyn Runner, they administered low doses of each hormone at December intervals of 48 hours to immature female mice to induce oocyte maturation, ovulation, and mating (Gates & Bozarth, 1978).

There were many opinions that exogenous hormones such as PMS and hCG stimulate follicle growth and ovulation in immature female mammals, while in adults these hormones are inconvenient because they can interact poorly with the natural cycle. But later studies have revealed ideas that support the opposite. In one of the Beleki studies, PMS at a dose of 1-3 IU induced the growth of a large number of follicles and an estrous cycle and ovulation were initiated after 6 hours in almost all female animal models after HCG was administered after 42 hours. About 70 oocytes whose fertilization has been initiated in the ampulla region have progressed to blastocysts (Fowler & Edwards, 1957; Gates & Bozarth, 1978).

The Birth of LOUISE BROWN

The weight of the project, which Edwards, Steptoe, and Purdy walked together in 1969, was not easy, given the information efficiency of those years. The first embryo transfer attempt was made in December 1971 (Johnson & Elder, 2015).

Between 1969 and 1971, the MRC reported that although laparoscopy was performed in 97 women, they had no chance of pregnancy and were assigned as a control group. Moreover, 76 of these women had not had an embryo transfer before 1978. However, all evidence shows that these patients were better informed about risks and benefits, but Edwards, Steptoe, and Purdy deserve recognition for their pioneering role in the development of IVF.

By 1978, 112 embryo transfers had been performed. The last transfer, which was made in July 1978, resulted in pregnancy, and the first IVF baby was born in the history of ECO (Johnson & Elder, 2015).

Principles of Assisted Fertilization

There are several ways to create and launch a successful laboratory of assisted reproductive technologies (ART). ART fields range from a temporary laboratory with minimal equipment to fully equipped laboratories with a large area.

When designing an integrated institution, special attention is paid to the environment and physical equipment. The staff is important for the success of the entire operation. Success in clinical practice depends almost entirely on the qualifications and experience of medical and laboratory personnel. The laboratory manager and staff, as well as embryologists, must make good use of their experience and work toward a goal. The number and qualifications of laboratory personnel are critical factors for maintaining stability in the laboratory.

Programs should develop a reliable system to monitor individual data for important clinical and laboratory procedures, such as embryo transfer, ICSI, and biopsy.

As is the case with each discipline, performance monitoring is necessary to verify the correctness and optimal execution of the procedure. They must not deviate from the protocol so that everything goes smoothly (Go, 2015).

By the end of the 1980s, a series of methods had been developed, the most famous of which were partial zone dissection (PZD) and subzonal sperm insemination (SUZI). A technical accident in 1992 led to the achievement of clinical success by microinjecting one sperm directly into the ooplasm of the oocyte, and thus to the discovery that successful in vitro fertilization can be achieved.

Timing and Process of Conventional Insemination

The idea of fertilizing oocytes outside the body was tested in infertile women with closed fallopian tubes. Convective fertilization simulates the process in vivo.Oocytes obtained from a natural cycle or after induction are placed in a Petri dish or test tube and mixed with processed sperm. Gametes are left in a Petri dish for several hours, usually overnight. The next morning, the cumulus and coronary cells are removed and the oocyte(s) are examined for the presence of pronuclei. If there is, it indicates fertilization (Hull, 1990; Thatcher & DeCherney, 1989).

The correct time for insemination corresponds approximately 4-5 hours after receiving oocytes. The collected CACs must be morphologically mature; otherwise, it may be advisable to extend the period one more time. A culture medium is placed in a culture dish in the form of drops and poured with oil. Semen in concentrations of 100,000 to 250,000 / ml is injected into the medium. Then, the cumulus oocyte complexes (CCOCs) are added to the medium. Usually, 2-6 CCOC are placed in a drop of approximately 100 μl (≈25 μl of medium per CCOC). The incubation period of gametes lasts 15-17 hours (Gardner et al., 2013).

Some studies have shown that a shorter incubation period may be sufficient to achieve a high fertilization rate with conventional IVF. For fertilization, one sperm must pass through the cumulus cells to interact with the transparent zone and merge with the olemma. This method can be used in patients who are not related to the malefactor, but also in patients with the malefactor (Dai et al., 2012; Gianaroli et al., 1996; Kattera & Chen, 2003).

In the early 1980s, controlled ovarian hyperstimulation (COH), although it did not affect normal fertilization, was of great importance because it provided a greater collection of oocytes (Fleming et al., 1982; Rogers et al., 1986; Trounson et al., 1981).

Furthermore, the introduction of follicle aspiration under ultrasound control provided a much more effective and reliable way to recruit oocytes (Lenz & Lauritsen, 1982).

Identification of Cumulus–Oocyte Complexes

Oocyte aspiration must be performed at the appropriate time. Based on physiological processes, decommunization of eggs is carried out within 34-38 hours after stimulation in a stimulated cycle (using a human chorionic gonadotropin agonist [hCG] or gonadotropin-releasing hormone [GnRH]) (Mauvais-Jarvis, 1967; Testart & Frydman, 1982; Zanartu et al., 1975).

In some cases, when the goal is to mature oocytes in vitro, for example, in cases of polycystic ovary syndrome [PCO], oocyte collection can be carried out without an HCG trigger (with or without "minimal stimulation") (Chian et al., 2004).

The aspirated follicular fluid is poured into a Petri dish and examined with a dissection microscope. Cumulus-oocyte complexes (CCOCS) are removed from blood clots. Then, after waiting for a certain time, it is cleaned from the dune cells by a denudation process (Daya et al., 1990).

Sperm Preparation

For IVF, fresh sperm is generally used, except for some special cases. Before sperm collection, the male patient is told to have an abstinence period of at least 3 days. Care should be taken to collect the ejaculate in a sterile container. To have the potential to fertilize the oocyte, it must be in a certain period that it spends in the female genital system, which is called capacitation. In IVF treatments, many processes are applied to complete the capacitation process outside the confines, so it is beyond the scope of this section to go into more detail on sperm capacitation. The sample is kept at room temperature after collection. The sample is kept at room temperature to undergo lichenification. If the sample is not liquified after 20 minutes, 5 mg of chymotrypsin can be added. Samples should be processed in the laboratory within one hour after receipt. Semen samples should be evaluated based on the evaluation guidelines of the World Health Organization (WHO) for basic sperm parameters before and after preparation (World Health Organization, 2001).

There are different techniques for preparing sperm for IVF, of which the most commonly used are (1) the buoyancy method and (2) the gradient density centrifuge. These two methods provide similar sperm yields in terms of concentration and mobility, but the gradient density centrifuge is more advantageous in removing residues from the ejaculate and largely preventing morphologically abnormal sperm selection (Henkel & Schill, 2003; Ricci et al., 2009).

Assisted Fertilization and Intracytoplasmic Sperm Injection (ICSI) Development of the Micro-Injection Technique

Due to the contradictory and poor results of IVF, where there was a heavy male factor, a new fertilization technique using microinjection was needed. In the early 1900s, Kite performed the first microinjection of sperm in starfish eggs, and the results obtained were inconclusive (Lillie, 1914).

Half a century later, Hiramoto, in his research, which studied the activation of the egg, tried to make microinjections of live sperm into unfertilized sea urchin eggs (Hiramoto, 1962).

Uehara and Yanagimachi studied the method of sperm injection to determine whether pronuclei develop in a hamster egg after sperm cells or sperm nuclei are injected into the cytoplasm (Uehara & Yanagimachi, 1977).

It was also found that the nuclei of fresh and frozen-thawed human spermatozoa can develop into pronuclei in hamster oocytes. This led to the idea that the cytoplasmic factors that control the transformation of sperm nuclei into male pronuclei are not species-specific (Naish et al., 1987a; Naish et al., 1987b).

In one of the studies, mouse sperm was injected into rat oocytes and found a high proportion of activation and formation of both pronuclei. The fact that the capacitated and non-capacitated spermatozoa reacted the same way suggests that when sperm is injected directly into the cytoplasm, sperm capacitation may be optional (Thadani, 1980).

in 1992, a technical accident led to the formation of clinical success by microinjection of a single sperm directly into the ooplasm of an oocyte, and thus to the discovery that successful in vitro fertilization can be achieved. The most widely used Intracytoplasmic Sperm Injection (ICSI) technique today is.

Indications for Assisted Reproductive Techniques

Infertility poses a significant challenge for modern reproductive medicine (Szamatowicz, 2016). Infertility, which is believed to affect 186 million people worldwide, is accepted as a disease by the World Health Organization. It also poses a social problem due to its prevalence in society (Szamatowicz, 2016).

The only real treatment for infertility is a healthy pregnancy and live birth. Three main treatment strategies have been determined for possible causes of infertility: pharmacological, surgical, and assisted reproductive techniques. And in recent years, great advances have been made in assisted reproductive techniques (Kamel, 2013). Assisted reproductive techniques refer to the entire process, including in vitro manipulations of human oocytes, spermatozoa, and embryos for reproductive purposes.

Classical in vitro fertilization (IVF), intracytoplasmic sperm injection (ICSI), and intrauterine insemination (IUI) are included in these processes (Geyter et al., 2019). In this section, the medical indications of these applications will be explained.

In Vitro Fertilization Indications

In vitro fertilization is a set of procedures that involve extracorporeal fertilization of gametes. It includes traditional in vitro insemination and ICSI (Zegers-Hochschild et al., 2017).

The in vitro fertilization method was first used in infertile individuals with tuba uterine dysfunction. With the change and development of assisted reproductive techniques over time, IVF has begun to be used for a wide variety of indications.

Tubal Factor

Tubal infertility causes account for 30% of female infertility causes and 14% of couples receiving ART treatment in the USA. (Huang & Rosenwaks, 2014) Tubal obstructions can be caused by intrinsic and extrinsic causes. Ascending salpantige and salpingitis isthmic nodosa as intrinsic causes, surgical sterilization, endometriosis, and peritonitis as extrinsic causes can be given as examples. Tubal damage is usually caused by chlamydia trachomatis and gonorrhea infections.

Before in vitro fertilization treatments, tube surgery was the only solution to these problems, but now IVF is the first treatment option recommended for female infertility due to tubal factors (Benadiva et al., 1995; Practice Committee of the American Society for Reproductive Medicine, 2015). The presence of hydrosalpinx is a risk factor that can reduce the success of the application by 50% in patients undergoing IVF treatment (N. Johnson et al., 2010; Strandell et al., 1999). Hydrosalpinge fluid is known to be a toxic fluid that disrupts embryo implantation (Strandell & Lindhard, 2002). Therefore, it is recommended to treat with surgical procedures prior to IVF treatment (N. Johnson et al., 2010).

Male Factor

Male physiological disorders, such as low testosterone concentrations or low sperm count, occur in 35% of infertile couples (Odisho et al., 2014). After the developments in ART and the use of ICSI, ART applications with the male factor have increased. In the treatment of infertility in individuals with mild male factors, ART treatments, including IUI, are recommended if medical and surgical treatment cannot improve sperm parameters (Lee et al., 2002).

Endometriosis

Endometriosis is an estrogen-dependent disease defined as the presence of endometrial tissue outside the uterine cavity. It is one of the leading causes of infertility and its prevalence has increased in infertile women. Affecting

0.5-5% of fertile women, endometriosis is seen in 25-40% of infertile women. Treatment for infertility remains unclear. Suppression of endometriosis with medical treatments and surgical removal of accumulated tissue are the main steps of treatment. Additionally, according to available evidence, medical treatment does not provide fertility benefits. Surgical treatment is considered effective at all stages of the disease. Controlled ovarian hyperstimulation with IUI is recommended in cases of early stage surgically treated endometriosis. In advanced cases, in vitro fertilization is recommended (Ozkan et al., 2008).

Ovulatory Dysfunction

Ovulatory dysfunction is a very common cause of infertility, accounting for 25% of female infertility (Carson & Kallen, 2021). These patients come to the hospital with complaints of oligomenorrhea or amenorrhea. The most common cause of anovulation is polycystic ovary syndrome (Rotterdam ESHRE / ASRM-sponsored PCOS consensus workshop group, 2004). Additionally, ovulatory dysfunction may be caused by thyroid diseases and hyperprolactinemia. For this reason, TSH screening should be performed for this etiology and thyroid hormone should be replaced if necessary. For hyperprolactinemia, screening for pituitary adenoma should be performed and evaluated together with thyroid function tests. Exogenous gonadotropin treatments are recommended for patients with hypogonadotropic hypogonadism (Martin et al., 1993).

Unexplained Infertility

Normal tubal patency, normal ovulation, normal semen analysis, normal ovarian reserve, and normal uterine cavity, that is, infertility cannot be determined by research. Its incidence is between 10-30% (Templeton & Penney, 1982). Treatment options include expectation management, IUI, empirical therapy with clomiphene citrate, clomiphene citrate therapy with IUI, gonadotropins/IUI, and IVF. IVF is the most effective treatment option for couples with unexplained infertility and provides the highest pregnancy rate per cycle in the shortest time frame (Guzick et al., 1994).

Preimplantation Genetic Diagnosis and Screening

Oocyte polar bodies, embryo blastomeres, and blastocyst trophectoderm can be evaluated postbiopsy and analyzed for single gene defects and used for aneuploidy screening. It enables the detection of genetic diseases such as sickle cell anemia and cystic fibrosis before pregnancy (Simpson, 2010).

Preservation of Fertility

Cancer treatments such as chemotherapy, radiotherapy, or combination therapy are highly toxic to the gonads. Causes girls and young women to develop early ovarian failure and subsequently become infertile. In addition to the causes of oncological disease, some treatments can cause this condition. Therefore, fertility preservation treatments should be offered to patients with these conditions (Dolmans & Manavella, 2019).

Intracytoplasmic Sperm Injection Indications

Approximately one third of couples diagnosed with subfertility in reproductive age are affected by the malefactor, and ICSI treatment is very valuable in patients with the malefactor. Indications for ICSI therapy, which was introduced in 1992, have evolved to include patients with normal and mild semen analysis defects (Babayev et al., 2014).

Although the debate on accepting many indications as definite indications continues, we can currently accept the following reasons as indications.

a. None or insufficient fertilization in two IVF cycles
b. Epididymis / testesicular spermatozoa
c. Globozoospermia
d. Immobile spermatozoa
e. Frozen-thawed spermatozoa with poor survival
f. Preimplantation genetic diagnosis (Hamberger et al., 1998).

Intra-Uterine Insemination Indications

Intrauterine insemination (IUI) is a relatively inexpensive and easily accessible assisted reproductive technique that is used as the first choice for infertile couples to achieve pregnancy within certain indications (Kandavel & Cheong, 2018). It includes the procedures for processing sperm in vitro and placing them directly in the uterus during the ovulation period. This procedure can be performed with ovarian stimulation or in a natural cycle (Fauque et al., 2014; Kandavel & Cheong, 2018). In couples with infertility due to intrauterine insemination, male factors, cervical factors, minimal or mild endometriosis, as well as unexplained subfertility (Kim et al., 2014). Bhattacharya et al. In an article published in 2008, stated that in couples with unexplained infertility, IUI after ovarian stimulation with clomiphene citrate and IUI without ovarian stimulation did not increase live birth rates compared to waiting for therapy (Bhattacharya et al., 2008). In addition, the results of a study (FASST) investigating the success of gonadotropin/IUI (FSH/IUI) administration in women aged 21-39 years with unexplained infertility were published in 2010. In this study, couples were randomized to the conventional treatment arm, which included 3 cycles of clomiphene citrate (CS)/IUI and 3 cycles of FSH/IUI, and up to 6 cycles of IVF, and the accelerated arm, in which 3 cycles of FSH / IUI were skipped. Pregnancy rates per cycle were 7.6% with KS/IUI, 9.8% with FSH / IUI and 30.7% with in vitro fertilization (IVF). Moreover, costs were lower in the accelerated treatment arm (Reindollar et al., 2010). Based on these results, IVF treatment was recommended instead of IUI as the first choice in 2013 in the NICE guideline for infertile couples with unexplained infertility, male factor, and mild endometriosis, unless there is a religious, social and cultural barrier (Kandavel & Cheong, 2018). After this recommendation, the place of IUI in practice has been variable with supporting evidence for its clinical use.

In the NICE's guide published in 2013 and updated in 2017;

- If pregnancy cannot be achieved by vaginal intercourse for psychosexual or physical reasons,
- If assisted reproductive techniques are used to reduce the risk of transmission of viral diseases such as HIV,
- If a donor is used for pregnancy in both homosexual and heterosexual couples, non-stimulation IUI is recommended as a treatment option.
- Couples who cannot conceive due to reasons such as unexplained infertility, low sperm count and low sperm quality, or mild endometriosis are said not to be offered IUI with or without ovarian stimulation, and it is recommended to try to get pregnant for 2 years before IVF is recommended (Fertility Problems: Assessment and Treatment, 2013).

Studies on IUI are ongoing and it is controversial how much the NICE guideline is applied by clinicians in clinical practice (Cohlen et al., 2018). In recent studies, especially in couples with unexplained infertility, it has been observed that IUI applied together with ovarian stimulation provides close success to IVF (Bensdorp et al., 2015; Nandi et al., 2017). In the current approach, IUI with ovarian stimulation (OS) is the first choice in men with a total motile sperm count of more than 10 million and a spontaneous pregnancy prognosis of <30% in 1 year in couples with unexplained infertility. It is recommended as a treatment, but treatment with IUI remains uncertain in couples with male factor-related infertility and low sperm quality. More data and more studies are needed on the use of IUIs (Cohlen et al., 2018).

Ethical Problems of Assisted Reproductive Techniques

Rapid developments in in vitro fertilization have also generated ethical debates. There is a complex relationship between in vitro fertilization practices and social values. These ethical problems include parental upper age limit, gametes and embryo owners, IVF requests of single women and homosexual couples, pre-implantation genetic diagnosis, oocyte freezing for social reasons, etc. there are situations. In other words, the decision to treat with assisted reproductive techniques includes not only clinical and economic reasons, but also a decision-making process intertwined with ethical values (Asplund, 2020).

Conclusion

Since the successful in vitro fertilization that began with the birth of Louise Brown in 1978, IVF has become the treatment option for infertility due to various indications. However, it should be emphasized that IVF is not always successful and has low results, especially in patients with a male factor present. Researchers who are always looking to increase the success results have also produced other techniques using micromanipulations of gametes.

None of these approaches helped to improve the outcome in severe cases. In 1988, the technique of gamete micromanipulation directly into the cytoplasm was proposed. This was carried out by the Norfolk IVF center laboratory team. Although we say that the end was successful by introducing a single sperm into the cytoplasm of the oocyte after crossing the boundaries of the zona pellucida and the oolemma and providing fertilization, the pregnancy did not continue. We know that this method, called intracytoplasmic sperm injection, was included in daily laboratory practice at the Free University of Brussels in 1991, and that the first pregnancy formed by this method was achieved. such as inserting spermatozoa into a hole created on the PZD-zona pellucida or in the perivitelline cavity under the SUZI-zona pellucid.

Although the point at which assisted reproduction has come in the recent period gives face-smiling results, studies are continuing to make it come to a better place in the future.

References

Asplund, K. (2020). Use of in vitro fertilization-ethical issues. *Upsala Journal of Medical Sciences*, *125*(2), 192–199. https://doi.org/10.1080/03009734.2019.1684405

Babayev, S. N., Park, C. W., & Bukulmez, O. (2014). Intracytoplasmic sperm injection indications: how rigorous? *Seminars in Reproductive Medicine*, *32*(4), 283–290. https://doi.org/10.1055/s-0034-1375180

Benadiva, C. A., Kligman, I., Davis, O., & Rosenwaks, Z. (1995). In vitro fertilization versus tubal surgery: is pelvic reconstructive surgery obsolete? *Fertility and Sterility*, *64*(6), 1051–1061. https://doi.org/10.1016/s0015-0282(16)57958-8

Bensdorp, A. J., Tjon-Kon-Fat, R. I., Bossuyt, P. M. M., Koks, C. A. M., Oosterhuis, G. J. E., Hoek, A., Hompes, P. G. A., Broekmans, F. J. M., Verhoeve, H. R., de Bruin, J. P., van Golde, R., Repping, S., Cohlen, B. J., Lambers, M. D. A., van Bommel, P. F., Slappendel, E., Perquin, D., Smeenk, J. M., Pelinck, M van Wely, M. (2015). Prevention of multiple pregnancies in couples with unexplained or mild male subfertility: a randomized controlled trial of in vitro fertilization with single embryo transfer or in vitro fertilization in the modified natural cycle compared with intrauterine insemination with controlled ovarian hyperstimulation. *BMJ (Clinical Research Ed.)*, *350*, g7771. https://doi.org/10.1136/bmj.g7771

Bhattacharya, S., Harrild, K., Mollison, J., Wordsworth, S., Tay, C., Harrold, A., McQueen, D., Lyall, H., Johnston, L., Burrage, J., Grossett, S., Walton, H., Lynch, J., Johnstone, A., Kini, S., Raja, A., & Templeton, A. (2008). Clomifene citrate or unstimulated intrauterine insemination compared with expectant management for unexplained infertility: a pragmatic randomized controlled trial. *BMJ (Clinical Research Ed.)*, *337*, a716. https://doi.org/10.1136/bmj.a716

Carson, S. A., & Kallen, A. N. (2021). Diagnosis and Management of Infertility: A Review. *JAMA*, *326*(1), 65–76. https://doi.org/10.1001/jama.2021.4788

Chian, R.-C., Buckett, W. M., Abdul Jalil, A. K., Son, W.-Y., Sylvestre, C., Rao, D., & Tan, S. L. (2004). Natural-cycle in vitro fertilization combined with in vitro maturation of immature oocytes is a potential approach in infertility treatment. *Fertility and Sterility*, *82*(6), 1675–1678. https://doi.org/10.1016/j.fertnstert.2004.04.060

Cohlen, B., Bijkerk, A., van der Poel, S., & Ombelet, W. (2018). IUI: review and systematic assessment of the evidence that supports global recommendations. *Human Reproduction Update*, *24*(3), 300–319. https://doi.org/10.1093/humupd/dmx041

Dai, S.-J., Qiao, Y.-H., Jin, H.-X., Xin, Z.-M., Su, Y.-C., Sun, Y.-P., & Chian, R.-C. (2012). Effect of coincubation time of sperm-oocytes on fertilization, embryonic development, and subsequent pregnancy outcome. *Systems Biology in Reproductive Medicine*, *58*(6), 348–353. https://doi.org/10.3109/19396368.2012.708087

Daya, S., Kohut, J., Gunby, J., & Younglai, E. (1990). Influence of blood clots in the cumulus complex on oocyte fertilization and cleavage. *Human Reproduction (Oxford, England)*, *5*(6), 744–746. https://doi.org/10.1093/oxfordjournals.humrep.a137179

de Geyter, C. (2019). Assisted reproductive technology: Impact on society and need for surveillance. *Best Practice & Research. Clinical Endocrinology & Metabolism*, *33*(1), 3–8. https://doi.org/10.1016/j.beem.2019.01.004

Dolmans, M.-M., & Manavella, D. D. (2019). Recent advances in fertility preservation. *The Journal of Obstetrics and Gynaecology Research*, *45*(2), 266–279. https://doi.org/10.1111/jog.13818

Fauque, P., Lehert, P., Lamotte, M., Bettahar-Lebugle, K., Bailly, A., Diligent, C., Clédat, M., Pierrot, P., Guénédal, M.-L., & Sagot, P. (2014). The clinical success of intrauterine insemination cycles is affected by the sperm preparation time. *Fertility and Sterility*, *101*(6), 1618-23.e1-3. https://doi.org/10.1016/j.fertnstert.2014.03.015

Fertility Problems: Assessment and Treatment. (2013). *National Institute for Health and Care Excellence.* Retrieved Nov 14, 2022 from www.nice.org.uk/guidance/cg156

Fleming, R., Adam, A. H., Barlow, D. H., Black, W. P., MacNaughton, M. C., & Coutts, J. R. (1982). A new systematic treatment for infertile women with abnormal hormone profiles. *British Journal of Obstetrics and Gynaecology*, *89*(1), 80–83. https://doi.org/10.1111/j.1471-0528.1982.tb04642.x

Fowler, R. E., & Edwards, R. G. (1957). Induction of Superovulation and Pregnancy in Mature Mice by Gonadotropins. *Journal of Endocrinology*, *15*(4), 374–384. https://doi.org/10.1677/joe.0.0150374

Gardner, T. W., Fisher, D. M., Morell, K. D., & Cupper, M. L. (2013). Upper-plate deformation in response to flat slab subduction inboard of the aseismic Cocos Ridge, Osa Peninsula, Costa Rica. *Lithosphere*, *5*(3), 247–264.

Gates, A. H., & Bozarth, J. L. (1978). Ovulation in the PMSG-Treated Immature Mouse: Effect of Dose, Age, Weight, Puberty, Season and Strain (BALB/c, 129 and C129F1 Hybrid)1. *Biology of Reproduction*, *18*(3), 497–505. https://doi.org/10.1095/biolreprod18.3.497

Gianaroli, L., Magli, M. C., Ferraretti, A. P., Fiorentino, A., Tosti, E., Panzella, S., & Dale, B. (1996). Reducing the time of sperm-oocyte interaction in human in-vitro fertilization improves the implantation rate. *Human Reproduction*, *11*(1), 166–171. https://doi.org/10.1093/oxfordjournals.humrep.a019011

Go, K. J. (2015). 'By the work, one knows the workman': the practice and profession of the embryologist and its translation to quality in the embryology laboratory. *Reproductive BioMedicine Online*, *31*(4), 449–458. https://doi.org/10.1016/j.rbmo.2015.07.006

Guzick, D. S., Grefenstette, I., Baffone, K., Berga, S. L., Krasnow, J. S., Stovall, D. W., & Naus, G. J. (1994). Infertility evaluation in fertile women: a model for assessing the efficacy of infertility testing. *Human Reproduction (Oxford, England)*, *9*(12), 2306–2310. https://doi.org/10.1093/oxfordjournals.humrep.a138442

Hamberger, L., Lundin, K., Sjögren, A., & Söderlund, B. (1998). Indications for intracytoplasmic sperm injection. *Human Reproduction (Oxford, England)*, *13 Suppl 1*, 128–133. https://doi.org/10.1093/humrep/13.suppl_1.128

Henkel, R. R., & Schill, W.-B. (2003). Sperm preparation for ART. *Reproductive Biology and Endocrinology: RB&E*, *1*, 108. https://doi.org/10.1186/1477-7827-1-108

Hiramoto, Y. (1962). Microinjection of the live spermatozoa into sea urchin eggs. *Experimental Cell Research*, *27*, 416–426. https://doi.org/10.1016/0014-4827(62)90006-x

Huang, J. Y. J., & Rosenwaks, Z. (2014). Assisted reproductive techniques. *Methods in Molecular Biology (Clifton, N.J.)*, *1154*, 171–231. https://doi.org/10.1007/978-1-4939-0659-8_8

Hull, M. G. (1990). Indications for assisted conception. *British Medical Bulletin*, *46*(3), 580–595. https://doi.org/10.1093/oxfordjournals.bmb.a072418

Johnson, M. H., & Elder, K. (2015). The Oldham Notebooks: an analysis of the development of IVF 1969–1978. IV. Ethical aspects. *Reproductive Biomedicine & Society Online*, *1*(1), 34–45. https://doi.org/10.1016/j.rbms.2015.04.002

Johnson, N., van Voorst, S., Sowter, M. C., Strandell, A., & Mol, B. W. J. (2010). Surgical treatment for tubal disease in women due to undergo in vitro fertilization. *The Cochrane Database of Systematic Reviews*, *1*, CD002125. https://doi.org/10.1002/14651858.CD002125.pub3

Kamel, R. M. (2013). Assisted reproductive technology after the birth of Louise brown. *Journal of Reproduction & Infertility*, *14*(3), 96–109.

Kandavel, V., & Cheong, Y. (2018). Does intra-uterine insemination have a place in modern ART practice? *Best Practice & Research. Clinical Obstetrics & Gynaecology*, *53*, 3–10. https://doi.org/10.1016/j.bpobgyn.2018.08.003

Kattera, S., & Chen, C. (2003). Short coincubation of gametes in in vitro fertilization improves implantation and pregnancy rates: a prospective, randomized, controlled study. *Fertility and Sterility*, *80*(4), 1017–1021. https://doi.org/10.1016/s0015-0282(03)01154-3

Kim, Y. J., Park, C. W., & Ku, S.-Y. (2014). Indications of intrauterine insemination for male and non-male factor infertility. *Seminars in Reproductive Medicine*, *32*(4), 306–312. https://doi.org/10.1055/s-0034-1375183

Lee, R. K.-K., Hou, J.-W., Ho, H.-Y., Hwu, Y.-M., Lin, M.-H., Tsai, Y.-C., & Su, J.-T. (2002). Sperm morphology analysis using strict criteria as a prognostic factor in intrauterine insemination. *International Journal of Andrology*, *25*(5), 277–280. https://doi.org/10.1046/j.1365-2605.2002.00355.x

Lenz, S., & Lauritsen, J. G. (1982). Ultrasonically guided percutaneous aspiration of human follicles under local anesthesia: a new method of collecting oocytes for in vitro fertilization. *Fertility and Sterility*, *38*(6), 673–677. https://doi.org/10.1016/s0015-0282(16)46692-6

Lillie, F. R. (1914). Studies of fertilization. VI. The mechanism of fertilization in arbacia. *Journal of Experimental Zoology*, *16*(4), 523–590. https://doi.org/10.1002/jez.1400160404

Martin, K. A., Hall, J. E., Adams, J. M., & Crowley, W. F. (1993). Comparison of exogenous gonadotropins and pulsatile gonadotropin-releasing hormone for induction of ovulation in hypogonadotropic amenorrhea. *The Journal of Clinical Endocrinology and Metabolism*, *77*(1), 125–129. https://doi.org/10.1210/jcem.77.1.8325934

Mauvais-Jarvis, P. (1967). Hypophyseal gonadotropins and control of ovulation. II. Hypothalamic control. Physiology of ovulation. *La Presse Medicale*, *75*(6), 283–287.

Naish, S. J., Perreault, S. D., Foehner, A. L., & Zirkin, B. R. (1987a). DNA synthesis in the fertilizing hamster sperm nucleus: sperm template availability and egg cytoplasmic control. *Biology of Reproduction*, *36*(1), 245–253. https://doi.org/10.1095/biolreprod36.1.245

Naish, S. J., Perreault, S. D., & Zirkin, B. R. (1987b). DNA synthesis following microinjection of heterologous sperm and somatic cell nuclei into hamster oocytes. *Gamete Research*, *18*(2), 109–120. https://doi.org/10.1002/mrd.1120180203

Nandi, A., Bhide, P., Hooper, R., Gudi, A., Shah, A., Khan, K., & Homburg, R. (2017). Intrauterine insemination with gonadotropin stimulation or in vitro fertilization for the treatment of unexplained subfertility: a randomized controlled trial. *Fertility and Sterility*, *107*(6), 1329-1335.e2. https://doi.org/10.1016/j.fertnstert.2017.03.028

Odisho, A. Y., Nangia, A. K., Katz, P. P., & Smith, J. F. (2014). Temporal and geospatial trends in male factor infertility with assisted reproductive technology in the United States from 1999-2010. *Fertility and Sterility*, *102*(2), 469–475. https://doi.org/10.1016/j.fertnstert.2014.05.006

Ozkan, S., Murk, W., & Arici, A. (2008). Endometriosis and infertility: epidemiology and evidence-based treatments. *Annals of the New York Academy of Sciences*, *1127*, 92–100. https://doi.org/10.1196/annals.1434.007

Pincus, G., & Chang, M. C. (1956). The effects of progesterone and related compounds on ovulation and early development in the rabbit. *Acta physiologica Latino Americana*, *3*, 177–183.

Practice Committee of the American Society for Reproductive Medicine. (2015). Role of tubal surgery in the era of assisted reproductive technology: a committee opinion. *Fertility and Sterility*, *103*(6), e37-43. https://doi.org/10.1016/j.fertnstert.2015.03.032

Reindollar, R. H., Regan, M. M., Neumann, P. J., Levine, B.-S., Thornton, K. L., Alper, M. M., & Goldman, M. B. (2010). A randomized clinical trial to evaluate optimal treatment for unexplained infertility: the fast track and standard treatment (FASTT) trial. *Fertility and Sterility*, *94*(3), 888–899. https://doi.org/10.1016/j.fertnstert.2009.04.022

Ricci, G., Perticarari, S., Boscolo, R., Montico, M., Guaschino, S., & Presani, G. (2009). Semen preparation methods and sperm apoptosis: swim-up versus gradient-density centrifugation technique. *Fertility and Sterility*, *91*(2), 632–638. https://doi.org/10.1016/j.fertnstert.2007.11.068

Rogers, P. A. W., Milne, B. J., & Trounson, A. O. (1986). A model to show human uterine receptivity and embryo viability following ovarian stimulation for in vitro fertilization. *Journal of In Vitro Fertilization and Embryo Transfer*, *3*(2), 93–98. https://doi.org/10.1007/BF01139353

Rotterdam ESHRE/ASRM-Sponsored PCOS consensus workshop group. (2004). Revised 2003 consensus on diagnostic criteria and long-term health risks related to polycystic ovary syndrome (PCOS). *Human Reproduction (Oxford, England)*, *19*(1), 41–47. https://doi.org/10.1093/humrep/deh098

Simpson, J. L. (2010). Preimplantation genetic diagnosis at 20 years. *Prenatal Diagnosis*, *30*(7), 682–695. https://doi.org/10.1002/pd.2552

Strandell, A., & Lindhard, A. (2002). Why does hydrosalpinx reduce fertility? The importance of hydrosalpinx fluid. *Human Reproduction (Oxford, England)*, *17*(5), 1141–1145. https://doi.org/10.1093/humrep/17.5.1141

Strandell, A., Lindhard, A., Waldenström, U., Thorburn, J., Janson, P. O., & Hamberger, L. (1999). Hydrosalpinx and IVF outcome: a prospective, randomized multicentre trial in Scandinavia on salpingectomy prior to IVF. *Human Reproduction (Oxford, England)*, *14*(11), 2762–2769. https://doi.org/10.1093/humrep/14.11.2762

Szamatowicz, M. (2016). Assisted reproductive technology in reproductive medicine — possibilities and limitations. *Ginekologia Polska*, *87*(12), 820–823. https://doi.org/10.5603/GP.2016.0095

Templeton, A. A., & Penney, G. C. (1982). The incidence, characteristics, and prognosis of patients whose infertility is unexplained. *Fertility and Sterility*, *37*(2), 175–182. https://doi.org/10.1016/s0015-0282(16)46035-8

Testart, J., & Frydman, R. (1982). Minimum time lapse between luteinizing hormone surge or human chorionic gonadotropin administration and follicular rupture. *Fertility and Sterility*, *37*(1), 50–53. https://doi.org/10.1016/S0015-0282(16)45976-5

Thadani, V. M. (1980). A study of hetero-specific sperm-egg interactions in the rat, mouse, and deer mouse using in vitro fertilization and sperm injection. *The Journal of Experimental Zoology*, *212*(3), 435–453. https://doi.org/10.1002/jez.1402120316

Thatcher, S. S., & DeCherney, A. H. (1989). A critical assessment of the indications for in-vitro fertilization and embryo transfer. *Human Reproduction*, *4*(suppl 1), 11–16. https://doi.org/10.1093/humrep/4.suppl_1.11

Toyoda, Y., & Chang, M. C. (1974). Fertilization of rat eggs in vitro by epididymal spermatozoa and the development of eggs following transfer. *Journal of reproduction and fertility*, *36*(1), 9–22. https://doi.org/10.1530/jrf.0.0360009

Trounson, A. O., Leeton, J. F., Wood, C., Webb, J., & Wood, J. (1981). Pregnancies in humans by fertilization in vitro and embryo transfer in the controlled ovulatory cycle. *Science (New York, N.Y.)*, *212*(4495), 681–682. https://doi.org/10.1126/science.7221557

Uehara, T., & Yanagimachi, R. (1977). Behavior of Nuclei of Testicular, Caput and Cauda Epididymal Spermatozoa Injected into Hamster Eggs. *Biology of Reproduction*, *16*(3), 315–321. https://doi.org/10.1095/biolreprod16.3.315

World Health Organization. (2001). Laboratory manual of the WHO for the examination of human semen and sperm-cervical mucus interaction. *Annali Dell'Istituto Superiore Di Sanita*, *37*(1), I–XII, 1–123.

Zanartu, J., Rosner, J. M., Guiloff, E., Ibarra-Polo, A. A., Croxatto, H. D., Croxatto, H. B., Aguilera, E., Coy, D. H., & Schally, A. v. (1975). Attempts to programme ovulation with exogenous oestrogens and LH-RH analogue. *BMJ*, *2*(5970), 527–529. https://doi.org/10.1136/bmj.2.5970.527

Zegers-Hochschild, F., Adamson, G. D., Dyer, S., Racowsky, C., de Mouzon, J., Sokol, R., Rienzi, L., Sunde, A., Schmidt, L., Cooke, I. D., Simpson, J. L., & van der Poel, S. (2017). The International Glossary on Infertility and Fertility Care, 2017. *Fertility and Sterility*, *108*(3), 393–406. https://doi.org/10.1016/j.fertnstert.2017.06.005

Chapter 13

Analysis of Fertilization

Elif Önder, MD*
Department of Medicine, Pamukkale University, Denizli, Turkiye

Abstract

Fertilization is a complex molecular cellular process in which gametes come together to form a new organism (Bing & Ouellette, 2009). Reproduction consists of steps that begin with postcoital sperm entry into the female reproductive system, followed by sperm capacitation and acrosome reaction, activation of the oocyte, attachment to the zona pellucida (ZP) and penetration. Disruption of the synchronization between these events, which are regulated by various substances secreted by the oviduct, can cause infertility (Mahutte & Arici, 2003). In vitro fertilization (IVF) is a technical process in which oocytes are fertilized outside the body and the resulting embryos are grown in the laboratory and transferred to the woman's uterus (Bing & Ouellette, 2009). Implantation rates of embryos resulting from IVF remain low at ~30 per cent. Transferring multiple embryos increases the pregnancy rate, but the risk of multiple pregnancy increases too and causes maternal and neonatal health problems. Therefore, transfer of a single healthy embryo avoids these problems (Kirkegaard et al., 2012). Given this success, the mechanisms of fertilization appear to be understood, but the precise details of many steps remain to be discovered (Siu et al., 2021). Here, we aim to explain what fertilization is, its stages, how to evaluate fertilization after IVF, and the factors that cause fertilization failure.

Key Words: Fertilization, IVF, Capacitation, Acrosome reaction, Fertilization failure, Pronucleus (PN)

---

* Corresponding Author's E-mail: elfndr16@gmail.com

In: Holistic Approach to Assisted Reproductive Technology
Editor: Kenan Demir and Rümeysa Yılmaz Göç
ISBN: 979-8-89113-017-3
© 2023 Nova Science Publishers, Inc.

Introduction

Approximately 15% of couples worldwide are affected by infertility, and in one third of these, the etiology is unknown. Although rapid advances in assisted reproductive technology have offered new opportunities to infertile couples, the epigenetic side effects they will face in the future are not known for certain. In addition, only 40% of couples can have a child despite two years of prolonged treatment. The safety and efficacy of contraceptives used to protect against pregnancy are also important, and many women find it difficult to use contraception for a long time due to the many side effects. Male contraceptive methods are limited. Therefore, a better understanding of the mechanism of fertilization and the molecules involved will lead to rapid progress in both assisted reproductive technologies and contraception (Siu et al., 2021). Since single embryo transfer is important for the health of both mother and child, single embryo transfer is the priority of assisted reproductive treatment, regardless of the stage of embryo development and the day of transfer that is accepted in any clinic (Gardner & Balaban, 2016). Embryo selection reduces the couple's time to conception, the number of transfers the patient has to undergo, and consequently the patient's financial and emotional suffering. Each transfer and subsequent pregnancy test affect the patient's psychology of infertility. 17% of IVF treatment is abandoned for this reason (Gardner et al., 2015). At certain times, there is a close relationship between the morphological appearance of the embryo and its stage of development and competence (Kirkegaard et al., 2012). Fertilization in mammals contains multiple numerous sequential stages, including capacitation, acrosome and zona pellucida reaction, sperm-egg attachment, and membrane fusion. Given the success of IVF, the fertilization mechanisms appear to be understood, but the precise details of many steps remain to be discovered (Siu et al., 2021). The elucidation of the molecular mechanisms of fertilization has attracted the interest of many researchers. Several molecules have been determined that play an important role in every phase of the very interesting step of fertilization (oocyte sperm attraction, sperm maturation, sperm and oocyte fusion, fusion of two gamete pronuclei leading to zygote formation). A better understanding of the molecular mechanisms of cellular interaction between sperm and oocyte will help us better understand the causes of infertility due to fertilization defects and will support the development of new contraceptive methods (Georgadaki et al., 2016).

Fertilization

Fertilization is a molecular process by which the gamete cells, oocytes, and sperm unite, fuse, and intermingle their chromosomes to form a new individual. The zygote, a diploid cell, is the first human form. Millions of sperm are released into the vagina with sexual intercourse. Some of these die in the vagina, which is an acidic environment, while others remain viable for 3-5 days in the mucosa of the female genital tract. Although a single live sperm is sufficient for fertilization, many sperm can remain alive in the fluids that protect them. Sperm then travel (in the mucus that keeps them alive) first into the uterus and then into the fallopian tubes. During this journey, the number of viable sperm decreases. contractions in the uterus allow the sperm to reach the egg, and fertilization occurs in the ampulla of the oviduct (Georgadaki et al., 2016). The sperm that encounter the egg in the ampulla must then overcome some physical and biochemical barriers. Activated by capacitation and acrosome reaction, the sperm binds to the egg and passes through the cumulus oophorous and zona pellucida to the perivitelline space. Here it encounters the oolemma and the membranes of these two cells start to fuse. The nucleus of sperm and organelles then passes into the egg and is incorporated into the oocyte cytoplasm (Siu et al., 2021). If the oocyte is not fertilized here, it migrates into the uterus, degenerates, and is absorbed within 24 hours. For fertilization, sperm activation and oocyte maturation are required. However, for egg and sperm fusion, both the egg and the cytoplasm must undergo various metabolic and biochemical changes (Georgadaki et al., 2016). IVF is a process that starts with ovarian stimulation, followed by oocyte retrieval, fertilization, incubation, and transfer of the embryos into the uterus. Fertilization of eggs occurs in two ways in this process. Sperm and egg are cultured together or intracytoplasmic sperm injection is performed (Van Voorhis, 2007).

Sperm

Although oogenesis is completed before birth, spermatogenesis begins at puberty and is a continuous process. In order for spermatogenesis, which lasts 74 days in humans, to be continuous, there must be more than one spermatogenesis process at the same time. For the duration of spermatogenesis, mitosis results in gene amplification, meiosis results in genome reduction, and maturation takes place. At this stage, the sperm is not motile and is not suitable for fertilization. The sperm continues to mature in two places outside the testes. Firstly, it undergoes post-translational modification as it passes through the epididymis and enters the maturation process. Second, it undergoes capacitation in the female genital tract and prepares for the acrosomal reaction (Siu et al., 2021).

Epididymal Maturation

The exchange of substances between the sperm and the epididymal epithelium occurs directly through interaction with epithelial cells, by exosome-like vesicles secreted from epithelial cells, or through the interaction of soluble proteins in the epididymal fluid. The purpose of this exchange is to change the composition and lipid balance of the membrane of sperm by redistributing sperm proteins. These events occur during the passage of the sperm through the epididymal compartments, the caput-corpus-cauda. Since fertilization does not occur immediately, the fertilization capacity of sperm is maintained by decapacitation factors active in the epididymis. Epididymal plasma and sperm comprise only 5% of semen, while the rest of semen is composed of fluid from the prostate and seminal vesicles, which protects the sperm and prevents premature maturation (Cornwall, 2009; Siu et al., 2021; Zalazar et al., 2020).

Sperm Capacitation

Sperm capacitation or activation is the stage of sperm maturation. It occurs in the female genitalia and prepares the sperm for the acrosome reaction. Proteolytic enzymes are important in capacitation, and no morphological changes are observed in the sperm. In mammals, sperm in the ejaculate are motile but have little ability to fertilize the oocyte. during capacitation, decapacitation factors are removed from the sperm plasma membrane. Energy substrates, electrolytes, and proteins such as albumin or seminal plasma protein initiate the removal of decapacitation factors. This increases sperm membrane fluidity and increases sperm permeability to calcium, chloride, and bicarbonate ions. The balance of intracellular ions, intracellular pH, and membrane potential regulate sperm motility. Ca++ is the most important ion for this function and for this secondary messenger that regulate sperm motility. This final state of active sperm is known as hyperactivation and is a high-energy phase in which strong flagellar movement is seen. Acrosome reaction, sperm hyperactivation, and protein phosphorylation are used to assess capacitation in vitro. Incubation in media, including bicarbonate ions, calcium, and serum albumin, can induce capacitation in vitro (Gangwar & Atreja, 2015; Georgadaki et al., 2016).

Acrosome Reaction

The acrosome, located in the anterior part of the sperm, is a secretory vesicle and originates from the Golgi apparatus of the spermatid. The acrosome reaction is the exocytosis of the acrosome contents as a result of the fusion of the plasma membrane with the outer membrane of the acrosome and is driven by SNARE complexes. So, the acrosome reaction changes the morphology of the sperm. The acrosome reaction time is critical and only spermatozoa that undergo this reaction are capable of fertilization. Sperm that undergo the acrosome reaction early have low fertilization success in vitro. Only some of the sperm can undergo a spontaneous acrosome reaction. At the same time, Inoue et al. showed that mouse spermatozoa obtained by recovering acrosome-reacting spermatozoa in the perivitelline space can fertilize other eggs.

Although some studies have argued that the acrosome reaction begins when the sperm specifically contacts the ZP3 protein, others have shown in mouse experiments that most mouse spermatozoa capable of fertilization undergo an acrosome reaction before contact with the ZP of the oocyte. The acrosome and the acrosome reaction are important for fertilization because low fertilization rates are observed after intracytoplasmic sperm injection with sperm without acrosomes (Inoue et al., 2011; Nakanishi et al., 2001; Okabe, 2018; Siu et al., 2021).

ZP Penetration

ZP is a glycoprotein and a physical barrier between the oocyte membrane and granulosa cells, synthesized in the primary follicle stage. Consisting of 4 glycoproteins, hZP1, hZP3, and hZP4 have been shown to induce sperm binding and the acrosome reaction, which has gained capacitation ability. It also prevents polyspermy during fertilization (Siu et al., 2021).

Sperm/oocyte Fusion

After attachment to the ZP, the sperm pass into the perivitelline space and approach the oolemma. Following the acrosome reaction, the inner acrosomal membrane of the sperm is exposed, and this inner part contacts the oocyte membrane. Electron microscopy has shown that the outermost membrane of human oocytes is variably covered with microvilli, either evenly and abundantly, in sparse patches, or absent. The microvilli of the oolemma surround the sperm and are involved in the fusion of sperm and oocytes. Then, through a multimolecular process, the sperm membrane adheres to the oocyte membrane and fusion takes place. The adhesion is mediated by pairs of receptor ligands. A conformational change in a fusion peptide is then initiated, resulting in the opening and expansion of a fusion pore that enters the opposite gamete bilayer. Sperm-specific protein IZUMO-1 is present in both the outer and inner acrosomal membranes. During the acrosome reaction, IZUMO-1 was observed to translocate towards the plasma membrane, accumulating in high density throughout the head, especially in the equatorial segment.

During fusion, IZUMO-1 in the equatorial region diffused into the oolemma, whereas IZUMO-1 in the inner acrosomal membrane maintained its localization. Fertilization cannot be achieved by a single fusion. Fertilization involves an initial sperm-egg fusion followed by a phagocytosis step. Ingestion of the inner acrosomal membrane takes place in the second step. Two different fusion processes are observed during fertilization in mammals. The first process involves the IZUMO1-JUNO system, as indicated by the IZUMO-1 membrane movement. The CRISPR-Cas9 system, which has revolutionized gene disruption experiments, also plays a role in oocyte sperm fusion. At the same time, CD9, which is an integrin-associated protein in the oocyte, is essential for sperm–egg interactions (Georgadaki et al., 2016; Okabe, 2018; Siu et al., 2021; Swain & Pool, 2008).

Oocyte Activation

Oocyte activation is a series of morphological and biochemical changes in the oocyte cell after sperm-oocyte fusion. Oocyte activation is an enigmatic process that involves two main events: first, zona pellucida reactions to prevent polyspermy and second, recovery from MII arrest and completion of the second meiotic division. In addition to these mechanical changes, oocytes undergo changes in protein synthesis necessary for the next fertilization events. One of the first indicators of oocyte activation is the increase in intracellular Ca++ and its rapid and repetitive oscillations, following sperm oocyte fusion. Ca++ starts to release a few minutes after gamete fusion and ends during PN formation. The increase, release, frequency, and duration of Ca++ ion have dramatic effects on both fertilization and embryo development (Marangos et al., 2003; Swain & Pool, 2008).

Cortical and Zona Reaction

When oocyte and sperm meet, sperm movement stops immediately. The fusion of oocyte and sperm causes elongation of the microvillus and polymerization of actin. Sperm are attracted to the oocyte by the elongation and fusion of microvillus in the oocyte. As a result, the sperm is incorporated into the oocyte with its nucleus and all organelles. The cytoplasm swells to form a colliculus that is called the cone of fertilization. Seconds after fertilization, the oocyte is depolarized by a high influx of Na^+ ions. It takes an average of one minute for the oocyte to depolarize due to K^+ ion leakage. This is rapid blockage of the polyspermy. another process that prevents polyspermy is the cortical reaction. The fast blockage of polyspermy rapidly inhibits additional sperm attachment to the oocyte. At the same time, the cortical reaction, which creates a permanent barrier against sperm entry, causes slow polyspermy blockage as shown in many animals. The cortical reaction is generated by a Ca++ wave on the surface of the oocyte. In this process, secretory vesicles under the plasma membrane of the oocyte fuse with the plasma membrane of the oocyte. As a result, the contents of the cortical granules are released into the extracellular matrix, altering its contents and preventing the passage of sperm into the oocyte. The cortical granules contain hydrolytic enzymes such as proteases that degrade proteins in the perivitelline space, peroxidases that stiffen the vitelline envelope, and glycosaminoglycans that draw water into the perivitelline space to form the hyaline layer. Ca++ ions from the cortical smooth endoplasmic reticulum are responsible for the breakdown of cortical granules. The cortical reaction modifies the zona pellucida, leading to polysperm block in mammals. Several enzymes released from cortical granules cause digestion of the glycoproteins ZP2 and ZP3, which are sperm receptors, preventing further attachment of spermatozoa (Georgadaki et al., 2016).

Completion of Meiosis II

Another step in oocyte activation is the completion of the second meiotic division. To complete meiosis, the oocyte in the MII stage must start dividing again, sister chromatids must separate, and the second polar body (PB) must be extruded. Ca^{2+} ions are involved in the completion of the second meiotic division. Improper completion of these processes, i.e., inappropriate segregation, leads to IVF failures, resulting in the formation of 3PN or 1PN zygotes (Swain & Pool, 2008).

Assessing Fertilization and Zygotes (Day 1)

At the time of oocyte activation, spermatozoa also undergo biochemical remodeling due to endogenous substances within the cytoplasm of oocytes. This process leads to the reorganization and even segregation of sperm components while paternal chromatin is redesigned. The first sperm processing is the decondensation of the sperm heads, which releases the sperm nucleus contents into the oolemma. Before PN formation, decondensation occurs in three main stages. The first is the removal of unpaired sperm nuclear membranes, the second is disassembly of the underlying structural lamina and the last decondensation of chromatin. The oocyte processes the centrosome brought by the sperm and provides essential proteins such as gamma tubulin to aid in the formation of the sperm aster. And sperm aster is important for the next organization of the spindle apparatus required for PN migration. Time-lapse imaging of oocytes has shown that these events occur before the second polar body is extruded. Little is known about the initial events of the oocyte-controlled sperm process. However, more information about the remodeling of sperm chromatin is known. In mammals, spermatozoa chromatin of is highly compact because it is organized by protamines and is transcriptionally inactive. Decondensation of paternal chromatin is facilitated by oocyte-derived factors by reducing protamine disulfide bonds. Through reversible phosphorylation, sperm chromatin is subsequently recondensed as protamines are displaced by maternally derived histones present in the oolemma. The maturation state of oocytes influences the processing of the sperm components and the remodeling of chromatin. The concentration of oocyte glutathione increases with maturation and is required for the formation of male pronuclei and decondensation of the sperm. Premature sperm chromatin condensation is a common cause of failure of fertilization in human assisted reproductive technology (ART) and is related to oocyte maturation. Ca^{2+} is involved in the exchange of sperm protamines with histones in the oocyte, and Ca^{2+} release is a characteristic of oocyte maturity. Even if the first steps of fertilization are bypassed by the intracytoplasmic sperm injection (ICSI) process, the lack of proteins such as histones and glutathione in the oocyte can lead to incorrect processing of sperm components and failure of fertilization (Swain & Pool, 2008).

PN Formation

The formation of female and male PN that indicates the completion of mammalian fertilization. The formation of PN formation contains the rebuilding of the nuclear envelope around the relevant genetic material from the oocyte and sperm. This process starts with membrane vesicles containing lamina receptors, continues with the addition of nuclear pore complexes to the nuclear envelope (NE), and finally culminates in the passage of these lamins through these pores to form the nuclear lamina skeleton. Time-lapse cinematography has shown that the male PN forms either earlier or almost simultaneously with the female PN. While the male PN begins to form in the center, the female PN begins to form adjacent to the second polar body. The female PN is then pulled to the side of the male PN by microtubules via male centrosomes. The male PN then becomes slightly larger than the female PN. The nuclear envelope consists of an inner and outer membrane covering a filamentous protein network known as nuclear lamins, and its formation is closely related to chromatin interaction. In mammals, the nuclear envelope contains all three types of lamins, A, B, and C, and the integrity of the nuclear envelope is maintained by the phosphorylation and dephosphorylation of these lamins. The nuclear envelope maintains its integrity when nuclear lamins are hypophosphorylated. Enzymes such as MAPK, PKC, CDK 1 kinase, and PP1 have been found to affect the integrity of the nuclear envelope in various animal studies. Therefore, these enzymes may affect the reassembly of the nuclear envelope during PN formation. In addition to multiple PN formation as a result of polyspermy penetration, evaluation of abnormal fertilization indicates that PN cannot form, migrate, or grow. The failure of PN formation may result from a defect in chromatin segregation during meiotic division and dysregulation of signalling pathways in lamin assembly. PN arrest may result from a defect in the composition of the nuclear envelope such as nuclear pore complexes. Oocyte-derived protein deficiency or protein deficiency such as soluble lamin B also alters PN formation. Oocyte maturation delayed MI human oocytes, and it was found that they were deficient in some factors involved in PN formation, compared to MII oocytes. Again, even if PN occurs, the formation of defective sperm aster formation as a result of improper processing in the oocyte may affect PN migration and syngamy (Collas et al., 1997; Moos et al., 1995; Payne et al., 1997).

A fertilized oocyte should be spherical in shape, with two pronuclei of equal size and with different membranes. In the central position of the oocyte and two polar bodies. Pronuclei should have an equal number and size of nucleolar precursor bodies (NPB) in the region where the membranes are juxtaposed. Both PN size and localization are used to assess fertilization. Pronuclei that are widely separated from each other, micronuclei and widely different sizes are considered atypical. Pronuclear scoring assesses both the number, size, and localization of pronuclei and the number and position of NPBs. Ideally, each pronucleus should have 5-7 NPB and a similar distribution. The number and appearance of pronuclei, the presence of a cytoplasmic halo, and polarization are used as morphological parameters in zygote scoring. Fertilization is easy to assess because a fertilized oocyte should have two polar bodies and two pronuclei. The pronucleus formation time is about 1 hour later in IVF, compared to ICSI. Fertilization is assessed 16-18 hours after insemination, so this may not always be the best time. Another confusing situation is that polar bodies can sometimes disintegrate and disperse before fertilization check. In fertilization, the pronuclei are expected to be of equal number and equal size, centrally located, and close to each other. Scott et al. scored fertilization 17-18 hours after insemination according to the number and location of the PN and NPB morphology. Fertilized oocytes with an equal number of NPBs lined up at the junction of the PN were called Z1, those with equal numbers of diffuse NPBs were called Z2, those with unequal numbers or irregular localization were called Z3, and those with very unequal PN or PN that were not localized in a central position within the oocyte were called Z4. Consequently, it was

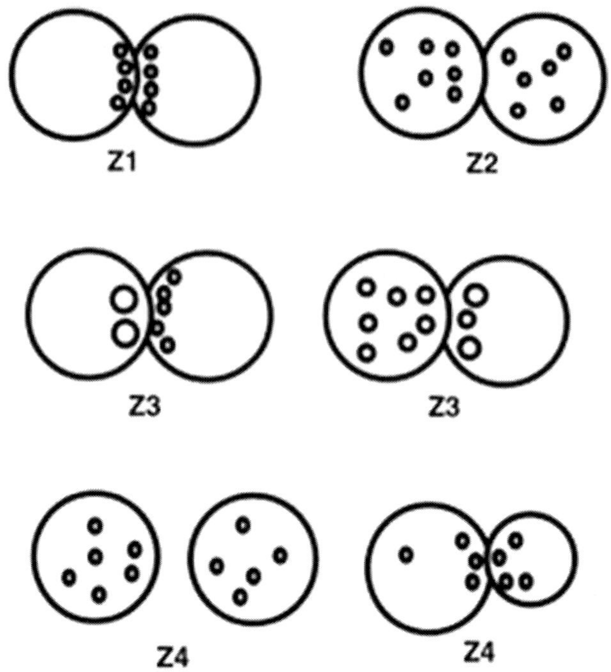

Figure 13.1 NPB numbers and sequences in pronuclei according to the Z scoring system (Scott et al., 2000).

Table 13.1 ALPHA/ESHRE consensus pronucleus classification (Medicine & Embryology, 2011)

Category	*Rating*	*Description*
1	Symmetrical	Equivalent to Z1and Z2
2	Non-Symmetrical	Other arrangements, including peripherally sited pronuclei
3	Abnormal	Pronuclei with 0 or 1 NPB

shown that embryos obtained from zygotes with Z1 and Z2 scores formed blastocysts at a higher rate and that implantation and pregnancy rates were higher (Medicine & Embryology, 2011; Scott et al., 2000) (Figure 13.1).

ALPHA and ESHRE created a simple assessment scheme for pro-nuclear scoring (Table 13.1). Consequently, as described by Scott and Smith, symmetric zygotes equivalent to Z1 and Z2 were defined as category 1, all other non-symmetric zygotes with pronuclear appearance as category 2, and abnormal zygotes containing 0 or 1 NPB in the pronucleus were defined as category 3 (Figure 13.2, Figure 13.3, Figure 13.4, Figure 13.5).

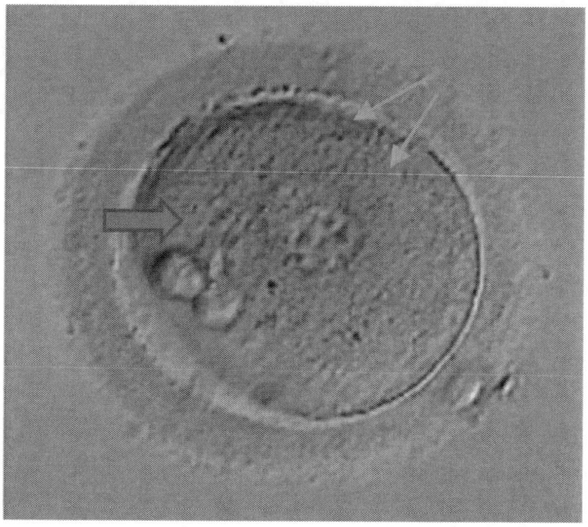

Figure 13.2 Fertilized oocyte with 2 pronuclei and 2 polar bodies (blue arrow PB, red arrow PN) (Pamukkale University IVF center archive, 2022) (Author's own archive).

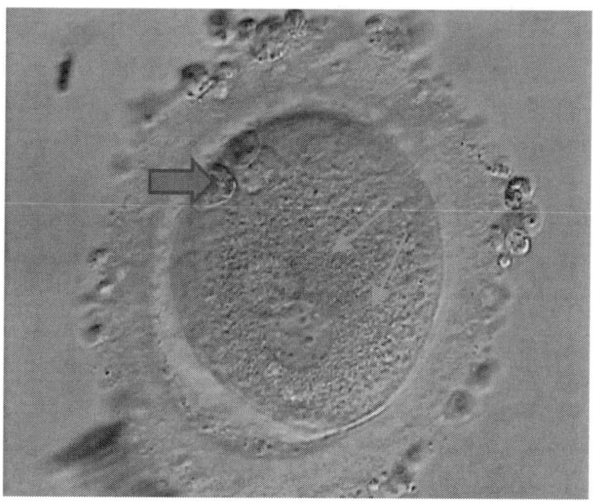

Figure 13.3 Fertilized oocyte with 2 pronuclei of different sizes and 2 polar bodies (blue arrow PB, red arrow PN) (Pamukkale University IVF center archive, 2022) (Author's own archive).

Failure of Fertilization

60-70% of oocytes retrieved with ART fertilize successfully. To be called failed fertilization, all available oocytes must fail to fertilize. In this case, emergency ICSI is performed and it is more effective to perform ICSI in the next ART cycle. Together, this leads to both emotional and financial distress for the patient. The actual incidence of the number of failed fertilizations is

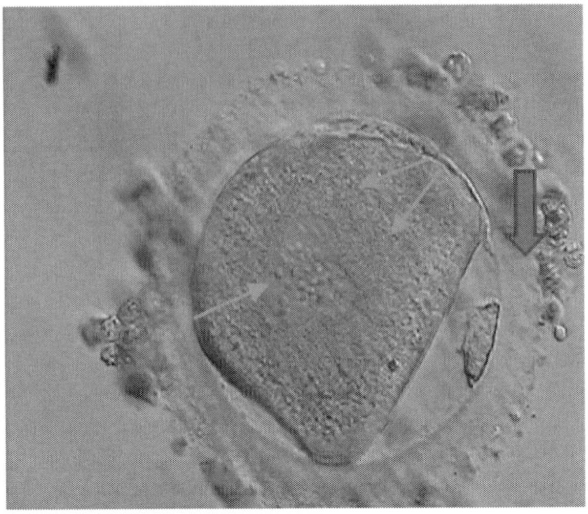

Figure 13.4 Fertilized oocyte with 3 pronuclei, 1 polar body (blue arrow PB, red arrow PN) (Pamukkale University IVF center archive, 2022) (Author's own archive).

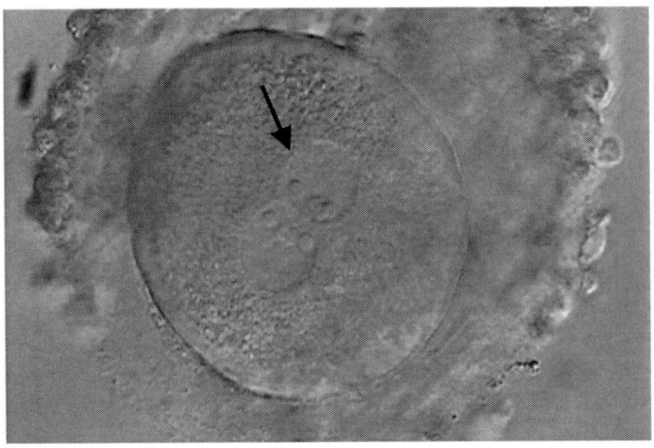

Figure 13.5 2 Pronuclei with equal number and size of nucleolar precursor bodies (black arrow NPB) (Pamukkale University IVF center archive, 2022) (Author's own archive).

between 5% and 10% in most in vitro fertilization programs and depends only on the number of available oocytes. If a couple experiences failure in the first IVF cycle, the risk is 30% in other cycles (Figure 13.6).

Causes of Failed Fertilization in In Vitro Fertilization

In general, the causes of fertilization failure may be due to defective or insufficient oocytes, defective or insufficient spermatozoa, or a lack of substances

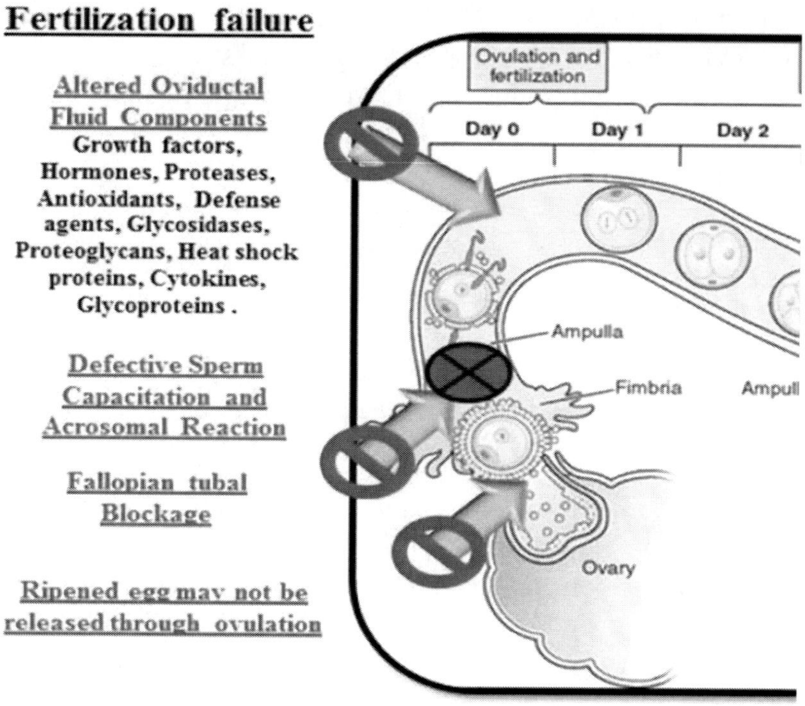

Figure 13.6 Factors affecting fertilization in humans (Budhwar et al., 2017).

that should be in the environment or toxic substances. The fact that fertilization is achieved by reincubation of unfertilized oocytes with donor spermatozoa supports this idea. Most cases of failed fertilization in IVF are due to a defect in the bonding surface between the sperm and oocyte, which may involve a problem in the attachment or fusion of the sperm to the zona pellucida. Although most of the causes of fertilization failure in IVF seem to be male factors, oocyte deficiencies and environmental factors also affect this process.

Causes of Failed Fertilization with Intracytoplasmic Sperm Injection

As with IVF, the fertilization rate with ICSI is 60-70%, but the total fertilization failure rate is 3%. This is remarkable in the types of patients that typically undergo ICSI, such as those with previous fertilization failure and/or severe oligo/astheno/teratospermia. Fertilization failure with ICSI is closely related to the number and maturation of existing oocytes, indicating that most causes of fertilization failure have been overcome. Clearly, in patients who undergo ICSI, several critical steps of normal fertilization are bypassed, namely the interactions between the zona pellucida and the sperm. Therefore, the outcome of ICSI is independent of typical sperm analysis and strict semen analysis. The most important cause of failure of fertilization in oocytes that 80% contain sperm after ICSI is inadequate activation of oocytes. Other causes of fertilization failure in oocytes subjected to ICSI are pronucleus fusion defects and metaphase arrest during the first mitotic division of the embryo. 50% of the cases of fertilization failure in oocytes subjected to ICSI have DNA fragmentation damage (Budhwar et al., 2017; Mahutte & Arici, 2003; Marcello et al., 2013; Swain & Pool, 2008).

Conclusion

Fertilization is a highly complex process in which male and female gamete cells fuse to form a new diploid cell, called the zygote. This process begins with sperm capacitation and an acrosomal reaction, followed by penetration and fusion of the zona pellucida. Biochemical and molecular rearrangements occur in the spermatozoa as the sperm pass into the oolemma. The oocyte is activated by sperm entry and undergoes cortical and zona reactions to prevent polyspermy. When fertilization occurs, two pronuclei are formed in the central region and two polar bodies in the perivitelline space. Any disruption or inadequacy at these stages results in fertilization failure. Because of many of these stages are bypassed by assisted reproductive techniques, many of the problems of fertilization failure are solved. However, failure of fertilization still affects many couples, causing both emotional and financial distress. Therefore, further studies to improve the quality of the environment in which the egg is incubated, especially to improve the quality of oocytes, and to investigate single cell and gene-based treatment solutions will be a hope for many patients.

References

Bing, Y., & Ouellette, R. J. (2009). Fertilization in vitro. *Methods Mol Biol*, *550*, 251-266. https://doi.org/10.1007/978-1-60327-009-0_16

Budhwar, S., Singh, V., Verma, P., & Singh, K. (2017). Fertilization failure and gamete health: Is there a link? *Front Biosci (Schol Ed)*, *9*(3), 395-419. https://doi.org/10.2741/s494

Collas, P., Thompson, L., Fields, A. P., Poccia, D. L., & Courvalin, J. C. (1997). Protein kinase C-mediated interphase lamin B phosphorylation and solubilization. *J Biol Chem*, *272*(34), 21274-21280. https://doi.org/10.1074/jbc.272.34.21274

Cornwall, G. A. (2009). New insights into epididymal biology and function. *Hum Reprod Update*, *15*(2), 213-227. https://doi.org/10.1093/humupd/dmn055
Gangwar, D. K., & Atreja, S. K. (2015). Signalling Events and Associated Pathways Related to the Mammalian Sperm Capacitation. *Reprod Domest Anim*, *50*(5), 705-711. https://doi.org/10.1111/rda.12541
Gardner, D. K., & Balaban, B. (2016). Assessment of human embryo development using morphological criteria in an era of time-lapse, algorithms and 'OMICS': is looking good still important? *Molecular Human Reproduction*, *22*(10), 704-718. https://doi.org/10.1093/molehr/gaw057 %J Molecular Human Reproduction
Gardner, D. K., Meseguer, M., Rubio, C., & Treff, N. R. (2015). Diagnosis of human preimplantation embryo viability. *Human Reproduction Update*, *21*(6), 727-747. https://doi.org/10.1093/humupd/dmu064 %J Human Reproduction Update
Georgadaki, K., Khoury, N., Spandidos, D. A., & Zoumpourlis, V. (2016). The molecular basis of fertilization (Review). *Int J Mol Med*, *38*(4), 979-986. https://doi.org/10.3892/ijmm.2016.2723
Inoue, N., Satouh, Y., Ikawa, M., Okabe, M., & Yanagimachi, R. (2011). Acrosome-reacted mouse spermatozoa recovered from the perivitelline space can fertilize other eggs. *Proc Natl Acad Sci U S A*, *108*(50), 20008-20011. https://doi.org/10.1073/pnas.1116965108
Kirkegaard, K., Agerholm, I. E., & Ingerslev, H. J. (2012). Time-lapse monitoring as a tool for clinical embryo assessment. *Human Reproduction*, *27*(5), 1277-1285. https://doi.org/10.1093/humrep/des079%J Human Reproduction
Mahutte, N. G., & Arici, A. (2003). Failed fertilization: is it predictable? *Curr Opin Obstet Gynecol*, *15*(3), 211-218. https://doi.org/10.1097/00001703-200306000-00001
Marangos, P., FitzHarris, G., & Carroll, J. (2003). Ca2+ oscillations at fertilization in mammals are regulated by the formation of pronuclei. *Development*, *130*(7), 1461-1472. https://doi.org/10.1242/dev.00340
Marcello, M. R., Singaravelu, G., & Singson, A. (2013). Fertilization. *Adv Exp Med Biol*, *757*, 321-350. https://doi.org/10.1007/978-1-4614-4015-4_11
Medicine, A. S. i. R., & Embryology, E. S. I. G. o. (2011). The Istanbul consensus workshop on embryo assessment: proceedings of an expert meeting†. *Human Reproduction*, *26*(6), 1270-1283. https://doi.org/10.1093/humrep/der037%J Human Reproduction
Moos, J., Visconti, P. E., Moore, G. D., Schultz, R. M., & Kopf, G. S. (1995). Potential role of mitogen-activated protein kinase in pronuclear envelope assembly and disassembly following fertilization of mouse eggs. *Biol Reprod*, *53*(3), 692-699. https://doi.org/10.1095/biolreprod53.3.692
Nakanishi, T., Ikawa, M., Yamada, S., Toshimori, K., & Okabe, M. (2001). Alkalinization of acrosome measured by GFP as a pH indicator and its relation to sperm capacitation. *Dev Biol*, *237*(1), 222-231. https://doi.org/10.1006/dbio.2001.0353
Okabe, M. (2018). Sperm-egg interaction and fertilization: past, present, and future. *Biol Reprod*, *99*(1), 134-146. https://doi.org/10.1093/biolre/ioy028
Payne, D., Flaherty, S. P., Barry, M. F., & Matthews, C. D. (1997). Preliminary observations on polar body extrusion and pronuclear formation in human

oocytes using time-lapse video cinematography. *Hum Reprod*, *12*(3), 532-541. https://doi.org/10.1093/humrep/12.3.532

Scott, L., Alvero, R., Leondires, M., & Miller, B. (2000). The morphology of human pronuclear embryos is positively related to blastocyst development and implantation*. *Human Reproduction*, *15*(11), 2394-2403. https://doi.org/10.1093/humrep/15.11.2394 %J Human Reproduction

Siu, K. K., Serrão, V. H. B., Ziyyat, A., & Lee, J. E. (2021). The cell biology of fertilization: Gamete attachment and fusion. *Journal of Cell Biology*, *220*(10). https://doi.org/10.1083/jcb.202102146

Swain, J. E., & Pool, T. B. (2008). ART failure: oocyte contributions to unsuccessful fertilization. *Human Reproduction Update*, *14*(5), 431-446. https://doi.org/10.1093/humupd/dmn025 %J Human Reproduction Update

Van Voorhis, B. J. (2007). In Vitro Fertilization. *356*(4), 379-386. https://doi.org/10.1056/NEJMcp065743

Zalazar, L., Stival, C., Nicolli, A. R., De Blas, G. A., Krapf, D., & Cesari, A. (2020). Male Decapacitation Factor SPINK3 Blocks Membrane Hyperpolarization and Calcium Entry in Mouse Sperm. *Front Cell Dev Biol*, *8*, 575126. https://doi.org/10.3389/fcell.2020.575126

Chapter 14

Micromanipulation Techniques in ART

Suleyman Erol, MD*
IVF Clinic, Etlik Zubeyde Hanim Women's Health Research Hospital, Ankara, Turkiye

Abstract

The contribution of micromanipulation techniques to the success of IVF applications is undeniable. The manipulation of sperm, oocytes and embryos is the mainstay of infertility treatment today. This journey, which started with the partial zona dissection technique, has undoubtedly reached advanced levels. These methods, which are based on cloning studies, will go further with technology development. In this section, micromanipulation techniques used before and recently in clinical embryology laboratories are mentioned. Our aim in this section is to introduce micromanipulation techniques.

Key Words: Micromanipulation, in vitro fertilization, Artificial reproductive techniques

Introduction

Since the birth of the first baby in 1978 (Dow, 2019), assisted reproductive techniques (ART) have advanced considerably. Today, the pregnancy rate of in vitro fertilization (IVF) treatment in women under the age of 35 is around 50%. Louise Brown was born (Steptoe & Edwards, 1978) as the first IVF baby in England in 1978 as a result of the knowledge we gained about the human oocyte and its fertilization in the 1960s. In this birth, physicians retrieved

* Corresponding Author's Email: drsuleymanerol@gmail.com

In: Holistic Approach to Assisted Reproductive Technology
Editor: Kenan Demir and Rümeysa Yılmaz Göç
ISBN: 979-8-89113-017-3
© 2023 Nova Science Publishers, Inc.

laparoscopically the oocyte formed during the mother's natural menstrual cycle and transferred the 8-cell embryo to the uterus after in vitro fertilization (Eskew & Jungheim, 2017). Twenty years later, thanks to the work of Refik Çapanoğlu and his colleagues, the first IVF baby in Turkey named Ece Çokar was born at Ege University. During the first 10 years of IVF treatment, the cumulus-oocyte complex was treated with sufficient motile sperm. When the husband was subfertile, great limitations remained in solving infertility problems. With the application of micromanipulation techniques, this situation has greatly improved (Laufer & Simon, 1992).

Partial Zona Dissection (PZD)

Partial zona dissection (PZD) is the process of opening the zona pellucida with mechanical force. Fertilization rates are high when conventional IVF is performed with semen with normal sperm parameters. However, the fertilization rate is low in patients with male factor. The aim of the PZD procedure is to create an artificial opening in the zona pellucida and to increase the success of fertilization in abnormal semen. During the procedure, sucrose is used to shrink the oocyte and reduce the risk of mechanical damage due to the microneedle. The oocyte is held by a pipette, the position of the pipette is at '9 o'clock. The polar body, or in other words, the largest area of the perivitelline space should come to the "12 o'clock" position. Openings are created in the pellucida zone using a microneedle (Malter & Cohen, 1989). However, its success is limited, especially in cases accompanied by teratozoospermia (Cohen et al., 1991).

As research on the PZD technique progressed, a consensus emerged that it was not superior to conventional IVF. These have resulted in skepticism about the clinical usefulness of PZD. Later, scientists performed the acrosome reaction by stimulating the spermatozoa and these spermatozoa were used after PZD. Nevertheless, it was seen that the fertilization rates did not increase significantly increase (Tarín, 1995). Today, the PZD technique has been abandoned in clinical practice.

Subzonal Insemination (SUZI)

The basics and purpose of the subzonal insemination technique (SUZI) are similar to those of the PZD technique. The procedure is completed by microinjection of prepared sperm into the perivitelline space to assist in fertilization in couples with severe male infertility (Ng et al., 1988). In the past, it was a promising method for couples who had previously failed conventional

IVF due to severe male infertility (Svalander et al., 1994). As with the PZD technique, the SUZI technique was not clinically superior to conventional IVF. Despite spermatozoa stimulation, the expected success was not achieved. Tarin reported that SUZI was superior to PZD in his meta-analysis. However, intracytoplasmic sperm injection (ICSI) was superior to both (Tarín, 1995).

Intracytoplasmic Sperm Injection (ICSI)

Intracytoplasmic sperm injection (ICSI) is widely used today because it provides fertilization with one sperm per oocyte and increases success in severe male infertility. The classical ICSI technique became the gold standard method after Palermo et al. achieved the first live birth in 1992 (Palermo et al., 1992). ICSI is basically a two-step procedure consisting of immobilization of spermatozoa and the latter placing them directly into the ooplasm by microinjection. The sperm immobilization process has two beneficial effects. First, theoretically motile sperm could damage the cytoskeleton of the oocyte. The second is that the sperm-related oocyte activation factor (Dozortsev et al., 1997), which passes into the oocyte by increasing the permeability of the spermatozoon membrane, increases the fertilization rate (Van Den Bergh et al., 1995). Sperm immobilization can be achieved by different methods. In the mechanical immobilization method, it is provided by touching the tail of the sperm with a microinjection pipette (Gerris et al., 1995). In the sperm immobilization process with the help of a laser, sperm immobilization is achieved by hitting the middle and last part of the sperm tail with a laser at a wavelength of 1.48 μm, without touching the sperm. There is no difference in fertilization rate between this method and the mechanical immobilization method. However, the laser-assisted immobilization method shortens the processing time and eliminates mechanical immobilization errors due to the position of the microinjection needle (Ebner et al., 2001). Another option is the immobilization method with a piezo-pulse application. A higher Ca^{2+} wave and a higher fertilization rate can be obtained compared to mechanical immobilization. However, piezo-assisted immobilization has no advantage in terms of pregnancy success. Reduce processing time considerably compared to the mechanical immobilization method. In this method, sperm immobility is ensured by hitting the upper third of the sperm tail with the needle of the piezo micromanipulator (Yanagida et al., 2001).

The oocyte supplies all the membrane and cytoplasm content necessary for embryo development. In fact, the gradual separation and small size of polar bodies are important for preserving the genetic material, the amount of cytoplasm, and membrane of the oocyte. The meiotic spindle of the oocyte is the manager of the maturation, fertilization, and embryo development (Gitlin et al., 2003). The meiotic spindle always displaces towards the pole closest to the polar body during meiosis I (Brunet & Verlhac, 2011). Theoretically, the meiosis spindle realigns the chromosomes and forms the meiosis II plate. Thus, it is customary to perform the microinjection at 3 o'clock in the ICSI application in order not to damage the meiotic spindle. The polar body can be placed at 6 or 12 o'clock. Some researchers suggested that the microneedle tip points towards 6 o'clock; therefore, the cytoplasm content close to the meiotic spindle may be damaged during aspiration (Figure 14.1). However, studies have shown that placing the polar body at 6 (Van Der Westerlaken et al., 1999) o'clock, or even at 7 and 11 o'clock, increases the fertilization rate. Researchers hypothesized that if the sperm is aligned to the meiotic spindle closely, higher success is achieved (Anifandis et al., 2010). Injecting the sperm head-first or tail-first does not change the fertilization rate and embryo quality (Woodward et al., 2008).

Intracytoplasmic sperm injection (ICSI) is widely used today. Because ICSI allows fertilization with one sperm per oocyte. It also increases the success of IVF in severe male infertility cases (Palermo et al., 1992). According to Pinheiro et al., no statistically significant differences were found between couples who performed ICSI for severe male infertility and those who performed classical IVF (cIVF) for tubal factor with normal sperm parameters (Pinheiro et al., 1999). Song et al. reported that the application of ICSI in unexplained infertility cases was not different from the classical application of IVF in terms of clinical pregnancy (ICSI: 47.2%- cIVF: 45.9%) and live birth rate (ICSI: 33.3%- cIVF: 35.2), even reported that the transfer cancellation rate is higher in ICSI cases (ICSI: 19.1%- cIVF: 11.1%) (Song et al., 2021). Apart from the success of the ICSI method in severe male infertility (Bathwal et al., 2018), it would be appropriate to apply it in selected group of patients, considering its

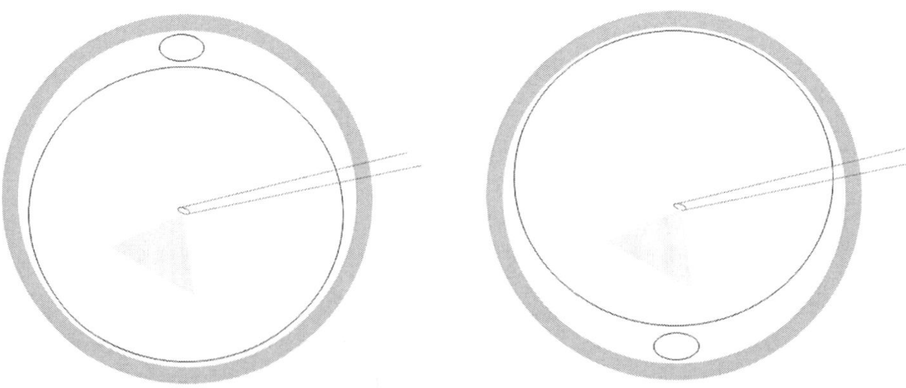

Figure 14.1 Field of view of the ICSI needle mouth when the polar body is placed at 12 o'clock and 6 o'clock during microinjection (Van Der Westerlaken et al., 1999).

declining superiority in mild male infertility and unexplained infertility cases, and its economic efficiency, especially for developing countries.

Laser-Assisted ICSI

The researchers observed that the rate of oocyte degeneration increased when the zona pellucida was resistant, as the ICSI method became more widespread. Because when the resistant zona is punctured, the oocyte is exposed to sudden and strong penetration by a microinjection needle. To avoid this, the zona pellucida should be weaker. Thus, the microinjection needle can easily and slightly enter the ooplasm. The laser is very beneficial for this purpose. Making a hole in the zona pellucida at 3 or 9 o'clock and performing ICSI here rescue fragile oocytes from degeneration caused by sudden penetration of the ICSI needle (Abdelmassih et al., 2002). Consequently, laser-assisted ICSI (LA-ICSI) improves oocyte survival, as well as the number of fertilized oocytes (Fawzy et al., 2020). Theoretically, the blastocyst can escape different spots if assisted hatching is performed or the trap in the small hole. Therefore, monozygotic twinning can occur. The hole drilled in the zona pellucida should be as small as possible to avoid adverse effects of the procedure such as blastomere loss and monozygotic twinning (Abdelmassih et al., 2002). Furthermore, researchers suggested that zona pellucida thinning may be more reliable than zona drilling in oocytes with resistant zona pellucida (Blake et al., 2001). However, LA-ICSI does not improve ongoing pregnancy rates (Fawzy et al., 2020).

Piezo-ICSI

The mechanical forces that occur on the oocyte during the ICSI procedure were mentioned before. Especially in oocytes with fragile oolemma and/or resistant zone pellucida, the rate of degeneration due to ICSI treatment increases. To avoid this situation, Kimura et al. developed the piezo-ICSI method. In this method, the ICSI needle enters the ooplasm with minimal distortion on the oocyte (Kimura & Yanagimachi, 1995). Later, researches were shown in humans that the fertilization rate increased with the piezo-ICSI method (Yanagida et al., 1999). A microinjection needle (ICSI pipette) is attached to the tip of a piezo drill (Figure 14.2). The piezo-drill creates lateral oscillations at the tip of the micro-injection needle. These mechanical forces serve to puncture the zona pellucida and oolemma without the need for the stabbing force of ICSI pipette (Ediz & Olgac, 2004). Thus, the oocyte is protected from the mechanical forces caused by stabbing. Piezo-ICSI may be beneficial because

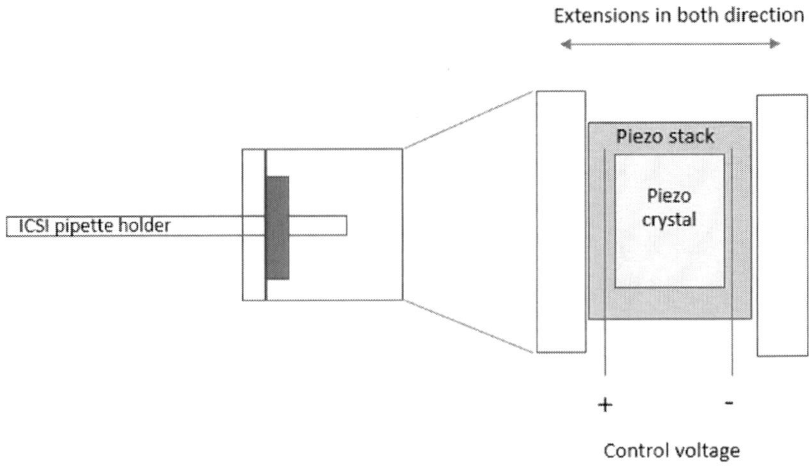

Figure 14.2 Schematic diagram of the piezo-ICSI drill (Ediz & Olgac, 2004).

it increases fertilization and blastocyst development rates in older women's (>35 years old) oocytes. However, there were no significant differences in fertilization, survival and blastocyst development rates in younger women's (≤35 years) oocyte (Furuhashi et al., 2019).

Assisted Hatching

The occurrence of pregnancy in humans depends on a healthy embryo and its implantation. The embryo must hatch from the zona pellucida for implantation. The hatching process is accompanied by hydrostatic pressure of expanded blastocyst and is promoted by secretions of zonalytic proteases such as strypsin, hepsin, and cathepsin. Observations on in vitro cultured embryos show that the embryo can hatch without the support of proteases (Seshagiri et al., 2016). However, a substantial number of healthy IVF embryos according to morphology criteria are impaired in their ability to hatch from the zona pellucida. Therefore, Cohen et al. described the assisted hatching method. Theoretically, this method would increase the rate of implantation and reduce the risk of necrosis at 5 and 6 days (Cohen et al., 1990). Indeed, assisted hatching increases the rates of implantation and clinical pregnancy. Nowadays, there are several methods to apply assisted hatching. In the mechanical method, an opening is created in zona pellucida with the help of a microneedle using a micromanipulator. Then the hatch occurs during the natural expansion of the embryo with the effect of hydrostatic pressure. Assisted hatching using acid Tyrode's solution is also applied on micromanipulator. The embryo is secured on a holding pipette. Tyrode's solution that was loaded into the microneedle before is gently expelled over a small area until the zona is cracked. Suction should be applied immediately to prevent excess acid from entering the perivitelline space. Acid may be detrimental to blastomeres. This method requires very quick handling. Laser-assisted zona drilling is a safe and quick way to make a hole in the zona pellucida. Laser-assisted hatching technique provides significant increase in hatching of in vitro embryos even when zona thinned rather than drilling.

Assisted hatching especially has important beneficial effects in patients with a poor prognosis, such as those two or more failed IVF cycles, poor embryo quality, and older women (>38 years of age). However, there are specific complications, including damage to the embryo or blastomeres. Furthermore, it has been associated with an increased risk of monozygotic twinning (Hammadeh et al., 2011).

Artificial Shrinkage of Blastocoel Cavity

The survival rate after cryopreservation has been shown to be negatively related to expansion. Morula and early blastocyst have a higher survival rate after thawing than expanded blastocyst. The survival rate after cryopreservation depends on the stage of the embryo. It reduces the chances of transferring viable embryos in the frozen embryo transfer cycle, especially for blastocysts. The hypothesis that could explain the differences in the efficiency between different stages of embryos is based on the water content of the blastocoel cavity. The large amount of water in the expanded blastocyst may be detrimental to the embryo during freezing due to ice crystal formation. Therefore, researchers suggested that artificial shrinkage (AS) of the blastocoel cavity may improve embryo survival after cryopreservation. In this method, the blastocyst is clutched by holding a pipette. The inner cell mass is placed at 6 or 12 o'clock. A glass micro-needle is pushed into the blastocoele cavity until it shrinks. Then the freezing protocol is applied (Vanderzwalmen et al., 2002). Some researchers consider that AS of the blastocoel cavity also creates a large hole in the zona pellucida (Hur et al., 2011). In other words, when the AS of the blastocoel cavity is applied, assisted hatching is also generated. AS of the blastocoel cavity prior to vitrification improves implantation, pregnancy, and delivery rates (Levi-Setti et al., 2016). However, prospective randomized trials are needed to confirm this information.

Conclusion

The clinical utility of some techniques needs to be further studied on a large-scale prospective basis. However, many techniques are fundamental to increasing IVF success in the world. These techniques will be cost effective when used in selected patient groups, considering the economic situation of the country. In addition, this journey that began with the development of technology opens us up for the future. For example, the technical possibility of transfer of ooplasms and nuclei raises ideas in the field of in vitro fertilization.

Administration to the content of oocyte or zygote by ooplasm transfer or nuclear transfer is a challenging and impressive idea for low quality oocytes. With plasma transfer, it is desired to transfer organelles and other cell elements, especially mitochondria, from the healthy donor cell to the low-quality cell. Research shows that it will work, but there is still a long way to go before it can be put into clinical practice (Darbandi et al., 2017). Who knows, maybe in the future we will transfer the genome to a commercially available artificial oocyte and obtain healthy oocytes (Oqani et al., 2022).

References

Abdelmassih, S., Cardoso, J., Abdelmassih, V., Dias, J. A., Abdelmassih, R., & Nagy, Z. P. (2002). Laser-assisted ICSI: a novel approach to obtain higher oocyte survival and embryo quality rates. *Human Reproduction*, *17*(10), 2694–2699. https://doi.org/10.1093/HUMREP/17.10.2694

Anifandis, G., Dafopoulos, K., Messini, C. I., Chalvatzas, N., & Messinis, I. E. (2010). Effect of the position of the polar body during ICSI on fertilization rate and embryo development. *Reproductive Sciences (Thousand Oaks, Calif.)*, *17*(9), 849–853. https://doi.org/10.1177/1933719110372421

Bathwal, S., Bhattacharya, R., Sharma, S., Chattopadhyay, R., Saha, I., & Chakravarty, B. (2018). Is ICSI superior to conventional IVF in severe male factor infertility: a 3 year prospective observational study. *Fertility and Sterility*, *110*(4), e288. https://doi.org/10.1016/j.fertnstert.2018.07.813

Blake, D. A., Forsberg, A. S., Johansson, B. R., & Wikland, M. (2001). Laser zona pellucida thinning—an alternative approach to assisted hatching. *Human Reproduction*, *16*(9), 1959–1964. https://doi.org/10.1093/HUMREP/16.9.1959

Brunet, S., & Verlhac, M. H. (2011). Positioning to get out of meiosis: the asymmetry of division. *Human Reproduction Update*, *17*(1), 68–75. https://doi.org/10.1093/HUMUPD/DMQ044

Cohen, J., Alikani, M., Malter, H. E., Adler, A., Talansky, B. E., & Rosenwaks, Z. (1991). Partial zona dissection or subzonal sperm insertion: microsurgical fertilization alternatives based on evaluation of sperm and embryo morphology. *Fertility and Sterility*, *56*(4), 696–706. https://doi.org/10.1016/S0015-0282(16)54602-0

Cohen, J., Elsner, C., Kort, H., Malter, H., Massey, J., Mayer, M. P., & Wiemer, K. (1990). Impairment of the hatching process following IVF in the human and improvement of implantation by assisting hatching using micromanipulation. *Human Reproduction*, *5*(1), 7–13. https://doi.org/10.1093/OXFORDJOURNALS.HUMREP.A137044/2/5-1-7.PDF.GIF

Darbandi, S., Darbandi, M., Khorram Khorshid, H. R., Sadeghi, M. R., Agarwal, A., Sengupta, P., Al-Hasani, S., & Akhondi, M. M. (2017). Ooplasmic transfer in human oocytes: efficacy and concerns in assisted reproduction. *Reproductive Biology and Endocrinology : RB&E*, *15*(1). https://doi.org/10.1186/S12958-017-0292-Z

Dow, K. (2019). Looking into the Test Tube: The Birth of IVF on British Television. *Medical History*, *63*(2), 189. https://doi.org/10.1017/MDH.2019.6

Dozortsev, D., Qian, C., Ermilov, A., Rybouchkin, A., De Sutter, P., & Dhont, M. (1997). Sperm-associated oocyte-activating factor is released from the spermatozoon within 30 minutes after injection as a result of the sperm-oocyte interaction. *Human Reproduction (Oxford, England)*, *12*(12), 2792–2796. https://doi.org/10.1093/HUMREP/12.12.2792

Ebner, T., Yaman, C., Moser, M., Sommergruber, M., Hartl, J., & Tews, G. (2001). Laser assisted immobilization of spermatozoa prior to intracytoplasmic sperm injection in humans. *Human Reproduction*, *16*(12), 2628–2631. https://doi.org/10.1093/HUMREP/16.12.2628

Ediz, K., & Olgac, N. (2004). Microdynamics of the piezo-driven pipettes in ICSI. *IEEE Transactions on Biomedical Engineering*, *51*(7), 1262–1268. https://doi.org/10.1109/TBME.2004.827346

Eskew, A. M., & Jungheim, E. S. (2017). A History of Developments to Improve in vitro Fertilization. *Missouri Medicine*, *114*(3), 156.

Fawzy, M., Emad, M., Mahran, A., Abdelrahman, M. Y., Fetih, A. N., Abdelghafar, H., Elsuity, M. A., Rashed, H., & Sabry, M. (2020). A randomized controlled trial of laser-assisted ICSI. *Human Reproduction (Oxford, England)*, *35*(12), 2692–2700. https://doi.org/10.1093/HUMREP/DEAA160

Furuhashi, K., Saeki, Y., Enatsu, N., Iwasaki, T., Ito, K., Mizusawa, Y., Matsumoto, Y., Kokeguchi, S., & Shiotani, M. (2019). Piezo-assisted ICSI improves fertilization and blastocyst development rates compared with conventional ICSI in women aged more than 35 years. *Reproductive Medicine and Biology*, *18*(4), 357–361. https://doi.org/10.1002/RMB2.12290

Gerris, J., Mangelschots, K., Royen, E. Van, Joostens, M., Eestermans, W., & Ryckaert, G. (1995). ICSI and severe male-factor infertility: Breaking the sperm tail prior to injection. *Human Reproduction*, *10*(3), 484–485. https://doi.org/10.1093/OXFORDJOURNALS.HUMREP.A135968/2/10-3-484.PDF.GIF

Gitlin, S. A., Gibbons, W. E., & Gosden, R. G. (2003). Oocyte biology and genetics revelations from polar bodies. *Reproductive Biomedicine Online*, *6*(4), 403–409. https://doi.org/10.1016/S1472-6483(10)62158-X

Hammadeh, M. E., Fischer-Hammadeh, C., & Ali, K. R. (2011). Assisted hatching in assisted reproduction: a state of the art. *Journal of Assisted Reproduction and Genetics*, *28*(2), 119. https://doi.org/10.1007/S10815-010-9495-3

Hur, Y. S., Park, J. H., Ryu, E. K., Yoon, H. J., Yoon, S. H., Hur, C. Y., Lee, W. D., & Lim, J. H. (2011). Effect of artificial shrinkage on clinical outcome in fresh blastocyst transfer cycles. *Clinical and Experimental Reproductive Medicine*, *38*(2), 87. https://doi.org/10.5653/CERM.2011.38.2.87

Kimura, Y., & Yanagimachi, R. (1995). Intracytoplasmic sperm injection in the mouse. *Biology of Reproduction*, *52*(4), 709–720. https://doi.org/10.1095/BIOLREPROD52.4.709

Laufer, N., & Simon, A. (1992). Treatment of male infertility by gamete micromanipulation. *Human Reproduction (Oxford, England)*, *7 Suppl 1*, 73–80. https://doi.org/10.1093/HUMREP/7.SUPPL_1.73

Levi-Setti, P. E., Menduni, F., Smeraldi, A., Patrizio, P., Morenghi, E., & Albani, E. (2016). Artificial shrinkage of blastocysts prior to vitrification improves pregnancy outcome: analysis of 1028 consecutive warming cycles. *Journal of Assisted Reproduction and Genetics*, *33*(4), 461. https://doi.org/10.1007/S10815-016-0655-Y

Malter, H. E., & Cohen, J. (1989). Partial zona dissection of the human oocyte: a nontraumatic method using micromanipulation to assist zona pellucida penetration. *Fertility and Sterility*, *51*(1), 139–148. https://doi.org/10.1016/S0015-0282(16)60443-0

Ng, S. C., Bongso, A., Ratnam, S. S., Sathananthan, H., Chan, C. L. K., Wong, P. C., Hagglund, L., Anandakumar, C., Wong, Y. C., & Goh, V. H. H. (1988). Pregnancy after transfer of sperm under zona. *Lancet (London, England)*, *2*(8614), 790. https://doi.org/10.1016/S0140-6736(88)92433-6

Oqani, R. K., So, S., Lee, Y., Ko, J. J., & Kang, E. (2022). Artificial Oocyte: Development and Potential Application. *Cells*, *11*(7). https://doi.org/10.3390/CELLS11071135

Palermo, G., Joris, H., Devroey, P., & Van Steirteghem, A. C. (1992). Pregnancies after intracytoplasmic injection of single spermatozoon into an oocyte. *Lancet (London, England)*, *340*(8810), 17–18. https://doi.org/10.1016/0140-6736(92)92425-F

Pinheiro, R. C., Lambert, J., Bénard, F., Mauffette, F., & Miron, P. (1999). Effectiveness of in vitro fertilization with intracytoplasmic sperm injection for severe male infertility. *CMAJ: Canadian Medical Association Journal*, *161*(11), 1397. /pmc/articles/PMC1230827/?report=abstract

Seshagiri, P. B., Vani, V., & Madhulika, P. (2016). Cytokines and Blastocyst Hatching. *American Journal of Reproductive Immunology*, *75*(3), 208–217. https://doi.org/10.1111/AJI.12464

Song, J., Liao, T., Fu, K., & Xu, J. (2021). ICSI Does Not Improve Live Birth Rates but Yields Higher Cancellation Rates Than Conventional IVF in Unexplained Infertility. *Frontiers in Medicine*, *7*, 960. https://doi.org/10.3389/FMED.2020.614118/BIBTEX

Steptoe, P. C., & Edwards, R. G. (1978). Birth after the reimplantation of a human embryo. *Lancet (London, England)*, *2*(8085), 366. https://doi.org/10.1016/S0140-6736(78)92957-4

Svalander, P., Wikland, M., Jakobsson, A. H., & Forsberg, A. S. (1994). Subzonal insemination (SUZI) or in vitro fertilization (IVF) in microdroplets for the treatment of male-factor infertility. *Journal of Assisted Reproduction and Genetics*, *11*(3), 149–155. https://doi.org/10.1007/BF02332092

Tarín, J. J. (1995). Subzonal insemination, partial zona dissection or intracytoplasmic sperm injection? An easy decision? *Human Reproduction*, *10*(1), 165–170. https://doi.org/10.1093/HUMREP/10.1.165

Van Den Bergh, M., Bertrand, E., Biramane, J., & Englert, Y. (1995). Importance of breaking a spermatozoon's tail before intracytoplasmic injection: a prospective randomized trial. *Human Reproduction (Oxford, England)*, *10*(11), 2819–2820. https://doi.org/10.1093/OXFORDJOURNALS.HUMREP.A135798

Van Der Westerlaken, L. A. J., Helmerhorst, F. M., Hermans, J., & Naaktgeboren, N. (1999). Intracytoplasmic sperm injection: position of the polar body affects pregnancy rate. *Human Reproduction (Oxford, England)*, *14*(10), 2565–2569. https://doi.org/10.1093/HUMREP/14.10.2565

Vanderzwalmen, P., Bertin, G., Debauche, C., Standaert, V., Van Roosendaal, E., Vandervorst, M., Bollen, N., Zech, H., Mukaida, T., Takahashi, K., & Schoysman, R. (2002). Births after vitrification at morula and blastocyst stages: effect of artificial reduction of the blastocoelic cavity before vitrification. *Human Reproduction*, *17*(3), 744–751. https://doi.org/10.1093/HUMREP/17.3.744

Woodward, B. J., Campbell, K. H. S., & Ramsewak, S. S. (2008). A comparison of headfirst and tailfirst microinjection of sperm at intracytoplasmic sperm injection. *Fertility and Sterility*, *89*(3), 711–714. https://doi.org/10.1016/J.FERTNSTERT.2007.03.087

Yanagida, K., Katayose, H., Hirata, S., Yazawa, H., Hayashi, S., & Sato, A. (2001). Influence of sperm immobilization on onset of Ca2+ oscillations after ICSI. *Human Reproduction*, *16*(1), 148–152. https://doi.org/10.1093/HUMREP/16.1.148

Yanagida, K., Katayose, H., Yazawa, H., Kimura, Y., Konnai, K., & Sato, A. (1999). The usefulness of a piezo-micromanipulator in intracytoplasmic sperm injection in humans. *Human Reproduction*, *14*(2), 448–453. https://doi.org/10.1093/HUMREP/14.2.448

Chapter 15

Ovulation Induction

Ismet Hortu[1], MD.*, Ph.D and
Elif Yagmur Erdem[2], MD
[1,2]Department of Obstetrics and Gynecology, School of Medicine, Ege University, Izmir, Turkiye

Abstract

Ovulation and the ovarian cycle occur through these two physiological activities of the ovary, periodic release of oocytes and steroid hormone production. And it is the gonadotropic hormones of the pituitary gland that control the repetitive process of follicle maturation, ovulation, corpus luteum formation, and regression in the ovarian cycle. Failure of ovulation (amenorrhea or oligomenorrhoea) can be identified in 18 to 25% of couples with infertility. The purpose of ovulation induction is to achieve monofollicular development that will improve the outcome of pregnancy by obtaining normo/mono-ovulatory cycles in these women. In this chapter, we aim to review different regiments used for ovulation induction and to provide the best approach in the management of women with anovulation as the cause of infertility.

Key Words: Ovulation Induction, Gonadotropins, Ovarian stimulation, GnRH, FSH, LH

Introduction

The first principle of anovulatory infertility management should be to determine the underlying cause. Ovulatory disorders are classified into three

* Corresponding Author's Email: ismethortu@yahoo.com

In: Holistic Approach to Assisted Reproductive Technology
Editor: Kenan Demir and Rümeysa Yılmaz Göç
ISBN: 979-8-89113-017-3
© 2023 Nova Science Publishers, Inc.

Table 15.1 WHO Classification of Anovulation

WHO class 1	Hypogonadotropic hypogonadal anovulation (hypothalamic amenorrhea) *Examples: Kallmann's synd., Amenorrhea ass. With weight loss, stress, Sheehan synd., Idiopathic hypogonadotropic hypogonadism, Pituitary tumor*
WHO class 2	Normogonadotropic normoestrogenic anovulation *Example: Polycystic ovarian syndrome*
WHO class 3	Hypergonadotropic hypoestrogenic anovulation *Example: Turner syndrome, premature/autoimmune ovarian failure, iatrogenic (chemotherapy, radiotherapy), Primary ovarian insufficiency*

categories according to the World Health Organization (WHO). Table 15.1 presents these three categories.

Hypogonadotropic hypogonadism (WHO Classes 1); In this group, which represents 5-10% of women suffering from anovulatory infertility, ovarian sex hormones cannot be produced due to anatomical or functional defects in the hypophysis or hypothalamus (Woodward, 2020). Functional hypothalamic amenorrhea (FHA); refers to secondary amenorrhea in which factors such as eating disorders (anorexia nervosa), excessive exercise, and stress contribute to the pathogenesis. Hypogonadotropic hypogonadism should be suspected if gonadotropin concentrations are below normal (less than 5 IU/L) in the presence of estrogen deficiency (A. Balen, 2008). With hypothalamic amenorrhea secondary to low weight or excessive exercise, LH levels are generally suppressed more than FSH. Reversing lifestyle factors (low weight, excessive exercise, stress) that contribute to anovulation should be attempted before induction of ovulation with medication is planned.

GnRH-producing neurons originate in the olfactory region in embryogenesis; defective migration of olfactory neurons and GnRH along cranial nerves through embryological development causes Kallmann syndrome. Although this syndrome is rarely seen, it progresses with hypogonadotropic hypogonadism and anosmia due to congenital GnRH deficiency. Irreversible delayed puberty and subsequent infertility are seen in these individuals (Lee & Leonard, 1994).

Polycystic ovary syndrome (PCOS) (WHO Class 2) affects 5-10% of women of reproductive age and is related to 75% of all anovulation disorders that cause subfertility (Homburg, 2005). Polycystic ovary syndrome is the most prevalent cause of clinically significant androgen excess, and these women typically have irregular anovulatory menstrual cycles, along with symptoms of excessive androgen effect, such as hirsuitism and acne (Homburg, 2005). Concentration of luteinizing hormone (LH) may be normal or high, while serum estradiol and FSH concentrations are normal (Laven et al., 2002).

Ovarian function is affected by various factors, and being overweight and high serum LH concentrations of the individual with PCOS are conditions that negatively affect fertility (Badawy et al., 2009). In women with PCOS accompanied by overweight, losing weight that can restore spontaneous ovulation should be attempted before ovulation induction therapy is planned; lifestyle changes to enhance fecundity, together with exercise, reducing drinking alcohol, and smoking cessation, should be recommended. (Norman et al., 2002).

In addition to induction of ovulation, the use of assisted reproductive techniques (ART) is also common in the treatment of infertile women with PCOS. However, there are not enough potent randomized trials to resolve which of these treatments provides the best chance of healthy fertilization. Ovarian hyperstimulation syndrome (OHSS) and multiple pregnancies are among the main complications of infertility treatment in women with PCOS, and therefore serial ultrasonography should be maintained for induction of ovulation (A. H. Balen, 2013).

Primary ovarian insufficiency (POI) *(WHO Class 3)* is the decrease/ loss of ovarian activity before the age of 40 and occurs in only 1% of all women but accounts for 5% to 10% of anovulation cases (Woodward, 2020). Gonadal dysgenesis can also be seen as a result of chromosomal abnormalities such as Fragile X and Turner syndrome (Iwase et al., 2016). Turner syndrome, which can be diagnosed with typical body structure such as webbed neck, cubitus valgus, and short stature, can be seen as a cause of amenorrhea (Homburg, 2005). Mutations in the FMR1 gene cause Fragile X syndrome, while premutations in this gene can cause other diseases in women, such as fragile x-associated tremor/ataxia syndrome (FXTAS) and primary ovarian failure (Mila et al., 2018). Autoimmune oophoritis; may be seen as a cause of early menopause, is responsible for infertility in up to 5% of women with POI (La Marca et al., 2009). Autoimmune oophoritis is often associated with other autoimmune endocrinopathies, particularly autoimmune Addison's disease, but rarely occurs in isolated premature ovarian failure (Lee & Leonard, 1994). Iatrogenic causes of premature ovarian failure include radiation to the abdomen / pelvis, or chemotherapy, and other indications such as bilateral oophorectomy for borderline or malignant ovarian tumors. The probability of developing ovarian failure in such cases is difficult to predict, but when the patient is young and the follicle pool is larger, there is a better chance of preserving ovarian function (A. Balen, 2008). For POI, the only efficient choice is IVF with donor oocytes, but an experimental approach including in vitro activation (IVA) of the patient's own ovarian tissue/oocytes has been started to be tested in these patients (Kawamura et al., 2020).

Hyperprolactinemic anovulation, ; In this group, which comprises 5-10% of women with anovulation , hyperprolactinemia inhibits the pulsatility of

GnRH through a short feedback loop and causes sexual dysfunction (Lee & Leonard, 1994). The reason for hyperprolactinemia may be drug-induced (neuroleptic drugs, antidepressants), pathological (prolactinomas, pituitary or sellar tumors) or physiological (pregnancy, lactation, stress).

Overview of the Approach

Purpose; the aim of ovulation induction in a patient with anovulatory infertility is to develop monofollicular instead of multifollicular development in anovulatory disorder, thus achieving a singleton pregnancy. In order to achieve this goal, the low-cost, slightest invasive, and simplest treatment choice should be initially focused, and the method to be chosen should be directed to the underlying cause of anovulation. Ovulation induction strategies must be considered before attempting assisted reproductive technologies (ART) in women with ovulatory disorders due to low complication rates and good success rates.

Prepregnancy counseling; Like every couple planning a pregnancy, couples who are planning ovarian induction should also receive preconception counseling. This includes, in addition to medical history and physical examination, an accurate anamnesis aimed at addressing individual risk factors, a review of lifestyle habits, a family history of infertility, and a variety of laboratory assesment and genetic tests. Serum anti-Müllerian hormone (AMH) concentration is seen as an early and reliable indicator of the quality and quantity of available oocytes, i.e. ovarian reserve (Iwase et al., 2016).

Patient-specific approach; Most infertile anovulatory women are in class 2 WHO (normogonadotropic anovulation) and most of these women are diagnosed with PCOS. These women are well estrogenized and have normal levels of FSH, but LH may be elevated; in contrast, decreased hypothalamic/pituitary activity in women with hypogonadotropic hypogonadism (HH) (WHO class 1) results in abnormally low concentrations of FSH and LH and a hypoestrogenic course. These hypoestrogenic women are unlikely to respond to antiestrogen clomiphene citrate; although, since clomiphene citrate is easier to apply, it may be rational to administer clomiphene before starting pulsatile gonadotropin-releasing hormone (GnRH) or gonadotropin therapy, and if ovulation occurs, treatment can continue. If ovulation does not occur, pulsatile GnRH is switched to primary treatment, and in the absence of pulsatile GnRH, gonadotropin treatment with both LH and FSH should be started because these women do not respond to FSH alone. In women with PCOS, the approach starts with weight loss exercise and continues with induction of ovulation. First-line therapy in women with PCOS (especially if obesity is present) is now considered letrozole, an aromatase inhibitor. As in both groups of patients in this sample; Women with different causes of anovulation have different gonadotropin requirements for ovulation induction and a separate treatment approach should be planned for each patient.

Oral Agents

Letrozole, a third-generation aromatase inhibitor, has started to replace clomiphene citrate, which has been the best approach to induction of ovulation for more than 50 years. Letrozole was originally used to treat postmenopausal breast cancer. It should be noted that letrozole, which is currently approved by the FDA as a first-line adjuvant therapy in the management of estrogen receptor positive breast cancer, is not approved by the FDA in the management of ovulation induction. However, the American College of Obstetrics and Gynecology (ACOG) now recommends letrozole as the first-line choice for the selection of ovulation induction agents in women with PCOS. Aromatase is responsible for the conversion of androgen to estrogen; by inhibiting this enzyme, aromatase inhibitors lower the level of circulating estrogen. This hypoestrogenic state reduces the negative estrogenic feedback in the pituitary and thereby increases FSH output, leading to enhanced growth of ovarian follicles. (Woodward, 2020). The starting dose of letrozole is 2.5mg/day from days 3 to 7 of the cycle following spontaneous menstruation or bleeding induced by progestin. If the cycle has resulted in ovulation, but pregnancy has not occurred, the same dose should be used in the next cycle; if ovulation has not occurred, the dose should be elevated to 5 mg/day (to a maximum of 7.5 mg/day) (Al-Fadhli et al., 2006).

Clomiphene citrate, Clomiphene citrate (CC) has been the most commonly used and best known choice for ovulation stimulation since the early 1960s. It has been the first choice in the treatment of anovulation due to the fact that it does not require close follow-up, ease of patient compliance, and low cost. In normogonadotropic anovulatory infertile patients, 75% of ovulatory cycles are achieved with clomiphene citrate treatment (Laven et al., 2002). While it results in pregnancy in 35-40% of patients; 20-25% of patients do not respond at all and are considered ‘clomiphene resistant’ (Homburg, 2005).

Clomiphene is structurally related to the potent synthetic estrogen diethylstilbestrol, this similarity allows clomiphene citrate to bind to estrogen receptors (ER) throughout the reproductive tract; although, unlike estrogen, CC binds to the nuclear ER for a long time and affects the normal ER regeneration process, ultimately depleting ER concentrations (Rabe, 2000). Clomiphene citrate binds to estrogen receptors in the pituitary and hypothalamus, eliminating the negative feedback effect of endogenous estrogens; stimulates pituitary gonadotropins by increasing the secretion of GnRH, and increased gonadotropins stimulate follicle growth (Fıçıcıoğlu & Özcan, 2017).

On day 3 of the cycle, clomiphene citrate is started orally 50 mg/ day and continued for 5 days. In the 10-day period following the last dose of clomiphene citrate, the patient should be encouraged to have sexual intercourse every other day. A second course of 100 mg per day for 5 days can be started if follicular development does not occur after the first course of treatment. (Lee & Leonard, 1994).

Metformin, with the understanding that insulin resistance plays an important role in the pathophysiology of PCOS; the use of insulin-lowering metformin in anovulatory women with PCOS has increased. In these women, metformin plays a positive role in correcting hyperinsulinemia, increasing the menstrual cycle, and improving spontaneous ovulation. Still, metformin does not seem to increase live birth rates when given in combination with clomiphene citrate or alone and is not recommended as first-line therapy for ovulation induction in women with PCOS.

The main effect of metformin is to inhibit hepatitis glucose production, reduce lipid synthesis, inhibit gluconeogenesis, and increase fatty acid oxidation, thus reducing circulating insulin and glucose (A. H. Balen, 2013). Primary studies of metformin in the management of PCOS showed that metformin showed benefit in the reduction of serum androgens, weight loss, and restoration of the menstrual cycle in these patients. However, most of these studies were observational and involved small study groups. Conflicting results were found in larger randomized studies conducted afterward, and these early positive findings could not be confirmed (Impact & No, 2017).

Dopamine agonists, Dopamine agonists are the treatment of choice for hyperprolactinemic anovulatory women. For example, most women with lactotroph adenomas have anovulatory infertility, and pregnancy can occur when lactotroph adenoma has been treated and serum prolactin concentration is reduced to normal. Bromocriptine is an ergot alkaloid that tries to restore the balance of dopamine; it also lowers growth hormone and prolactin levels. Several other compounds have been shown to bind to the dopamine d2 receptor with greater affinity and reduce prolactin levels, the benefit of many of these newly discovered dopamine agonists is longer half-life, ease of once daily dosage, and fewer side effects (Rabe, 2000). For example, patients who are more concerned about nausea from bromocriptine often opt for cabergoline. Although the fetal safety of bromocriptine is greater than that of cabergoline, cabergoline is also considered safe (Molitch, 2015). Since the safety of continued use of dopamine agonists has not been fully established, treatment should be stopped after the diagnosis of pregnancy. Although rare, if the size of the adenoma becomes large enough to affect vision, dopamine agonist treatment is continued during pregnancy. The outcome of pregnancy after induction of ovulation with prolactin-lowering drugs is similar to that of the normal population. (Homburg, 2005).

If hyperprolactinemia is due to a drug, the related preparation should be discontinued. However, if this drug is a psychotropic drug that needs to continue, a low-dose combined oral contraceptive can be started to continue the drug and counteract the symptoms of estrogen deficiency after imaging the pituitary fossa (A. Balen, 2008). However, the use of dopamine agonists with antipsychotics must be used very carefully, in consultation with a psychiatrist, as it may reduce serum prolactin levels and at the same time antagonize the therapeutic effects of the antipsychotic.

In the treatment of women with lactotroph microadenoma who want to have a pregnancy, preconception counseling should first be provided first; to restore ovulation, serum prolactin should be normalized with cabergoline. Cabergoline treatment can start at 0.25 mg orally twice a week. When the serum prolactin level is measured again after 2-3 months, if it is not normal or close to normal, the dose should increase by 0.5 mg/week. Further dosage may be increased at monthly intervals (e.g. up to 1 mg orally per week if necessary and tolerated) until the prolactin level decreases to normal or near normal and the cycles are ovulatory. When the level of prolactin is normal/close to normal, if the cycles are not ovulatory, an ovulation induction agent such as clomiphene citrate can be added to treatment. If pregnancy is achieved in 6 to 12 months, cabergoline treatment should be stopped and adenoma growth should be monitored throughout pregnancy.

Pulsatile GnRH Therapy

Pulsatile GnRH therapy is used for the induction of ovulation in patients with hypogonadotropic hypogonadism (hypothalamic amenorrhea) with normal pituitary function (Shoham et al., 1990). The reason why pulsatile GnRH therapy is preferred in hypogonadotropic amenorrhea is that pulsatile GnRH produces more physiological preovulatory estradiol levels and luteal phase progesterone levels compared to exogenous gonadotropin therapy. In this way, a high ovulation and conception rate is achieved, most cycles are successful with a single dominant follicle, and the risk of many folliculogenesis and multiple pregnancy is reduced (Martin et al., 1993).

While continuous GnRH treatment reduces gonadotropin release; pulsatile administration of gonadotropin releasing hormone using an infusion pump stimulates endogenous LH and FSH production. When GnRH administration began to be used clinically, it was first administered intravenously, using a dose of 2.5-10 μg per pulse, with a pulse interval of 60-90 minutes to mimic the normal pulsatile release of GnRH. However, pulsatile GnRH therapy is now mostly applied to the adipose tissue of the lower abdominal wall, to eliminate possible side effects of prolonged intravenous application, including local venous thrombosis or infection (Mattle et al., 2008). Though, delayed resorption of GnRH from subcutaneous adipose tissue may result in inadequate serum GnRH levels for adequate stimulation of gonadotropes. Dosage starts at a minimum to prevent multifollicular growth and is increased until follicular growth and ovulation are induced and continued until pregnancy is achieved (Bruna-Catalán & Menabrito, 2011). Pulsatile GnRH was maintained throughout the entire cycle in published studies. In the clinical setting, pulsatile GnRH administration can be discontinued after ovulation and corpus luteum supplemented with hCG. The potential regimen for luteal phase hCG administration combined with gonadotropin treatment is 500 units administered on days 7, 10 and 13 after ovulation (Martin et al., 1993).

Gonadotropin Therapy

Human menopausal gonadotropin, which was extracted from the urine of postmenopausal women in the 1960s, was the first gonadotropin to be obtained. The first preparations of the resulting hMG were not as pure; purified urinary FSH (uFSH) perperate was developed by reducing the amount of inactive protein with the purification techniques developed in the 1980s (Zwart-Van Rijkom et al., 2002). Pure preparations available; cause less hypersensitivity reaction and provide ease of administration (subcutaneous instead of intramuscular). With the advances of recombinant DNA technology, large-scale production of human recombinant follicle stimulating hormone (rFSH) has been made possible (Fauser, 1998). Consistent and large-scale usability can be achieved through recombinant products.

The indications for the use of gonadotropins are; women with PCOS who cannot ovulate or become pregnant despite weight loss, clomiphene citrate and letrozol therapy; and hypogonadotropic anovulatory women with hypothalamic amenorrhea (HA) or hypopituitarism who cannot approach pulsatile GnRH therapy.

Preparations; hMG and FSH ; The extent to which rFSH and urinary gonadotropins used affect the outcome of ovulation induction is controversial. In a large-scale review, the following results were seen (Weiss et al., 2019); there may be slight or no difference in the incidence of multiple pregnancy, clinical pregnancy rate, miscarriage, or live birth rate between recombinant FSH and urinary-derived gonadotropins in women with PCOS. However, in women with clomiphene citrate failure, gonadotropins resulted in more live births than clomiphene citrate and did not increase the rate of multiple pregnancy. It is also unclear whether any of the interventions decrease the incidence of ovarian hyperstimulation syndrome. The latest advancement in urinary gonadotropins is highly purified menotropin (highly purified human menopausal gonadotropin) containing equal amounts of FSH and LH activity (Weiss et al., 2019) .When the ovarian follicles mature, at the minimum a follicle of at least 17mm in diameter develops, ovulation is triggered by injection of 5000 units of hCG (A. Balen, 2008).

Protocols; The point of induction of ovulation with gonadotropin is to obtain a single dominant follicle, which is provided by a temporary increase in FSH concentrations above the threshold value at the beginning of spontaneous cycles (Fauser & Van Heusden, 1997). Because each woman differs in ovarian sensitivity to FSH simulation, individual treatment and monitoring protocols are required to ensure the outcome of a single follicle. The initial dose of FSH in the conventional protocol is 150 international units/day. If this dose is insufficient for the ovarian response, the doses can be increased after 5 days (Fauser & Van Heusden, 1997). This regimen has been associated with multiple pregnancy rates of up to 36%. Low-dose step-up protocol can be preferred, especially in patients with PCOS who are at a certain risk of complications, to minimize the risk of over-stimulation and multiple follicle development. In the low-dose step-up protocol, the starting dose is 37.5 to 75 international units/ day. If the ovarian response is insufficient after 14 days, increments of 37.5 international units can be increased to a maximum of 225 international units/ day at weekly intervals. In the low-dose step-down protocol, which is closer to the physiology of normal cycles, treatment begins with 150 international units of FSH / day soon after progesterone-induced or spontaneous bleeding. The dose is continued until the dominant follicle (>10mm) is seen in transvaginal USG and then reduced to 112.5 international units of FSH / day. It is then reduced to 75 international units/day three days later and continued through hCG administration.

Laparoscopic Ovarian Diathermy

In the past, the standard treatment for infertility in women with PCOS was wedge resection of the ovaries. However, this approach was abandoned due to both the efficacy of clomiphene and the high incidence of pelvic adhesions caused by wedge resection. Today, laparoscopic ovarian diathermy (ovarian drilling) is a possible second-line treatment for women with PCOS. When ovulation is still not achieved despite adequate trials of clomiphene citrate, an alternative treatment option after gonadotropins is laparoscopic surgery with laser or electrocautery. Compared to gonadotropin theapy, the potential advantage of ovarian drilling is its lower risk of OHSS and lower cost (Farquhar et al., 2004).

It was revealed that testosterone and LH levels decreased significantly in follow-up after successful laparoscopic ovarian drilling, while the FSH level remained unchanged after the procedure (Elnaggar et al., 2016). It has been shown that those who are thin and have high basal LH concentrations have a greater clinical and endocrine response to treatment. The main concern with laparoscopic treatment is the danger of diathermy damage to the pelvic and other internal organs and the risk of adhesion formation. Therefore, the lowest effective dose of diathermy, three to six punctures per ovary at 40 W of coagulating (modulated) current for four seconds per puncture seems reasonable (Flyckt & Goldberg, 2011). It has also been shown that LOD offers a lower risk of adhesion formation (10-20% of cases) and that those that form are generally fine and of little clinical significance (A. H. Balen et al., 2016). Irrigation with 500-1000 ml isotonic saline solution can be tried to reduce the risk of adhesion formation and to prevent heat dissipation in adjacent tissues (El-Sayed et al., 2017). Finally, in published studies, approximately 80% of patients with a range of 30 to 90 percent achieved spontaneous ovulation after LOD (Seow et al., 2008).

Conclusion

Clomiphene citrate is one of the most widely accepted drugs for ovulation induction by clinicians because it is easy to use, effective, and largely safe. Close follow-up is not required, and the cost is low. Aromatase inhibitors, on the other hand, have a more suitable profile in the treatment of infertility than clomiphene citrate, as they have a short half-life and are not an estrogen receptor antagonist. Today, a fertility practitioner can choose from a wide range of gonadotropin preparations. It is known that there are many different FSH isoforms in gonadotropin preparations, and these preparations may differ in terms of purity and LH activity. Which agent will be administered according to which protocol should be evaluated on a patient basis, depending on the experience of the clinician, the availability of the preparation, the ease of use, and the cost. Long-acting GnRH agonists; Although receptor down-regulation desensitizes gonadotropes to GnRH, first stimulating and then inhibiting pituitary gonadotropin secretion, antagonists competitively block the GnRH receptor and gonadotropin suppression occurs almost immediately. In general, although antagonist protocols are more widely used than GnRH agonist protocols worldwide due to their ease of use and comparable results, more studies are needed to claim superiority over each other in terms of pregnancy outcomes.

References

Al-Fadhli, R., Sylvestre, C., Buckett, W., Tan, S. L., & Tulandi, T. (2006). A randomized trial of superovulation with two different doses of letrozole. *Fertility and Sterility*, *85*(1), 161–164. https://doi.org/10.1016/j.fertnstert.2005.07.1283

Badawy, A., Mosbah, A., Tharwat, A., & Eid, M. (2009). Extended letrozole therapy for ovulation induction in clomiphene-resistant women with polycystic ovary syndrome: a novel protocol. *Fertility and Sterility*, *92*(1), 236–239. https://doi.org/10.1016/j.fertnstert.2008.04.065

Balen, A. (2008). Infertility in Practice. In *Infertility in Practice*. https://doi.org/10.3109/9781439807224

Balen, A. H. (2013). Ovulation induction in the management of anovulatory polycystic ovary syndrome. *Molecular and Cellular Endocrinology*, *373*(1–2), 77–82. https://doi.org/10.1016/j.mce.2012.10.008

Balen, A. H., Morley, L. C., Misso, M., Franks, S., Legro, R. S., Wijeyaratne, C. N., Stener-Victorin, E., Fauser, B. C. J. M., Norman, R. J., & Teede, H. (2016). The management of anovulatory infertility in women with polycystic ovary syndrome: An analysis of the evidence to support the development of global WHO guidance. *Human Reproduction Update*, *22*(6), 687–708. https://doi.org/10.1093/humupd/dmw025

Bruna-Catalán, I., & Menabrito, M. (2011). Ovulation induction with minimal dose of follitropin alfa: A case series study. *Reproductive Biology and Endocrinology*, *9*, 5–10. https://doi.org/10.1186/1477-7827-9-142

El-Sayed, M. L. M., Ahmed, M. A., Mansour, M. A. A., & Mansour, S. A. A. (2017). Unilateral Versus Bilateral Laparoscopic Ovarian Drilling Using Thermal Dose Adjusted According to Ovarian Volume in CC-Resistant PCOS, A Randomized Study. *Journal of Obstetrics and Gynecology of India*, *67*(5), 356–362. https://doi.org/10.1007/s13224-017-1010-7

Elnaggar, E. A., Elwan, Y. A., Ibrahim, S. A., & Abdalla, M. M. (2016). Hormonal Changes After Laparoscopic Ovarian Diathermy in Patients with Polycystic Ovarian Syndrome. *Journal of Obstetrics and Gynecology of India*, *66*, 528–533. https://doi.org/10.1007/s13224-016-0882-2

Farquhar, C. M., Williamson, K., Brown, P. M., & Garland, J. (2004). An economic evaluation of laparoscopic ovarian diathermy versus gonadotrophin therapy for women with clomiphene citrate resistant polycystic ovary syndrome. *Human Reproduction*, *19*(5), 1110–1115. https://doi.org/10.1093/humrep/deh219

Fauser, B. C. J. M. (1998). Developments in human recombinant follicle stimulating hormone technology: Are we going in the right direction? *Human Reproduction*, *13*(SUPPL. 3), 36–51. https://doi.org/10.1093/humrep/13.suppl_3.36

Fauser, B. C. J. M., & Van Heusden, A. M. (1997). Manipulation of human ovarian function: Physiological concepts and clinical consequences. *Endocrine Reviews*, *18*(1), 71–106. https://doi.org/10.1210/er.18.1.71

Fıçıcıoğlu, C., & Özcan, P. (2017). First Line Agents for Ovulation Induction: Oral Agents. *Türk Üreme Tıbbı ve Cerrahisi Dergisi (Turkish Journal of Reproductive Medicine and Surgery)*, *1*(1), 29–35. https://doi.org/10.24074/tjrms.2016-54245

Flyckt, R. L., & Goldberg, J. M. (2011). Laparoscopic ovarian drilling for clomiphene-resistant polycystic ovary syndrome. *Seminars in Reproductive Medicine*, *29*(2), 138–146. https://doi.org/10.1055/s-0031-1272476

Homburg, R. (2005). Ovulation Induction and Controlled Ovarian Stimulation. In *Ovulation Induction and Controlled Ovarian Stimulation*. https://doi.org/10.1201/b14449

Impact, S., & No, P. (2017). Metformin Therapy for the Management of Infertility in Women with Polycystic Ovary Syndrome: Scientific Impact Paper No. 13. *BJOG: An International Journal of Obstetrics and Gynaecology*, *124*(12), e306–e313. https://doi.org/10.1111/1471-0528.14764

Iwase, A., Nakamura, T., Osuka, S., Takikawa, S., Goto, M., & Kikkawa, F. (2016). Anti-Müllerian hormone as a marker of ovarian reserve: What have we learned, and what should we know? *Reproductive Medicine and Biology*, *15*(3), 127–136. https://doi.org/10.1007/s12522-015-0227-3

Kawamura, K., Ishizuka, B., & Hsueh, A. J. W. (2020). Drug-free in-vitro activation of follicles for infertility treatment in poor ovarian response patients with decreased ovarian reserve. *Reproductive BioMedicine Online*, *40*(2), 245–253. https://doi.org/10.1016/j.rbmo.2019.09.007

La Marca, A., Marzotti, S., Brozzetti, A., Stabile, G., Artenisio, A. C., Bini, V., Giordano, R., De Bellis, A., Volpe, A., & Falorni, A. (2009). Primary ovarian insufficiency due to steroidogenic cell autoimmunity is associated with a preserved pool of functioning follicles. *Journal of Clinical Endocrinology and Metabolism*, *94*(10), 3816–3823. https://doi.org/10.1210/jc.2009-0817

Laven, J. S. E., Imani, B., Eijkemans, M. J. C., & Fauser, B. C. J. M. (2002). New approach to polycystic ovary syndrome and other forms of anovulatory infertility. *Obstetrical and Gynecological Survey*, *57*(11), 755–767. https://doi.org/10.1097/00006254-200211000-00022

Lee, P., & Leonard, J. (1994). Textbook on endocrinology. In *Bmj* (Vol. 308, Issue 6942). https://doi.org/10.1136/bmj.308.6942.1512c

Martin, A., Hall, J. E., & Adams, M. (1993). Comparison of Exogenous Gonadotropins and Pulsatile Gonadotropin-Releasing Hormone for Induction of Ovulation in Hypogonadotropic Amenorrhea. *Society*, *77*(1), 125-129. https://doi.org/10.1210/jcem.77.1.8325934

Mattle, V., Leyendecker, G., & Wildt, L. (2008). Side effects of pulsatile GnRH therapy for induction of ovulation. *Expert Review of Endocrinology and Metabolism*, *3*(5), 535–538. https://doi.org/10.1586/17446651.3.5.535

Mila, M., Alvarez-Mora, M. I., Madrigal, I., & Rodriguez-Revenga, L. (2018). Fragile X syndrome: An overview and update of the FMR1 gene. *Clinical Genetics*, *93*(2), 197–205. https://doi.org/10.1111/cge.13075

Molitch, M. E. (2015). Endocrinology in pregnancy: Management of the pregnant patient with a prolactinoma. *European Journal of Endocrinology, 172*(5), R205–R213. https://doi.org/10.1530/EJE-14-0848

Norman, R. J., Davies, M. J., Lord, J., & Moran, L. J. (2002). The role of lifestyle modification in polycystic ovary syndrome. *Trends in Endocrinology and Metabolism, 13*(6), 251–257. https://doi.org/10.1016/S1043-2760(02)00612-4

Rabe, T. (2000). Frontiers in gynecological endocrinology. In *International Journal of Gynecology & Obstetrics* (Vol. 70). https://doi.org/10.1016/s0020-7292(00)81433-2

Seow, K. M., Juan, C. C., Hwang, J. L., & Ho, L. T. (2008). Laparoscopic surgery in polycystic ovary syndrome: Reproductive and metabolic effects. *Seminars in Reproductive Medicine, 26*(1), 101–110. https://doi.org/10.1055/s-2007-992930

Shoham, Z., Homburg, R., & Jacobs, H. S. (1990). 11 Induction of ovulation with pulsatile GnRH. *Bailliere's Clinical Obstetrics and Gynaecology, 4*(3), 589–608. https://doi.org/10.1016/S0950-3552(05)80312-8

Weiss, N. S., Kostova, E., Nahuis, M., Mol, B. W. J., van der Veen, F., & van Wely, M. (2019). Gonadotrophins for ovulation induction in women with polycystic ovary syndrome. *Cochrane Database of Systematic Reviews, 2019*(1). https://doi.org/10.1002/14651858.CD010290.pub3

Woodward, B. J. (2020). Textbook of Assisted Reproduction. In *Textbook of Assisted Reproduction*. https://doi.org/10.1007/978-981-15-2377-9

Zwart-Van Rijkom, J. E. F., Broekmans, F. J., & Leufkens, H. G. M. (2002). From HMG through purified urinary FSH preparations to recombinant FSH: A substitution study. *Human Reproduction, 17*(4), 857–865. https://doi.org/10.1093/humrep/17.4.857

Chapter 16

Intrauterine Insemination

Işıl Tuğçe Turan, MD*

Department of Histology and Embryology, Erciyes University, Kayseri, Turkiye

Abstract

Intrauterine insemination is a first-line, noninvasive, and cost-effective assisted reproductive technique in selected cases. The sperm sample prepared from semen under laboratory conditions is transmitted directly to the upper uterine cavity. It can be applied in indications such as unexplained infertility, moderate male factor, and cervical factor. In the literature, the clinical success rate is stated to be between 10-20%. The purpose of sperm preparation is to isolate sperm from decapacitating factors, viral and bacterial residues in semen, to increase sperm motility and to provide sperm capacitation. A female patient can be subjected to a preapplication stimulation protocol. While stimulation increases the success rate of IUI, it also increases the risk of multiple pregnancy.

Key Words: Intrauterine insemination, Sperm preparation, Assisted reproductive technique

Introduction

Intrauterine insemination (IUI) is an assisted conception technique that consists of delivering a semen sample prepared in the laboratory to increase the number of motile sperm directly to the upper uterine cavity with a thin cannula.

* Corresponding Author's E-mail: isil.tc@gmail.com

In: Holistic Approach to Assisted Reproductive Technology
Editor: Kenan Demir and Rümeysa Yılmaz Göç
ISBN: 979-8-89113-017-3

© 2023 Nova Science Publishers, Inc.

IUI is the first-line treatment in cases of unexplained subfertility because it is cost-effective and relatively non-invasive. With IUI, some natural barriers are overcome that cause infertility, such as cervical factor, moderate male factor, immunological factors, and ejaculation disorders. The clinical pregnancy rates per cycle of the IUI method range from 10% to 20%. IUI is considered first-line therapy for patients with functionally normal tubes selected with appropriate indications such as cervical factor subfertility, retrograde ejaculation, anatomical factors, unexplained subfertility, moderate male factor subfertility. However, its use is limited in patients with endometriosis, severe male factor infertility, bilateral tubal block, and advanced maternal age ≥ 35. Important prognostic indicators of success with IUI include many female factors such as patient age, duration of infertility, stimulation protocol, infertility etiology, number of cycles, number of pre-ovulatory follicles on hCG day, endometrial thickness on hCG day, and male factors such as age, infertility etiology, sexual period of abstinence, total number of motile sperm after preparation, normal percentage of sperm and sperm motility, and other factors such as ovulation induction agents, sperm preparation techniques, insemination time (Allahbadia, 2017; Rizk & Montag, 2017).

IUI can be administered with ovarian stimulation or during the natural menstrual cycle. There is no evidence that unstimulated IUI results in a higher pregnancy rate compared to non-treatment. Therefore, ovarian stimulation is usually performed with agents such as clomiphene or gonadotropin before IUI. Thus, a higher success rate is achieved, but the risk of multiple pregnancy after stimulation also increases. If the duration of unexplained infertility is long, IVF should be preferred over IUI, as the success rate is higher and it is easier to control multiple pregnancy, especially when elective single embryo transfer is used (Kevin Coward, 2013).

Sperm Preparation for IUI

The purpose of sperm preparation for IUI is to increase the concentration of normal morphology and advanced motile sperm in semen, decapitation factors, separation of seminal plasma containing foreign cells, and capacitation of sperm. During the procedure, media that contains or can produce potentially toxic substances should not be used, and care should be taken not to create free oxygen radicals that are toxic to sperm.

There are various sperm preparation techniques. An ideal sperm preparation technique allows isolating a highly functional sperm population with preserved DNA from ROS produced by sperm and leukocytes (Björndahl & Brown, 2022).

Methods

Semen Collection

For IUI, the male patient should collect masturbated semen in a sterile disposable plastic container in a room adjacent to the laboratory. All plastics, glassware, and media should be checked for toxicity to sperm (e.g. sperm may become immobilized if they come into contact with rubber). Sperm should be prepared immediately after the liquefaction of seminal plasma.

Although the time difference between semen collection and preparation does not seem critical for good semen samples, studies have found a relationship between keeping the time short and pregnancy rates. In a study by Yavas et al., the relationship between semen collection with sperm washing, sperm washing with IUI time, and semen collection with IUI time in IUI and pregnancy outcomes was investigated. In this study, 62 couples consisting of women treated with clomiphene citrate and women treated with hMG were examined, and ultrasound detection of fetal heartbeat was taken as the basis for pregnancy outcome. As a result of the study, it was found that semen sample collection in the clinic in hMG-treated patients was more effective than collection at home, and it is recommended to be preferred. There were no significant differences in this regard in patients treated with clomiphene citrate. Delaying semen processing from 30 minutes to 1 hour and/or delaying IUI from 90 minutes to 2 hours after collection compromises pregnancy outcome in hMG-IUI cycles. Semen samples should be processed immediately after liquefaction and within 30 minutes of collection, and IUI should be performed immediately after processing and within 90 minutes of collection (Yavas & Selub, 2004).

Methods of Sperm Preparation

The choice of method in sperm preparation is determined by the characteristics of the semen sample and which assisted reproduction technique will be used. The ideal technique should cause minimal DNA damage, not induce dysfunction through ROS production by sperm or leukocytes, and restore maximum quality and number of sperm. When preparing sperm for IUI, indication and purpose of use should be considered in the selection of the method. For example, the technique that is useful in the selection of motile sperm is the direct floatation technique. This technique is usually used when semen samples are considered normal. In cases of oligozoospermia, asthenozoospermia or teratozoospermia, DGC is used because of the higher yield and therefore possibly a higher total number of motile sperm recovered. Although the pellet flotation technique includes centrifugation, which has the risk of adversely affecting other functional parameters of the sperm, it reduced the DNA fragmentation rate as in the direct flotation technique. Variables such as centrifugation time, volume, or density of gradients used can be rearranged according to the characteristics of the sample, thereby optimizing certain properties of the sample. For example, a longer centrifugation time may be preferred when working with high-viscosity samples. The total volume of garnet material can be reduced to maximize total recovery of motile sperm. Each laboratory should meticulously test its modifications in centrifugation time and centrifugal force before clinical application and determine the most appropriate preparation method according to the motility and viability characteristics of the recovered sperm (Björndahl & Brown, 2022).

The efficiency of separating sperm from seminal plasma is evaluated using absolute sperm count, morphologically normal motile sperm count, and total motile sperm count. The DGC method recovers 20% more motile spermatozoa than the swim-up method.

Sperm preparation techniques should ensure the elimination of low quality sperm as well as cells such as leukocytes and bacteria, toxic substances, and bioactive agents. However, these techniques cannot completely isolate infectious agents from semen, so when working with semen in the laboratory, samples should be considered biohazardous and safety precautions must be followed.

As with all therapeutic applications for IUI, semen should be collected in a sterile manner and prepared using sterile techniques and materials.

Simple Wash

A simple washing method, which may be preferred for good quality semen samples, can provide a large amount of spermatozoa, but residues or leukocytes are not removed. Proprietary and appropriately tested products should be used as media, preferably supplemented with human serum albumin or serum.

The semen sample is homogenized with a sterile pipette. The semen sample and the medium are mixed in a 1 / 1 ratio. The diluted sample is divided into tubes, preferably no more than 3 ml in each tube. It is centrifuged at 300-500 g for 5-10 minutes. Supernatants are aspirated and discarded. The pellets are then combined and resuspended in 1 ml of medium by gentle pipetting behavior. Centrifugation is repeated at 300-500g for 3-5 minutes. The supernatant is carefully aspirated and discarded. Sperm pellet is resuspended at the appropriate volume for IUI.

Direct Swim UP

Spermatozoa are selected on the basis of their motility and ability to enter culture media from seminal plasma. Sperm swim up directly from semen without dilution or centrifugation. This technique can be used to prepare sperm for procedures such as IVF, ICSI, in cases where the percentage of motile sperm in semen is low.

Discontinuous Density Gradient Method

The density gradient method is an effective and adaptable method for high-quality sperm recovery, free from other cells and residues. The method prepared with simple two-stage discontinuous density gradients is widely used.

One of the advantages of the density gradient method over the swim up method is that the semen preparation time is shorter. This period can be shortened further, provided that the sample parameters are sufficient. Although it is possible to apply the density gradient method with various agents, density gradients consisting of colloidal silica coated with silane are commonly used. The method works on the following principle: Two gradients and semen with different densities are placed in the same tube and centrifuged, then sperm and other materials form distinct bands. It has been stated that with this method, the isolation of motile and healthy sperm from abnormal and immobile sperm, various residues, and other seminal components is achieved quickly and efficiently (Björndahl & Brown, 2022). When studies comparing CSDG centrifugation with swim-up and other techniques related to sperm preparation were examined, it was concluded that the recovery of motile sperm was higher with gradient techniques. However, the percentage of sperm with progressive motility and the rate of sperm with good morphology are generally lower in the CSDG centrifugation method than in SWIM UP (Centola et al., 1998; Mortimer, 1994).

Example Method for Density Gradient Centrifugation

- 45% stock solution: 45x "SpermGrad" and 55x "SpermRinse" are prepared and heated in an oven at 37°C.
- 90% stock solution: 90x "SpermGrad" and 10x "SpermRinse" are prepared and heated in an oven at 37°C.
- 2.5 ml of "SpermRinse" is heated in a 37°C oven.
- 0.5 ml of "SpermRinse" is heated in a 37°C oven.
- Semen taken by masturbation is expected to liquefy. After liquefaction, semen is homogenized with a sterile pasteur pipette, and the total volume of semen is measured for use in calculations.
- Dispense 1.0 ml of 90% gradient stock solution in a 15 ml conical tube (Falcon 2095, Becton Dickinson, NJ) with a sterile Pasteur pipette.
- Add 1.0 ml of 45% gradient stock solution by leaking it from the side of the tube with a sterile Pasteur pipette (Figure 16.1).
- ~2 mL of semen (fresh or thawed) or sperm suspension is added by leaking it from the side of the tube with a sterile Pasteur pipette (Figure 16.2).

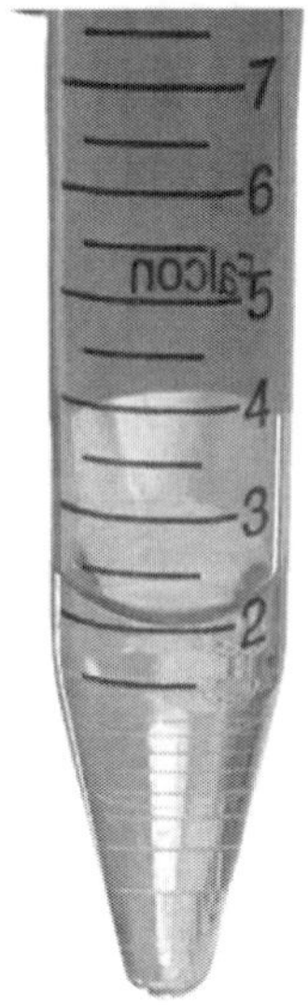

Figure 16.1 Gradients (Author's own archive).

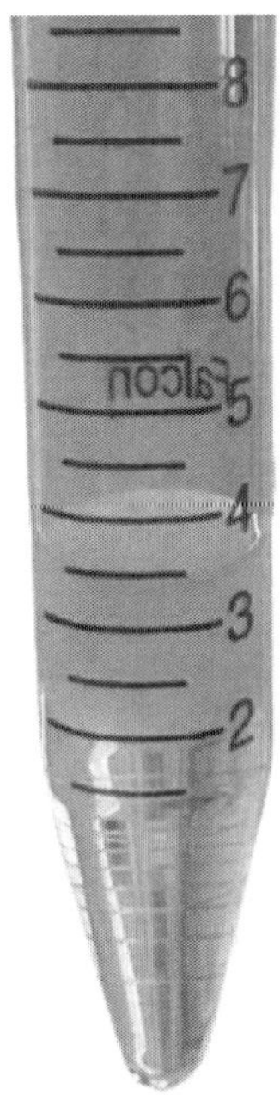

Figure 16.2 View before centrifugation (Author's own archive).

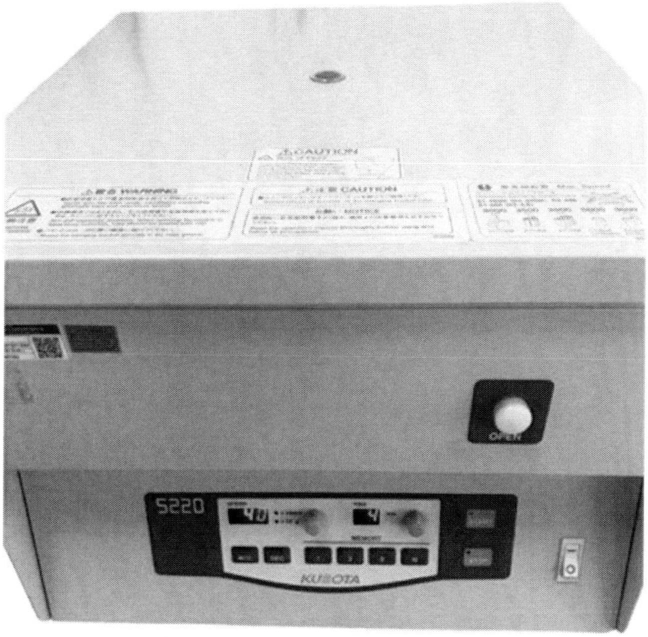

Figure 16.3 Centrifuge device (Author's own archive).

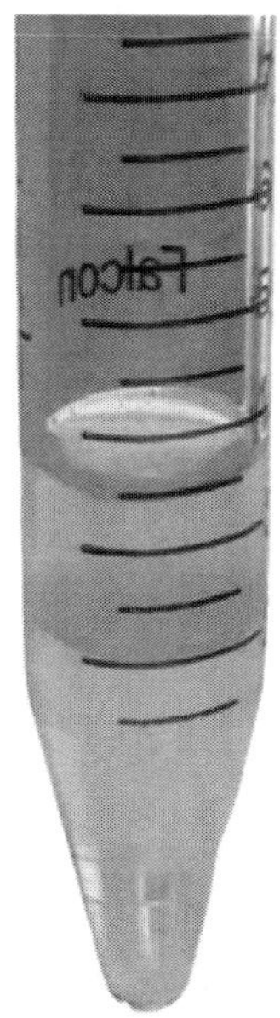

Figure 16.4 View after 1st centrifugation (Author's own archive).

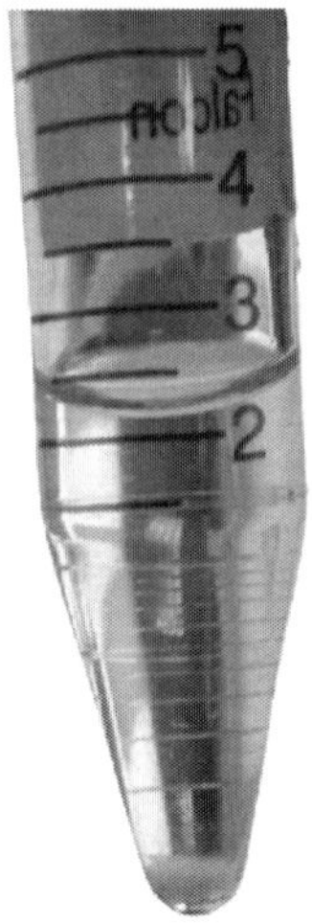

Figure 16.5 View after 2nd centrifugation (Author's own archive).

- Centrifugation can be performed on average for 10 minutes, 400 g, 1450 RPM in the centrifuge (Figure 16.3). After the first centrifugation, a stratified appearance occurs, with the sperm at the bottom and the semen at the top (Figure 16.4).
- After centrifugation, the upper supernatant is taken until approximately 0.5 ml of pellet remains at the bottom. The pellet is resuspended with 2.5 ml of SpermRinse.
- Centrifugation is repeated at an average of 10 minutes, 400 g, 1450 RPM (Figure 16.5).
- This time, the entire supernatant is withdrawn so that only the pellet remains at the bottom. It is desired to remove the residuals of the medium from the environment.
- Then, 0.5 ml of warmed SpermRinse is added to the tube and administered to the inoculation chamber (Gardner et al., 2018).

Conclusion

IUI is a simple, cost-effective noninvasive first-line treatment recommended for indications such as cervical infertility, moderate male factor, anovulatory infertility, disovulation, mild or moderate endometriosis, immunological factors, or unexplained infertility. IUI is an assisted reproductive technique that can be preferred, especially in centers where technological opportunities are limited. Ovarian stimulation is necessary in cases of disovulation, endometriosis, and unexplained infertility. To prevent complications such as multiple pregnancy and ovarian hyperstimulation syndrome (OHSS) and increase the success of IUI, patients should be closely monitored in terms of ovulation control, age, lifestyle and duration of infertility should be evaluated, infertility etiology should be investigated and treatment should be arranged accordingly.

References

Allahbadia, G. N. (2017). Intrauterine Insemination: Fundamentals Revisited. *J Obstet Gynaecol India*, *67*(6), 385-392. https://doi.org/10.1007/s13224-017-1060-x

Björndahl, L., & Brown, J. K. (2022). The sixth edition of the WHO Laboratory Manual for the Examination and Processing of Human Semen: ensuring quality and standardization in basic examination of human ejaculates. *Fertility and Sterility*, *117*(2), 246-251.

Centola, G. M., Herko, R., Andolina, E., & Weisensel, S. (1998). Comparison of sperm separation methods: effect on recovery, motility, motion parameters, and hyperactivation. *FertilSteril*, *70*(6), 1173-1175. https://doi.org/10.1016/s0015-0282 (98)00352-5

Gardner, D. K., Weissman, A., Howles, C. M., & Shoham, Z. (2018). *Textbook of Assisted Reproductive Techniques* (5th ed., Volume 1: Laboratory Perspectives). CRC Press.

Kevin Coward, D. W. (2013). *Textbook of Clinical Embryolog.* Cambridge University Press.

Mortimer, D. (1994). Sperm recovery techniques to maximize fertilizing capacity. *Reprod Fertil Dev*, *6*(1), 25-31. https://doi.org/10.1071/rd9940025

Rizk, B., & Montag, M. (2017). *Standard Operational Procedures in Reproductive Medicine: Laboratory and Clinical Practice.* CRC Press.

Yavas, Y., & Selub, M. R. (2004). Intrauterine insemination (IUI) pregnancy outcome is enhanced by shorter intervals from semen collection to sperm wash, from sperm wash to IUI time, and from semen collection to IUI time. *Fertil Steril*, *82*(6), 1638-1647. https://doi.org/10.1016/j.fertnstert.2004.04.061

Chapter 17

Conventional In Vitro Fertilization

Abdülkadir Kutlu[1], MD* and
Ayşe Firuze Biyik[2], MD

[1]Department of Histology and Embryology, Necip Fazıl City Hospital, Kahramanmaraş, Turkiye

[2]Department of Histology and Embryology, Kanuni Training and Research Hospital, Trabzon, Turkiye

Abstract

The history of reproductive medicine research dates back to ancient times. However, the fact that reproductive physiology is an extremely complex subject and the need for technological developments in this regard have made the discovery of the subject difficult and delayed its detailed explanation. So much so that even the knowledge that fertilization occurs as a result of penetration of a single sperm from the male into the oocyte from the female was only discovered by Hertwig in 1875. In the middle of the 20th century, Thibault achieved fertilization in vitro for the first time as a result of his studies in rabbits. The following year, Chang took this success a step further, succeeding in developing the rabbit embryos he had obtained, and even he transferred an oocyte that he had fertilized in vitro in 1959 and achieved the first live birth. In humans, this success was first achieved by Edwards with the birth of Louis Brown on July 25, 1978. Therefore, it has not been long since in vitro fertilization was first successful as a solution to human infertility, and it can be said that we are witnessing and contributing to a milestone in reproductive medicine.

Key Words: Conventional in vitro fertilization, Assisted reproductive techniques, Infertility, Reproductive medicine

---

* Corresponding Author's E-mail: drabdulkadirkutlu@gmail.com

In: Holistic Approach to Assisted Reproductive Technology
Editor: Kenan Demir and Rümeysa Yılmaz Göç
ISBN: 979-8-89113-017-3
© 2023 Nova Science Publishers, Inc.

Introduction

Conventional in vitro fertilization is of great importance as it forms the basis for assisted reproductive techniques. Because the first pregnancy that was successfully created and concluded in humans through in vitro fertilization was obtained with this method (Johnson, 2019). In this method, each oocyte is placed in an oil-coated culture medium with an optimal sperm concentration in a culture dish, and during incubation, a sperm naturally penetrates the oocyte to fertilize it (Weng, 2019).

Although new techniques have emerged with the rapidly developing technology of today, conventional IVF is still valid in case of indication and is an option that should be tried in suitable patients (tubal factor, endometriosis, male subfertility, unexplained infertility, etc.). It is important to note that, in addition to being cheap and easy to apply, it is a method more similar to the physiological process. In this method, sperm and oocyte are manipulated less, steps such as zona reaction and cortical reaction are not skipped.

On the other hand, the intracytoplasmic sperm injection (ICSI), which is commonly preferred today, is an invasive procedure. It is indicated mainly after severe male factor infertility and fertilization failure. But off-indication use of ICSI is increasing rapidly worldwide, despite evidence showing that, except for its indication, it has no superiority over conventional IVF (Sauerbrun-Cutler et al., 2020). It is forgotten that ICSI has some self-limiting features, such as bypassing the natural selection checkpoints of the oocyte and therefore incorporating potentially genetically defective materials into the process. Furthermore, the sperm to be used in ICSI applications are subjectively selected by the person applying the treatment, and it is not known whether the selected sperm has the capacity to fertilize the oocyte under physiological conditions. In addition, ICSI is a method that can damage meiotic spindles, trigger aneuploidies, cause weak oocyte activation, negatively affect sperm chromatin decompression, or inject unwanted substances into the oocyte together with sperm (Giacobbe et al., 2022). It must be a natural result of moving away from physiological functioning, even though it is not necessary, there are publications reporting that babies born after ICSI use are at higher risk of congenital malformations, are admitted to neonatal intensive care units at a higher rate, and have a higher risk of autism and intellectual disability (Liu et al., 2020).

For all these reasons, conventional IVF is an assisted reproductive technique that is still being applied by many centers and should never be ignored.

Methods

Ovarian Stimulation

First, by applying the appropriate protocol to the patient, early ovulation is prevented and controlled ovarian hyperstimulation is provided. The development of follicles is observed by monitoring serum estradiol levels and performing transvaginal USG for folliculometry (Zhu et al., 2022). The right time for ovulation induction is waited and when the appropriate follicle sizes and compatible estradiol levels are obtained, ovulation is triggered by human chorionic gonadotropin (hCG) injection. Oocyte pick-up (OPU) is performed 34-36 hours after hCG injection. Endometrial preparation and treatment with luteal support are started the next morning (Sauerbrun-Cutler et al., 2020).

The natural cycle method can also be used for the retrieval of oocytes. The oocyte used in the IVF experiment that resulted in the birth of Louis Brown was obtained by this method (Johnson, 2019). In this method, the patient's normal menstrual cycle is not affected and the date of ovulation can be estimated by monitoring serum or urinary levels of luteinizing hormone (LH). Approximately 36 hours after detection of the LH peak, the oocyte is collected by aspiration under the guidance of transvaginal USG. Although this method is positive in terms of purely physiological selection of the oocyte, it often has a low success rate because only one oocyte is obtained. Therefore, its use has been almost completely abandoned, except in rare places.

Oocyte Preparation

To keep the oocytes at 37°C, all the equipment to be used must be ready and collection tubes, dishes in which oocytes will be collected and evaluated, wash media, incubation media, mineral oils should be prewarmed. In addition, the pH of the incubation media and the mineral oils that will cover the media should be adjusted so that the oocytes are not damaged.

First, the obtained cumulus-oocyte complexes (COC) are transferred to the washing medium under a stereomicroscope and purified from unwanted structures such as blood, secretion, cell debris, etc. The cumulus cells are then mechanically partially loosened with a sterile needle tip (Kobayashi et al., 2021). Clearing large granulosa cell masses will facilitate evaluation of oocyte maturation and increase the ability of sperm to fertilize the oocyte during insemination. At this stage, of course, it is not possible to clearly determine the maturation of the oocytes, but an idea can still be obtained. After a rough evaluation of the maturation of oocytes under an inverted microscope with Hoffman modulation contrast or equivalent objective attachment, the cumulus-oocyte complexes are transferred to fertilization medium and incubated for approximately 3 hours in an incubator with 37°C, 5% O_2, 5-6% CO_2 (Goswami & Gouri, 2020). To be incubated in a media with a suitable pH for a while would be good for the oocytes that have been in the washing medium whose pH is adversely affected by blood, secretion, cell debris, etc. Cumulus-oocyte complexes can be incubated individually in microdroplets or collectively in a center-well or four-well dish preferably not more than 8 COCs in 1 ml of medium. The incubation period can be extended depending on the degree of maturation of the oocytes.

Sperm Preparation

Since conventional IVF is an effective and preferred method in infertility cases without severe male factor, the number of progressively motile spermatozoa to be used for insemination should be sufficient to prefer conventional IVF (0,1 – 0,5 x 10^6/ ml) (European Society of Human Reproduction and Embryology (ESHRE), 2016). Therefore, it is essential to perform at least one semen analysis before starting a treatment cycle to decide on the treatment protocol to be applied.

The ejaculate should be collected after 2-7 days of abstinence without loss of sample (World Health Organization, 2021). On the day of oocyte retrieval (OPU), the male semen sample is placed in a sterile plastic container, preferably 1-2 hours before insemination, in an oven (20-37°C) for liquefaction after macroscopic analysis. After liquefaction, the semen is evaluated under a phase contrast microscope and according to the results of this analysis an appropriate sperm preparation technique is applied. In this way, progressive motile sperm are substantially concentrated and purified from seminal plasma, dead and abnormal sperm, debris, and waste (ESHRE, 2016). The new concentration is determined by making a re-evaluation under the microscope. The sperm are then kept in an incubator at 37°C, 5% CO_2 in order to balance the pH until the time of insemination (van der Westerlaken et al., 2005; Kong et al., 2021). Waiting at room temperature after 30 minutes of incubation is also one of the preferred methods.

Insemination

Large-Volume Culture

Large-volume culture dishes such as center-well dish or four-well dish, are often preferred in the insemination process (Ten et al., 2022). In this way, the effect of the liquid containing concentrated sperm to be added to the culture medium for insemination is minimized on the temperature and pH of the fertilization medium, and also an area to move is provided for sperms. Preferably, 0.75-1 ml of fertilization medium is placed in the center-well dish compartment or in each compartment of the four-well dish and then covered with mineral oil. Care should be taken not to completely fill the compartments so that the liquids do not get on the lid of the dish with the force of adhesion. The dishes are incubated for a minimum of 4 hours in an incubator with 37°C, 5% O_2, 5-6% CO_2 to provide the temperature and pH balances of the fertilization media and mineral oils. A sufficient number of culture dishes should be prepared in advance according to the expected number of COC.

Just before the time of insemination, the prepared sperm sample is evaluated for the last time to ensure concentration. Then, the number of motile sperm required for insemination of each cumulus-oocyte complex is determined. It is important to determine this number carefully. Because a low number of sperm per oocyte can cause fertilization failures and an excess can cause polyploidies. Normally, it is appropriate to use 0.5-1 x 10^5 motile spermatozoa for each cumulus-oocyte complex (Goswami & Gouri, 2020). However, if necessary, this number can be increased to 5 x 10^5 per COC. The criterion to be taken as a basis for making the right decision about the number is the observed movement capacity of the sperm. After deciding on the number of sperm to be used per COC, the volume of fluid containing this number of motile sperm is calculated. In patients with high sperm concentration, this volume may appear as an extremely low value. In such cases, the liquid containing concentrated motile sperm is diluted as necessary.

The cumulus-oocyte complexes, which are incubated and stabilized, are transferred to preheated and pH-balanced mineral oil-coated fertilization media for insemination. It would be appropriate to ensure that the number of COCs placed in each compartment should preferably not exceed 8. Then, the calculated volume of liquid from the prepared sperm sample is gently dropped into the chambers at a 45° angle with the help of a micropipette. After a final microscope control, the culture dishes are removed to an incubator with 37°C, 5% O_2, 5-6% CO_2 for insemination.

Although 2-3 hours of incubation is often sufficient for insemination, overnight incubation may be preferred depending on the conditions of the center where the application is made (Isikoglu et al., 2021; Gunderson et al., 2021). If 2-3 hours of incubation is preferred, sperm must be removed from oocytes at the end of the insemination period and incubation should continue in clean culture media.

Droplet Culture

Another method of insemination is the droplet culture method. In this method, a sufficient number of microdroplets of 50-80 µl are formed with fertilization medium in Petri dishes (Zhu et al., 2022; Deng et al., 2020). Fertilization

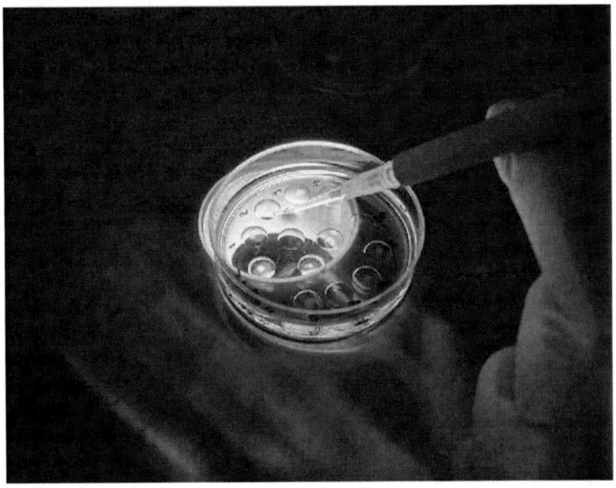

Figure 17.1 Insemination by the droplet culture method (Author's own archive).

mediums covered with mineral oil are incubated for sufficient time (min. 4 hours) in an incubator with 37°C, 5% O_2, 5-6% CO_2 for the temperature and pH balance to ensure that they are ready at the time of insemination. At the time of insemination, preferably, 1-2 cumulus-oocyte complexes are placed in each microdroplet. Then the liquid containing a sufficient number of sperm is added gently and the dishes are allowed to re-incubate, this time for insemination (Figure 17.1).

Fertilization Control

The addition of sperm to the fertilization medium containing cumulus-oocyte complexes is considered the beginning of insemination and fertilization control should be performed approximately 16-18 hours after this. As first, mechanical denudation is applied to the cumulus-oocyte complexes with the help of a pipette for this purpose. At this stage, it will be seen that the granulosa cells are spilled more easily compared to before incubation and denudation results in more success. In this way, pronucleus (PN) controls of oocytes will be easier to perform.

Since 2 PNs should be seen in oocytes fertilized with a single sperm as desired, oocytes with more than 2 PNs should be separated. If these oocytes pass to the division stage, it will no longer be possible to distinguish them. Rescue ICSI can be applied to oocytes without PN seen in fertilization control. Oocytes with 2 PNs and thus successfully pass the fertilization control are left to develop in previously prepared culture media coated with mineral oil with

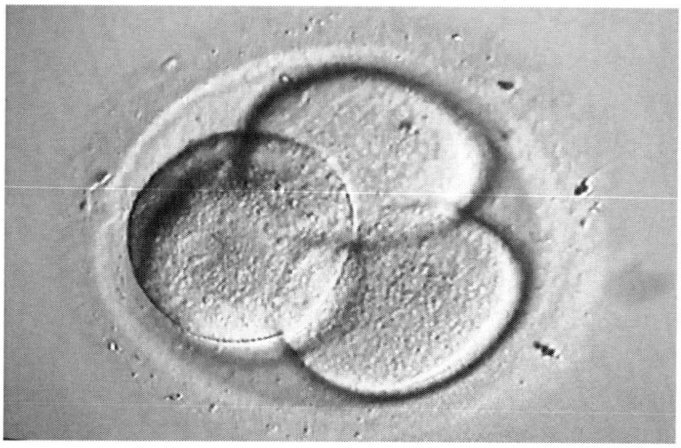

Figure 17.2 An embryo 45-46 hours after insemination with cIVF (Author's own archive).

temperature and pH balance in an incubator with 37°C, 5% O_2, 5-6% CO_2. At this stage, it would be more appropriate to follow the oocytes separately using the droplet culture method to avoid confusion in the follow-up of their development (Figure 17.2).

Conclusion

As we mentioned before, it has not been a long time since the success of assisted reproduction techniques in humans. Therefore, it is not possible to talk about definitive protocols on this subject yet. Each laboratory may have applications based on their own experience, different from the ones we have mentioned. However, it should never be forgotten that classical IVF is an assisted reproductive technique that should not be ignored if indicated.

References

Deng, J., Kuyoro, O., Zhao, Q., Behr, B., & Lathi, R. B. (2020). Comparison of aneuploidy rates between conventional in vitro fertilization and intracytoplasmic sperm injection in in vitro fertilization–intracytoplasmic sperm injection split insemination cycles. *F&S Reports*, 1(3), 277-281. https://doi.org/10.1016/j.xfre.2020.07.006

European Society of Human Reproduction and Embryology (ESHRE) Guideline Group on Good Practice in IVF Labs. (2016). Revised guidelines for good practice in IVF laboratories. Retrieved November 24, 2022 from https://www.eshre.eu/Guidelines-and-Legal/Guidelines/Revised-guidelines-for-good-practice-in-IVF-laboratories-(2015)

Giacobbe, M., Conatti, M., Gomes, A., Bonetti, T. C., & Monteleone, P. A. (2022). Effectivity of conventional in vitro fertilization (IVF) and intracytoplasmic sperm injection (ICSI) when male factor is absent: a perspective point of view. *JBRA assisted reproduction*, *26*(1), 123–128. https://doi.org/10.5935/1518-0557.20210031

Goswami, G., & Gouri, M. D. (2020). Relevance of Split In vitro Fertilization-Intracytoplasmic Sperm Injection Method of Insemination in Normozoospermic and Mildly Oligospermic Men: A Retrospective Study. *Journal of Human Reproductive Sciences*, 13(2), 145–149. https://doi.org/10.4103/jhrs.JHRS_19_19

Gunderson, S. J., Molina, L. C. P., Spies, N., Balestrini, P. A., Buffone, M. G., Jungheim, E. S., Riley, J., & Santi, C. M. (2021). Machine-learning algorithm incorporating capacitated sperm intracellular pH predicts conventional in vitro fertilization success in normospermic patients. *Fertility and Sterility*, 115(4), 930-939. https://doi.org/10.1016/j.fertnstert.2020.10.038

Isikoglu, M., Avci, A., Ceviren, A. K., Aydınuraz, B., & Ata, B. (2021). Conventional IVF revisited: Is ICSI better for non-male factor infertility? Randomized controlled double blind study. *Journal of Gynecology Obstetrics and Human Reproduction*, 50(7), 101990. https://doi.org/10.1016/j.jogoh.2020.101990

Johnson, M. H. (2019). A short history of in vitro fertilization (IVF). *International Journal of Developmental Biology*, *63*(3-4-5), 83-92. https://doi.org/10.1387/ijdb.180364mj

Kobayashi, T., Ishikawa, H., Ishii, K., Sato, A., Nakamura, N., Saito, Y., Hasegawa, H., Fujita, M., Mitsuhashi, A., & Shozu, M. (2021). Time-lapse monitoring of fertilized human oocytes focused on the incidence of 0PN embryos in conventional in vitro fertilization cycles. *Scientific reports*, *11*(1), 1-7. https://doi.org/10.1038/s41598-021-98312-1

Kong, P., Yin, M., Tang, C., Zhu, X., Bukulmez, O., Chen, M., & Teng, X. (2021). Effects of early cumulus cell removal on treatment outcomes in patients undergoing in vitro fertilization: a retrospective cohort study. *Frontiers in Endocrinology*, 12, 669507. https://doi.org/10.3389/fendo.2021.669507

Liu, L., Wang, H., Li, Z., Niu, J., & Tang, R. (2020). Obstetric and perinatal outcomes of intracytoplasmic sperm injection versus conventional in vitro fertilization in couples with nonsevere male infertility. *Fertility and Sterility*, *114*(4), 792-800. https://doi.org/10.1016/j.fertnstert.2020.04.058

Sauerbrun-Cutler, M. T., Huber, W. J., Has, P., Shen, C., Hackett, R., Alvero, R., & Wang, S. (2020). Is intracytoplasmic sperm (ICSI) better than traditional in vitro fertilization (IVF): confirmation of higher blastocyst rates per oocyte using a split insemination design. *Journal of Assisted Reproduction and Genetics*, *37*(7), 1661-1667. https://doi.org/10.1007/s10815-020-01819-1

Ten, J., Peinado, P., Guerrero, J., Bernabeu, A., Llácer, J., Orozco-Beltran, D., Carratala-Munuera, C., & Bernabeu, R. (2022). Comparison of the assisted reproductive technology outcomes between conventional IVF and ICSI with donor oocytes in normozoospermic patients. *Human Fertility*, 25(1), 56-62. https://doi.org/10.1080/14647273.2019.1686775

van der Westerlaken, L., Helmerhorst, F., Dieben, S., & Naaktgeboren, N. (2005). Intracytoplasmic sperm injection as a treatment for unexplained total fertilization failure or low fertilization after conventional in vitro fertilization. *Fertility and sterility*, *83*(3), 612-617. https://doi.org/10.1016/j.fertnstert.2004.08.029

Weng, L. (2019). IVF-on-a-Chip: recent advances in microfluidics technology for in vitro fertilization. *SLAS Technology: Translating Life Sciences Innovation*, *24*(4), 373-385. https://doi.org/10.1177/2472630319851765

World Health Organization. (2021). WHO laboratory manual for the examination and processing of human semen. Retrieved November 24, 2022 from https://apps.who.int/iris/rest/bitstreams/1358672/retrieve

Zhu, Y., Zhang, F., Cheng, H., Sun, X. X., & Jiang, F. (2022). Modified strict sperm morphology threshold aids in the clinical selection of conventional in vitro fertilization (IVF) or intracytoplasmic sperm injection (ICSI). *Asian Journal of Andrology*, 24(1), 62–66. https://doi.org/10.4103/aja.aja_45_21

Chapter 18

Human Embryo Development and Assessment of Viability

Yasemin Yuksel, MD*

Center for Assisted Reproduction, Obstetrics and Gynecology Clinics, Ankara City Hospital, Ankara, Turkiye

Abstract

The number of embryos transferred to patients has been recently limited in many countries in Europe to prevent complications that may occur as a result of multiple pregnancy. The main purpose of embryo selection is to reduce the number of transferred embryos for decreasing the incidence of multiple pregnancy and to increase success rates. Therefore, it is very important to evaluate the embryo at every stage of development and to choose the embryo with the highest potential for implantation.

Especially in the last 30 years, dynamic evaluation and imaging systems with time-lapse microscopy, comparative genomic hybridization sequence investigation, and metabolomics have been used in addition to morphological evaluations for embryo selection and evaluation. Morphological evaluation criteria are still the primary and most widely used method among these. To date, many embryo scoring systems have been developed and published in order to evaluate the developmental potential of embryos in assisted reproductive techniques. Due to the diversity of the methods for classifying embryos in different countries, criteria that can be used routinely in all IVF laboratories for oocyte, zygote, and embryo classification were determined by the Alpha and ESHRE consensus in 2011 to standardize the classification methods throughout the world. The aim is to select embryos with healthy pregnancy potential by evaluating the number and cleavage rate of blastomeres, percentage of fragmentation, blastomere size, nuclear status of blastomeres, degree of compaction of the embryo,

* Corresponding Author's Email: dryuksely@gmail.com

In: Holistic Approach to Assisted Reproductive Technology
Editor: Kenan Demir and Rümeysa Yılmaz Göç
ISBN: 979-8-89113-017-3
© 2023 Nova Science Publishers, Inc.

and then in the blastocyst stage, blastocoel width, inner cell mass, and trophectoderm development using these criteria, by an experienced embryologist along with an optimized embryo culture medium.

Key Words: Embryo viability, Embryo development, Embryo morphology, Embryo cleavage

Introduction

The main purpose of in vitro fertilization techniques is to select the best quality embryo with the highest implantation potential using non-invasive techniques and to obtain a healthy pregnancy and live birth. The quality of the developing embryo after a successful fertilization process is directly related to pregnancy. Many clinicians aim to increase pregnancy rates by transferring more than one embryo in one cycle. In many countries in Europe, it is recommended that the number of embryos transferred to the patient be single due to the high costs of multiple pregnancy, as well as the serious risks of multiple pregnancy-related conditions for the mother and baby. Transfer of one or two embryos with the highest quality is recommended both for avoiding these side effects of multiple pregnancy and increasing implantation, pregnancy, and live birth rates (Racowsky et al., 2010).

Gametes and embryos were evaluated since the beginning of IVF to define embryo development (R. G. Edwards et al., 1981) and afterward to select the embryo that has the highest implantation potential (Alpha & ESHRE, 2011; Desai et al., 2000; Hill et al., 1989; Racowsky et al., 2010). Morphological evaluation, time-lapse imaging systems and also metabolomic research are used to evaluate embryos in IVF laboratories and to select the embryo with the highest implantation potential (Marhuenda-Egea et al., 2010; Milewski et al., 2015). The most widely used method among these is noninvasive morphological evaluations (Maxwell et al., 2015; Racowsky et al., 2010). To date, many embryo scoring systems have been developed and published to rate the developmental potential of embryos in assisted reproductive techniques. Due to the diversity of the methods for classifying embryos in different countries, criteria that can be used routinely in all IVF laboratories for oocyte, zygote, and embryo classification were determined by the Alpha and ESHRE consensus in 2011 to standardize the classification methods throughout the world (Alpha & ESHRE, 2011). Embryos with healthy pregnancy potential are selected after determining various criteria such as the distribution of blastomeres and cytoplasmic features such as cell number, fragmentation rate, size, and cleavage rate of blastomeres, mononuclear or multinuclear condition of blastomeres based on morphological features of the embryo in a process that requires an experienced embryologist along with an optimized embryo culture medium (Brison et al., 2004; Meseguer et al., 2011).

In conventional morphological evaluations, evaluation of embryo development begins with fertilization control, and embryos are get out of the incubator at a certain time in every day, and the predefined morphological features are evaluated and scored under the invert microscope as soon as possible, and then the embryos are put back into the incubator again. This scoring process repeats until embryo transfer. Since embryo development is a dynamic process, embryos should be evaluated in the same time zone every day. The time of observation of the embryo and the developmental stages recommended by the consensus of Alpha and ESHRE are given in Table 18.1 (Alpha & ESHRE, 2011). After controlling for fertilization, the zygotes are numbered and individually followed up in different drops in culture dishes in an incubator until the transfer process. The first cleavage phase generally begins about 3 hours after the break down of pronuclear membranes (Borini et al., 2005; Dennis et al., 2006; Ebner et al., 2003; Lee et al., 2012). At the end of the embryo follow-up and scoring processes, the best quality embryo(s) is selected and transferred to the patient's uterus. If the patient has enough quality embryos to be frozen after transfer, the freezing procedure can be applied.

Time-lapse microscopy, comparative genomic hybridization sequence investigation, and metabolomic investigations can be used in addition to non-invasive morphological evaluation for embryo selection (Nel-Themaat & Nagy, 2011). Systems such as time-lapse microscopy are carried out with a monitor

Table 18.1 Timing of observation for fertilized oocytes and embryos, and expected stage of development at each time point (Alpha & ESHRE, 2011).

Type of observation	Timing (hours after insemination)	Expected stage of development
Fertilization check	17±1	Pronuclear stage
Syngamy check	23±1	Expect 50% to be in syngamy (up to 20% may be at the 2 cell stage)
Early cleavage check	26±1 (post ICSI) 28±1 (post-IVF)	2 cell stage
Day 2 embryo assessment	44±1	4 cell stage
Day 3 embryo assessment	68±1	8 cell stage
Day 4 embryo assessment	92±2	Morula
Day 5 embryo assessment	116±2	Blastocyt

ICSI = intracytoplazmic sperm injection. IVF = conventional in vitro fertilization.

placed in the incubator device without the need to remove the embryos from the incubator and an automated system that transfers the data to the computer environment. Embryo development is a dynamic process. Although these systems are costly, they are useful because they can provide more data about the embryo and optimize the selection parameters morphologically. Also, there is no time constraint when evaluating the embryos and there is no need to take embryos out of the incubator, which protects the cells from both heat loss and pH changes (Hnida et al., 2004).

Morphological Evaluation of the Embryo

Morphological Evaluation of Embryo at Cleavage Stage

Detection of early cleavage (EC), blastomere number and cleavage rate, shape and size of blastomeres, amount of fragmentation in embryos, nuclei, and cytoplasmic characteristics of blastomeres are taken into account when the cleavage stage in embryo selection and scoring is evaluated. A good-quality cleavage embryo has been associated with high implantation rates in all studies (Cheng-He et al., 2018; Gardner & Balaban, 2016).

Early Cleavage (EC)

The morphology of the pronucleus and early cleavage status are evaluated on the first day of embryo development. Some embryos progress to the early cleavage stage to form two sister blastomeres after fertilization (26±1 hours after ICSI and 28±1 hours after conventional IVF, are shown in Table 18.1). The timing of the first stage of cleavage has been the subject of research, and early cleavage has been identified as a positive indicator of embryo development. However, rapid cleavage of embryos before the 20th hour has been defined as a poor prognostic marker for the embryo (Hardarson et al., 2006; Lee et al., 2012). When early- and late-cleavage stage embryos are compared in studies, it has been shown that viability and quality are better, rate of development of blastocyst and pregnancy are higher, rate of miscarriage is lesser, and euploid rates are better in early-cleavage stage embryos (Giorgetti et al., 2007; Thurin et al., 2005; Van Montfoort et al., 2004). At the same time, it has not been recognized as a reliable predictor of implantation in good-quality embryo transfers in some studies. Early cleavage has been evaluated as one of the key performance criteria by Alpha consensus in 2017. In the Alpha survey, the competence and benchmark values ranged from 10 to 50% and 15 to 60%, respectively (Alpha & ESHRE, 2017) (Figure 18.1, Figure 18.2).

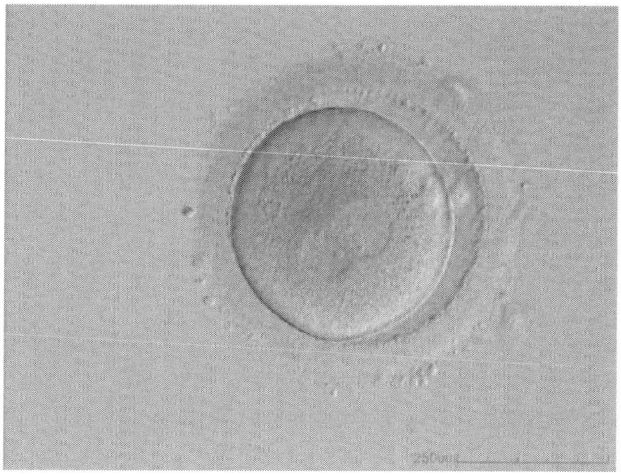

Figure 18.1 Two-pronucleus image after fertilization. (author's own archive)

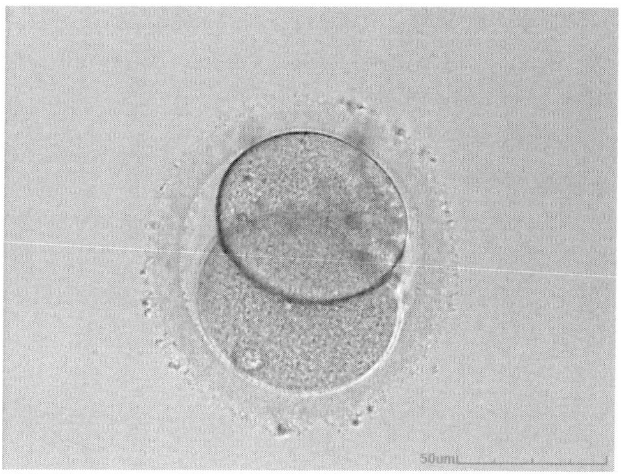

Figure 18.2 Early cleavage embryo (two cells) (author's own archive)

Blastomere Number and Cleavage Speed

Embryo cleavage status and speed are accepted as the most important indicators of embryo viability (Holte et al., 2007; Lee et al., 2012; MacHtinger & Racowsky, 2013). Blastomeres form two blastomeres of equal size, smaller than the original size, during embryo development by losing their volume as a result of mitosis. As a result, the number of blastomeres increases as a multiple of two. It is extremely important for the rate of cleavage to proceed at an optimal level.

According to the consensus criteria of Alpha and ESHRE, embryos with optimal cleavage rate (Table 18.1) and synchronous cleavage are expected to have 4 cells (blastomere) on day 2 and 8 cells on day 3 after fertilization, respectively (Alpha & ESHRE, 2011; Hossain et al., 2016). It was reported that when cleavage is too slow or too fast with nonoptimal cleavage speed, the incidence of chromosomal disorders is increased in correlation with lower quality embryo development, resulting with poor implantation and pregnancy when compared to embryos with optimal cleavage speed. It has also been shown that medium and culture conditions may also affect the rate of embryo development (M. Cristina Magli et al., 2007; Prados et al., 2012).

If the rate of cleavage does not occur simultaneously in all blastomeres, embryos with different blastomere numbers (five, six, or seven) may occur. For example, if an embryo with three blastomeres consists of one large and two small ones, it is understood that one blastomere was divided at the time of evaluation and the other is not yet divided. Contrary to this, if an embryo with 3 blastomeres consists of 3 blastomeres of equal size, this can be evaluated as a negative cleavage pattern for the embryo, and this is called direct cleavage (Direct Unequal Cleavage). The frequency of this cleavage pattern was found to be higher, especially in embryos inseminated with epididymal and testicular sperm, compared to inseminations with ejaculate sperm. The development of blastocysts and the rate of implantation are lower in embryos that undergo direct cleavage (Rubio et al., 2012; Sela et al., 2012).

The rate of pregnancy and aneuploidy was found to be lower in embryos with an odd number of asynchronously dividing blastomeres such as 3,5,7,9 compared to those with synchronous and optimal cleavage (Guerif et al., 2007; M. C. Magli et al., 2001; Prados et al., 2012) (Figure 18.3, Figure 18.4).

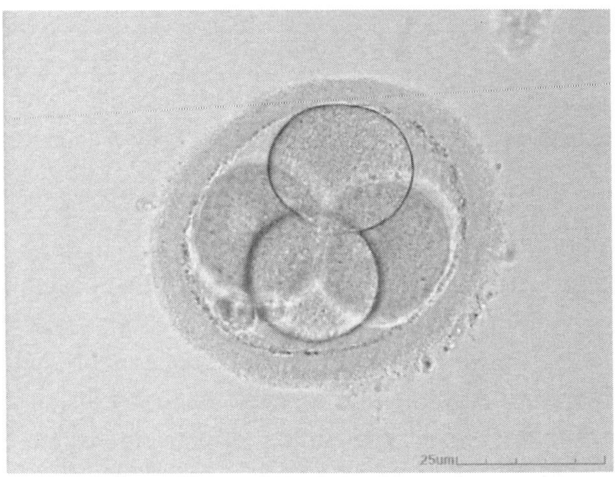

Figure 18.3 Consisted of 4-cells (even-equal size blastomeres, nucleus structure is clearly seen in the left blastomere) grade 1 embryo on day 2 after insemination (author's own archive).

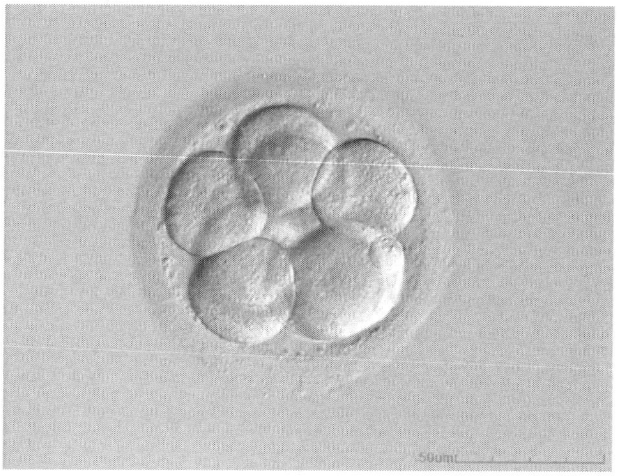

Figure 18.4 Grade 1 embryo with 8 cells (blastomeres of equal size) on day 3 after insemination (author's own archive).

Blastomere Symmetry

The symmetry of the blastomeres is also related to the developmental capacity of the embryo similar to the speed of cleavage and the number of the blastomeres. The size and shape of dividing cells are evaluated in blastomere symmetry (Rienzi et al., 2005). Equal blastomere sizes after cleavage are considered normal as even cleavage. If the size difference between the blastomeres is more than 25%, it is named an uneven cleavage (Paternot et al., 2011).

In case of uneven cleavage of blastomeres, embryo development is negatively affected since the distribution of mRNA, protein, mitochondria, and different cell organelles in sister blastomeres cannot be equal. For this reason, in the presence of a large blastomer, it should be defined whether the blastomere that has not yet entered the cleavage stage or blastomere formed after uneven cleavage by examining the cell count and status during embryo follow-up (Giorgetti et al., 1995). Studies have shown that uneven cleavage has negative effects on both implantation and pregnancy rates and contains higher aneuploidy and multinucleation than embryos with equal blastomeres (Hardarson et al., 2001; M. C. Magli et al., 2001) (Figure 18.5, Figure 18.6).

Fragmentation

Fragmentation is an important parameter among the evaluation criteria, since it greatly affects the development process and quality of embryos. Fragments are non-nuclear cytoplasmic particles originating from blastomeres that emerge during cell division. They are thought to originate from apoptosis (Dawson et al., 1995). To differentiate large fragmentations from blastomeres, annuclear

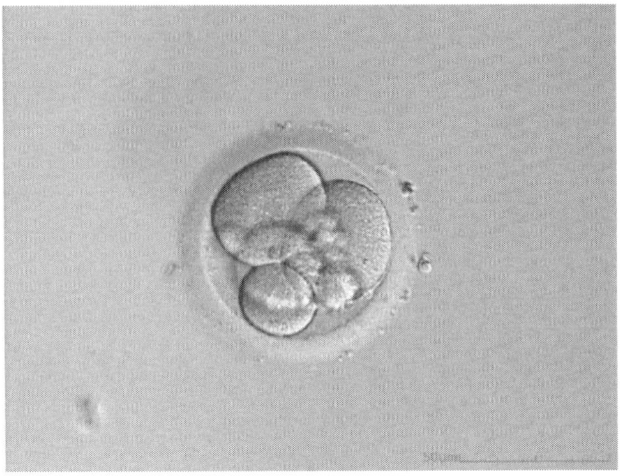

Figure 18.5 The embryo consisted of 4-cells (uneven-not equal-size blastomeres) on the second day (author's own archive).

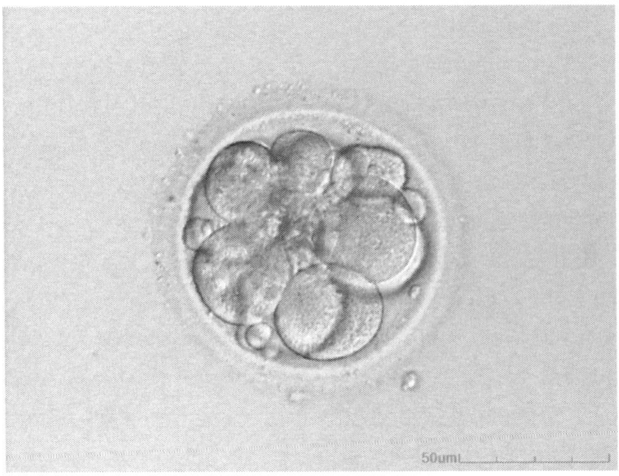

Figure 18.6 The embryo consisted of 9 cells (uneven-not equal-size blastomeres) on the third day (author's own archive).

structures smaller than 45 μm on the 2nd day and 40 μm on the 3rd day were named as fragmentation. Fragments often occur during embryo cleavage and are the result of defective embryogenesis. Fragmentation has been suggested to also occur as a result of abnormalities in cell division and metabolism, or as a result of damage to the cytoskeleton and mitotic network (Munné et al., 1994). Although the mechanism is not clear, some researchers have argued that the degree of fragmentation is reduced by the resorption of adjacent blastomeres (Hardarson et al., 2002).

As the degree of fragmentation (>25%) increases, there may be a decrease in the amount of cell organelles and important cytoplasmic structures such as mRNA, mitochondria, proteins. Therefore, large fragmentation results in blastomere formation that is quantitatively insufficient in terms of blastomeric volume (Johansson et al., 2003). In addition, excessive fragmentation can prevent the formation of tight junction complexes and desmosomes between blastomeres and also disrupt the cleavage plane, causing abnormal compaction and cavitation. Thus, it may impair blastocyst formation by negatively affecting embryo development (Alikani et al., 1999; Keltz et al., 2006). In the general evaluation of embryo fragmentation, subjective evaluations are performed based on the embryologist instead of clear objective measurements. The rate of fragmentation can be subjectively determined according to the volume of blastomere. Objective measurements are only possible with measurements made according to images obtained from different levels (Johansson et al., 2003; Vergouw et al., 2013).

The incidence of chromosomal disorders in embryos increases with increasing fragmentation. Large amounts of fragmentation have been associated with genetic abnormalities such as aneuploidy and mosaicism (Chavez et al., 2012; Munné, 1998). In addition to the amount of fragmentation, its pattern can also affect implantation. It was also observed in studies that the rates of implantation and pregnancy are decreased in embryos with large fragmentation asymmetrically located (Ebner et al., 2001; Giorgetti et al., 1995; Ziebe et al., 1997). It has been shown in studies that the presence of minimal fragmentation may be a part of normal embryo development and does not affect implantation (Fujimoto et al., 2011; Johansson et al., 2003). In other studies, fragmentation between the threshold value of 10-20% has been shown to not adversely affect pregnancy outcomes (Staessen et al., 1992; Van Royen et al., 2001; Ziebe et al., 1997). In a study, embryos on day 3 with less than 20% fragmentation had similar implantation with blastocyst transfers (Bungum et al., 2003).

According to the consensus of Alpha and ESHRE consensus, <10% fragmentation on day 2 and 3 reflects the viability and quality of the embryo. According to the Alpha questionnaire, the efficiency value for fragmentation ranges from 20-90% (mean 50%) and the expected value ranges from 30-90% (mean 70%). Since the determination of the amount of fragmentation is subjective, these value ranges are kept very wide and evaluated in the group of less important quality indicators (Alpha & ESHRE, 2017) (Figure 18.7, Figure 18.8).

Nucleus Structure and Multinucleation

One of the features that should be taken into account when evaluating embryos is the structure of the nucleus in the blastomeres. Since the structure of the

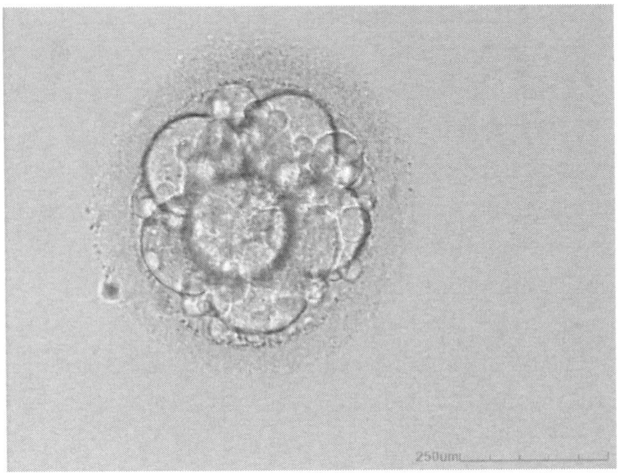

Figure 18.7 The embryo consisted of 8 cells, which had fragmentation on the 3rd day (author's own archive).

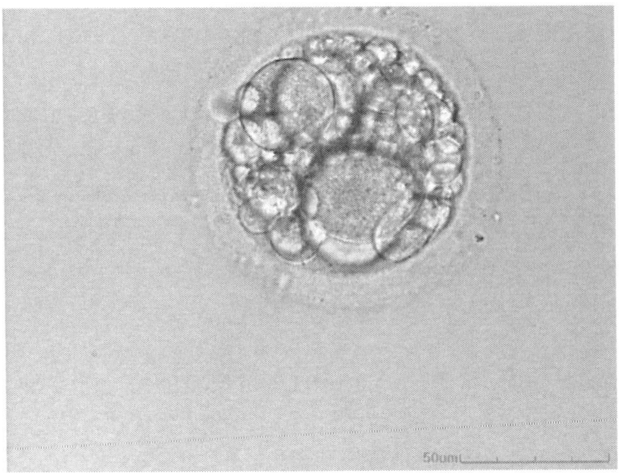

Figure 18.8 The embryo consisted of 5-cells has intense fragmentation on the 3rd day (author's own archive).

nucleus can only be observed in the interphase phase of cleavage, the nucleus may not be observed when evaluating the time of embryos. The number of enucleated embryos at the time of evaluation is generally higher than mononuclear or multinuclear embryos. Nuclei can be easily observed in blastomeres on the day 2 and day 3 controls. Since the number of blastomeres is low and the volume of blastomeres is larger in the 2nd day controls, the nuclear structure can be evaluated more clearly. A single nucleus should be observed in a normal blastomere structure. If karyokinesis occurs without cytokinesis during cleavage, multinucleation occurs in the blastomere. In such cases, nuclear structures with more than one nucleus or multiple fragmented nuclear structures are observed in a single blastomere. These blastomeres are generally larger than normal blastomeres. It is especially more common in embryos with uneven cleavage (Hardarson et al., 2001; Hnida et al., 2004).

The prevalence of multinucleation is lower in embryos with synchronous cleavage and normal development, which have 4 cells on day 2 and 8 cells on day 3. The presence of multinuclear embryos is 30% more frequent in asynchronous cleavage compared to synchronous embryos, for example, in 3-cell embryos compared to 2- or 4-cell embryos (Roux et al., 1995). Additionally, multinucleation has been suggested to result from errors during chromosome migrations in mitosis, mispackaging of chromosomes by nuclear membranes, nuclear fragmentation, or asymmetric cytokinesis (Hardy, 1999; Johansson et al., 2003; Pickering et al., 1995). Since multinucleation also affects embryo quality and implantation potential, it has been included in embryo evaluation criteria by the Alpha and ESHRE consensus indicator (Alpha & ESHRE, 2011). However, since the evaluation hours determined by the Alpha and ESHRE consensus (Table 18.1) do not coincide with the frequency of multinucleation in embryos, it may not be possible to determine the exact frequency of multinucleation for each embryo unless dynamic imaging systems are available.

The frequency of aneuploidy increases in multinuclear embryos. For this reason, multinucleation is carefully investigated, especially on the 2nd day of controls, and it is recommended to note the presence. Multinucleated embryos have been observed to compact by leaving out some blastomeres and repair themselves during the blastocyst development stage. Normal birth can also be seen after multinuclear embryo transfer. However, the embryo without multinucleation should be preferred when choosing embryos for transfer due to the lower implantation and pregnancy rates in multinuclear embryos compared to mononuclear embryos (Alpha & ESHRE, 2011; Desch et al., 2017; Jackson et al., 1998; Prados et al., 2012) (Figure 18.9, Figure 18.10).

Cytoplasmic Characteristics

A good blastomere should have a uniform shape, a lighter colored cytoplasm, and a homogeneous structure with less granulation (Hartshorne, 2000). Cytoplasmic granulation, cytoplasmic pits, and vacuoles can be evaluated as cytoplasmic anomalies. However, these characteristics are not included in the scoring systems, as there is no definite and clear information on the contribution of these characteristics to embryo development and their effect on implantation (Rienzi et al., 2003).

Some studies have shown that cytoplasmic pits can be associated with embryo culture media (Biggers & Racowsky, 2002). According to a study, rough and dark cytoplasmic granularity with central location of cortical halo

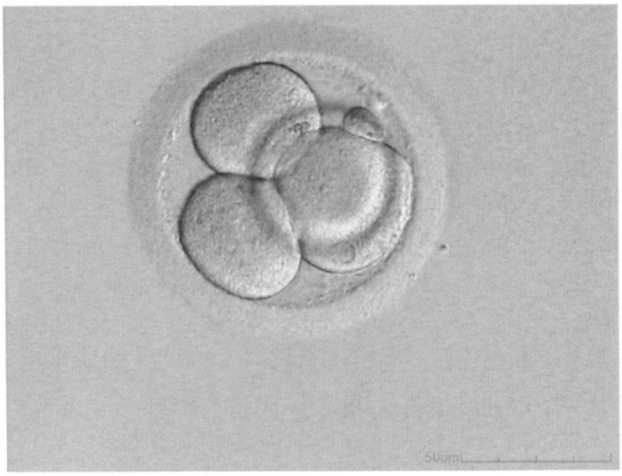

Figure 18.9 The mononuclear embryo (the single nucleus is prominent in the middle of each blastomer) consisted of 4-cells on the 2nd day (author's own archive).

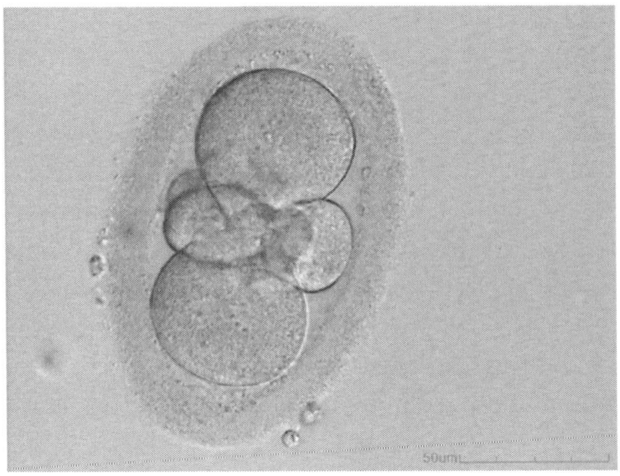

Figure 18.10 A multinuclear (there are two nuclei in every two big blastomers, nucleolus structure is observed inside the nucleus), uneven and ovoid embriyo consisted of 4-cell embryo on the 2nd day (author's own archive).

organelles has been shown to result in degeneration of embryo development and reduced implantation potential (Veeck, 1999).

Cytoplasmic vacuoles are the most common cytoplasmic abnormalities in oocytes and embryos. Vacuoles are membrane-enclosed structures filled with fluid-like content in the perivitelline space. They can be observed in varying numbers and sizes both in oocyte structure and in blastomeres. They are especially more common in compact embryos. Large vacuoles rather than small vacuoles have a poor prognostic value and should be noted in the scoring, as they can disrupt embryo development. In particular, the formation of large vacuoles can disrupt the developmental axis and three-dimensional structure of the embryo; thus blastocyst development may disturb (Ebner et al., 2005; Van Blerkom, 1990).

Planar Arrangement of Blastomeres

The cleavage planes have been believed to determine various aspects of embryo development in the future. Human oocytes have animal and vegetal pole regions from the earliest stages of their formation. There is some change in the oocyte axis after sperm entry into the oocyte. The fertilization cone formed by the sperm entry position determines the end of the short axis where cleavage will occur.

In the zygote, there is an animal pole close to the 2nd polar body and a vegetal pole opposite of the animal pole. Meiosis occurs in the animal pole region (Gray et al., 2004). It has been shown that the first cleavage begins at the polar body side where meiosis previously occurred and determines the embryonic and abembryonic poles of the blastocyst (Plusa et al., 2005). The axes of the first 2 cleavage are tightly controlled by genes. The first cleavage occurs on the meridian axis, and two sister blastomeres are formed with similar poles (in the same polarity) of the animal and vegetal cytoplasm after this cleavage. Since the second cleavage occurs on the equatorial axis, sister blastomeres have different polarity from each other after this cleavage (Robert G. Edwards & Hansis, 2005). Therefore, while two blastomeres formed after meridian cleavage have equal animal and vegetal poles; one of the blastomeres has the cytoplasm of the animal pole and the other has the cytoplasm of the vegetal pole in equatorial cleavage. Three blastomeres with animal cytoplasm located in association with the polar body and one blastomere with distantly located vegetal cytoplasm are formed as a result of this cleavage. As a result of this cleavage, a pyramidal or tetrahedral arranged cloverleaf embryo structure occurs (Gulyas, 1975; Prados et al., 2012).

In the study of Edwards and Beard, it was emphasized that the inner cell mass (ICM) of two blastomeres with complete animal and vegetal poles, the trophectoderm of the blastomere with animal cytoplasm, and the blastomere consisting of vegetal cytoplasm may be the germline precursor later (Robert G. Edwards & Beard, 1997). If embryo cleavage occurs differently from the meridian and equatorial cleavage planes; 4 blastomeres with non-tetrahedral appearance are formed since the distribution and placement of animal and vegetal poles will be different. Polarization is especially important in the development and regulation of the differentiation of trophectoderm cells in embryos. The area on the side where the ICM is located is called the polar trophectoderm, and the area where there is a thinner epithelium covering the cavity opposite this region is called the mural trophectoderm region. The polar trophectoderm regulates inner cell mass and embryonic development (Robert G. Edwards & Hansis, 2005).

In some cases, the shape of the oocytes may not be perfectly spherical. The cleavage plane will be abnormal and ovoid-shaped embryos can develop in a single plane, particularly in ovoid-shaped oocytes.

Reverse Cleavage

The reverse cleavage can be seen in two ways. The first way occurs after the embryo has completed cell division, when the blastomeres fuse and reintegrate. Another type of reverse cleavage is the reestablishment of cell borders before cytokinesis is fully realized during cell division. Reverse cleavage can be observed in the development process of embryos. The progression and aneuploidy rates of these embryos in the blastocyst have been shown to be not different from the others (Liu et al., 2014).

Scoring of Cleavage-Stage Embryos

Cell count, degree of fragmentation, blastomere symmetry, and multinucleation status are frequently used to describe the viability of embryos in the cleavage stage. More recently, a standard scoring system has been defined for cleavage-stage embryos by professionals in this field, namely the Society for Assisted Reproductive Technology (SART) and Alpha Scientists in Reproductive Medicine and the ESHRE Special Interest Group on Embryology after adding monitoring hours (Table 18.1) and additional standards (Table 18.2) (Alpha & ESHRE, 2011).

Table 18.2 Consensus scoring system for cleavage-stage embriyos (in addition to cell number), (Alpha & ESHRE, 2011)

Grade	Rating	Description
1	Good	• <10% fragmentation • Stage-specific cell size • No multinucleation
2	Fair	• 10-25% fragmentation • Stage-specific cell size for the majority of cells • There is no evidence of multinucleation
3	Poor	• Severe fragmentation (25%) • Cell size not stage-specific • Evidence of multinucleation

According to defined control times, an optimal day 2 embryo should have a mononuclear appearance, consisting of 4 equally sized blastomeres with a three-dimensional tetrahedral planar arrangement and fragmentation <10% at 44±1 hours after insemination. The optimal day 3 embryo should be composed of 8 equally sized mononuclear blastomeres and a <10% fragmentation at 68±1 hours after insemination. For embryos in the cleavage stage embryos, <10% fragmentation was considered mild, 10%-25% fragmentation moderate, and >25% severe. No definition of fragmentation location has been made (Alpha & ESHRE, 2011).

Appropriate performance indicators have been identified in the Vienna consensus (Alpha & ESHRE, 2017) to provide an adequate overview of the most important steps in the embryology laboratory process. As a result, 5 performance indicators, 12 key performance indicators, and 2 reference indicators were defined. Minimum performance levels and expected values were calculated for all of these indicators. It is recommended that each embryology laboratory determine their performance and reference values based on these values.

Key performance indicators used for cleavage-stage embryos are determined as early cleavage rate, cleavage speed, embryo development rate, embryo fragmentation rate, and good quality embryo rate. The cleavage rate is an indicator of embryo viability. It also reflects the state of culture systems. The cleavage speed is also an important parameter that can be followed to a large extent. The cleavage rate is defined as the zygote divided rate at 44±1 hours, in other words 2nd day after insemination. It is also recommended to classify the cleavage rate according to the indication of the patient. A decrease in cleavage rate can be observed as a result of negative changes in the culture environment.

In the Alpha survey, the competence values ranged from 80–95%, with a benchmark of 90–100% (Alpha & ESHRE, 2017). The embryo development rate is defined as the ratio of embryos with 4 cells (44±1-hour after insemination) on day 2, 8 cells (68±1 hour after insemination) on day 3, and morula stage embryos (92±2 hours post-insemination) on day 4 to zygotes with 2PN (Alpha & ESHRE, 2011). This ratio is extremely important, as it reflects the viability and quality of the 2nd and 3rd day embryos and the competence of all laboratory and culture systems.

Studies have shown that blastomere count, mononuclear cell ratio, degree of fragmentation, and blastomere size are the most important indicators in determining live birth rates and blastomere symmetry did not affect live birth as much as others. The minimum performance level and the expected value for the implantation rate of embryos in the cleavage stage are determined as ≥25% and ≥35%, respectively (Alpha & ESHRE, 2017).

Compaction

There are connection units between the blastomeres. Intracellular junction complexes begin to develop at the 8-cell stage from the 3rd day of the embryo, and the number of tight junction complexes between blastomeres increases and the embryo becomes a compact single-cell mass. This phenomenon is called compaction (Alikani, 2005). This phenomenon is found to be associated with embryonic genome activation (Desai et al., 2000). Compaction begins or is completed in the morula stage of the embryo at 92±2 hours after insemination on day 4 of development (Figure 18.11, Figure 18.12). For this reason, compaction is accepted as a good predictor of the evaluation of developmental capacity. The compaction process in embryos may occur earlier or later. The content of cultural media and other environmental factors have been shown to also play a role in early compaction. Compaction may begin at the stage where the embryo has 6-8 cells in some embryos without passing to the morula stage. Although some studies have evaluated early compaction on day 3 as a good prognostic factor (Le Cruguel et al., 2013), some studies argue that there is no definitive and clear study showing the effect on implantation and pregnancy (Desai et al., 2000).

A good quality morula is expected to consist of 16-32 blastomeres and all blastomeres are expected to participate in the compaction process. Compaction of the embryo is necessary for the development of the blastocyst. The cells gain polarity and the ability to differentiate into trophectoderm cells and inner cell mass with compaction. Sometimes, all blastomeres do not participate in the compaction of the embryo, and some blastomeres may be left out of the embryo. The increase in the number and volume of blastomeres that do not

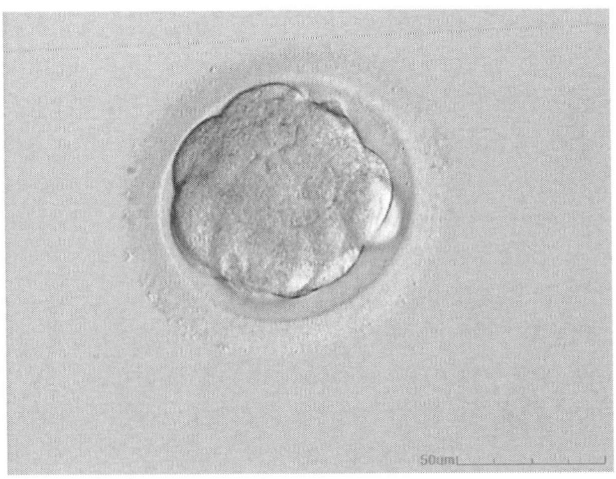

Figure 18.11 Partial compact embryo on the 4th day (author's own archive).

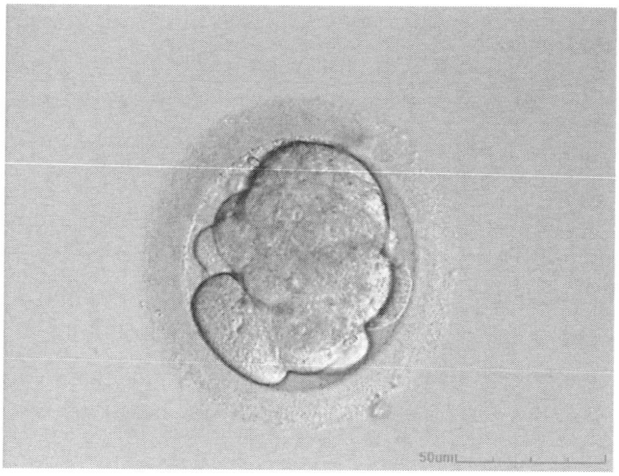

Figure 18.12 Compact embryo on the 4th day (author's own archive).

Table 18.3 Consensus scoring system for day-4 embryos (Alpha & ESHRE, 2011)

Grade	Rating	Description
1	Good	• Entered into a fourth round of cleavage. • Evidence of compaction that involves virtually all the embryo volume.
2	Fair	• Entered into a fourth round of cleavage. • Compaction involves most of the volume of the embryo.
3	Poor	• Disproportionate compaction involving less than half of the embryo, with two or three cells remaining as discrete blastomeres

participate in compaction is evaluated against the developing blastocyst. Cells that do not participate in compaction are thought to lose their trophectoderm-forming and totipotent properties or become abnormal (Cauffman et al., 2009; Prados et al., 2012). After completion of the compaction, cavitations occur in the embryo mass, and blastocyst development begins. The Alpha and ESHRE consensus published a scoring system for day 4 embryos, which is shown Table 18.3.

Blastocyst Development and Morphological Evaluation

Cavitation and fluid accumulation begin in an embryo after compaction has finished (at 115-117 hours after insemination, Table 18.1). Fluid accumulations in the form of separate foci then coalesce and completely fill the middle part of the embryo. This fluid is called the blastocoel fluid, and the space filled with this fluid is called the blastocoel cavity. Cells are tightly packed on one side of the embryo, forming the inner cell layer (ICM); cells line the remaining parts of the blastocoel cavity with a single layer of epithelium in the part called trophectoderm. The number of cells that line the ICM and trophectoderm and the diameter of the blastocyst increase with expansion of the blastocoel cavity. The zona pellucida becomes thinner at this stage and the embryo separation begins from the zona pellucida, this process being ‘hatching’. While the trophectoderm, consisting of a single layer of epithelium, contributes to implantation and is responsible for the development of the embryonic membranes and subsequently the formation of the placenta; the ICM, which consists of polygonal shaped cells, forms the embryoblast and the structure of the fetus in the future (Balaban et al., 2006; Hardarson et al., 2012). Although ICM plays an important role in implantation and fetal development, the main prognostic factor in implantation and live birth rates is emphasized as the trophectoderm (Ahlström et al., 2011; Alpha & ESHRE, 2011).

Scoring of Blastocyst Development

Morphological criteria are important in the evaluation and selection of blastocysts in embryos. Blastocyst structure was evaluated by Gardner in 1999 and this assessment was modified by Stephenson in 2007. Today, this scoring system is still widely used (Gardner & Schoolcraft, 1999; Stephenson et al., 2007) and is shown in Table 18.4. In blastocyst scoring, basically 3 parameters are considered. 1. Blastocoel cavity, 2. Inner Cell Mass (ICM) 3. Trophoectoderm. Based on this scoring, the structure of the trophectoderm cells, the state of the inner cell mass (ICM), the degree of the blastocoel cavity, and the hatching status of the embryo are scored. In addition, a common blastocyst scoring was determined in the Alpha and ESHRE consensus in 2011 by Alpha Scientists in Reproductive Medicine and the ESHRE Special Interest Group of Embryology is shown in Table 18.5. In this scoring, the number is used to identify ICM and trophectoderm different from the scoring system of Gardner (Gardner & Schoolcraft, 1999). The width and status of the blastocoel cavity was scored in 4 different stages. A good-quality blastocyst is expected to have an enlarged blastocoel cavity (at least half the volume) on day 5, have an inner cell mass consisting of prominent and well-structured cells, and have trophectoderm cells that are composed of regular single-layered squamous cells. The blastocysts at different stages are shown in the pictures (Figures 18.13, 18.14, 18.15, 18.16, 18.17, 18.18, 18.19).

Table 18.4 Gardner's scoring system of human blastocysts. Adapted from (Gardner & Schoolcraft, 1999)

Blastocyst stage	Grading	Description
Expansion of the embryo		
Early blastocyst	1	Blastocoele is less than half the volume of the embryo
Blastocyst	2	Blastocoele is greater than or equal to half of the volume of the embryo
Full blastocyst	3	Blastocoele completely fills the embryo
Expanded blastocyst	4	Blastocoele volume is larger than early embryo, and zona pellucida has begun to thin
Hatching blastocyst	5	Blastocyste begins to exit from zona pellucida is thinning
Hatched blastocyst	6	Blastocyst completely removed from zona pellucida
Trophectoderm	A B C	Many cells form a tightly knit epithelium Few cells Very few cells form a loose epithelium
Inner cell mass (ICM)	A B C	Tightly packed, many cells Various cells are loosely grouped. Very few cells

Table 18.5 Consensus scoring system for blastocysts (Alpha & ESHRE, 2011).

Blastocyst stage	Grading Rating	Description
Stage of development	1 2 3 4	Early Blastocyst Expanded Hatched/Hatching
Inner cell mass (ICM)	1 Good	Prominent, easily discernible, with many cells that are compacted and tightly adhered together
	2 Fair	Easily discernible, with many cells that are loosely grouped together
	3 Poor	Difficult to discern, with few cells
Trophectoderm	1 Good	Many cells form a cohesive epithelium
	2 Fair	Few cells form a loose epithelium
	3 Poor	Very few cells

The duration of reaching the expanded stage of the blastocyst is as important as the ICM and trophectoderm cells for the implantation potential of blastocyst embryos. The embryo may not reach this stage on the 5th day. In some embryos, blastocyst development can extend up to the 7th and 8th days. Embryos that reach the expanded blastocyst stage on day 5 have been shown to

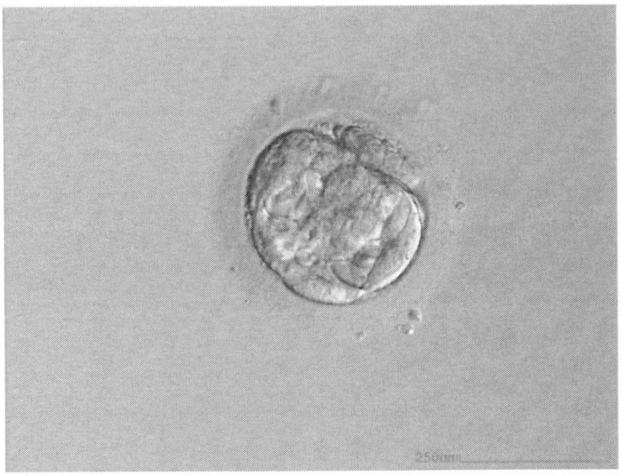

Figure 18.13 The blastocoele cavity and fluid begin to form in the embryo on the 5th day (author's own archive).

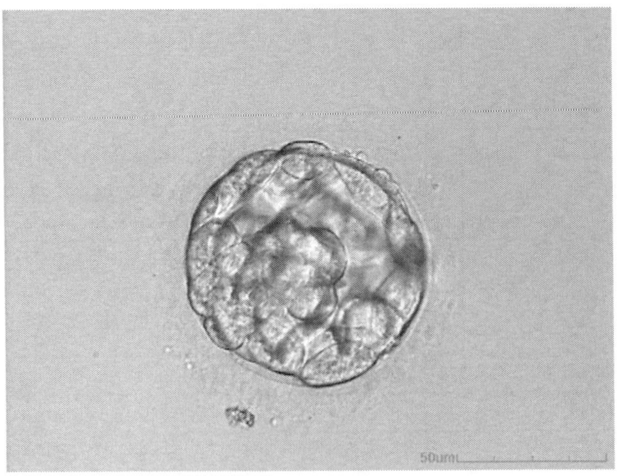

Figure 18.14 The blastocoele cavity and fluid filled the inside of the embryo on the 5th day (Early Blast) (author's own archive).

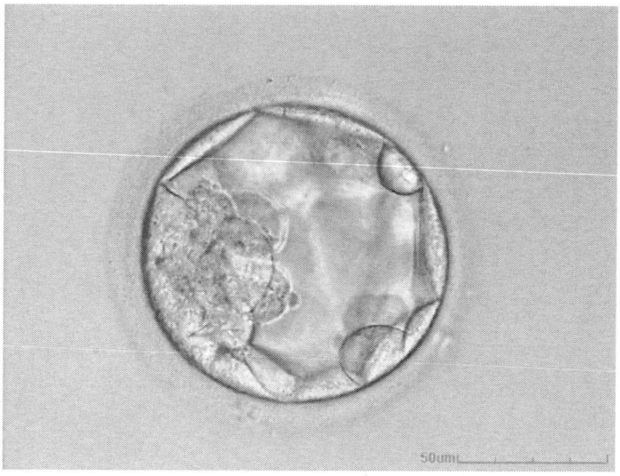

Figure 18.15 The blastocoele cavity and fluid completely filled the inside of the embryo and inner cell mass have started to become evident on the 5th day (full blastocyst) (author's own archive).

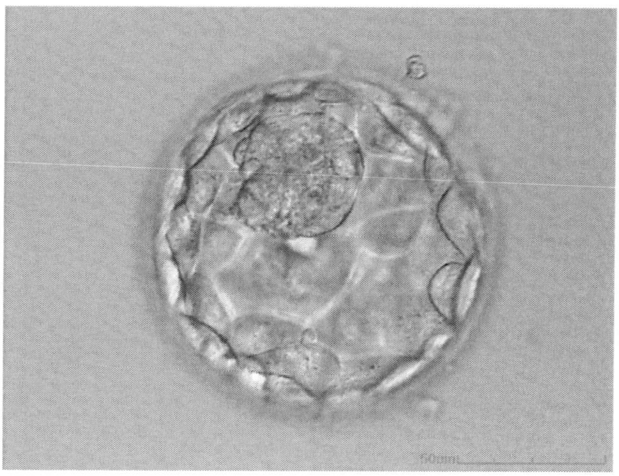

Figure 18.16 The embryo volume and the blastocoele cavity expanded and the number of cells increased in the embryo. Also, ICM (the side of 12 o'clock) clearly differentiated from trophectoderm cells (author's own archive).

have much higher implantation and live birth rates than those that reach later (Richter et al., 2001).

The collapse and expansion of the embryo during the development of the blastocyst can be considered a normal developmental process. Since ICM cannot be clearly selected when collapsed, re-evaluation of the embryo after a few hours is recommended.

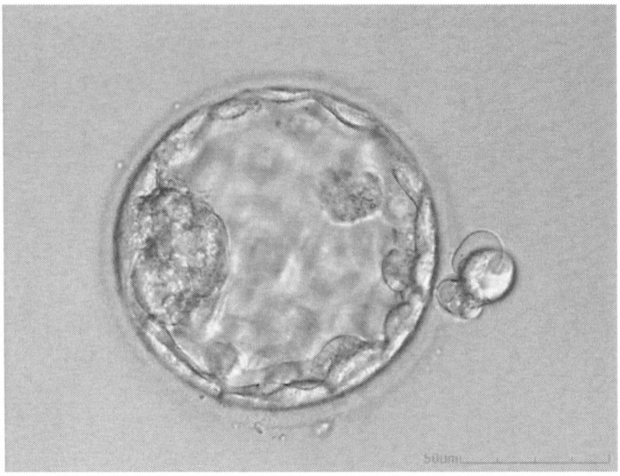

Figure 18.17 ICM is on the side of 9 o'clock. Hatching has started through the trophectoderm across the ICM (Author's own archive).

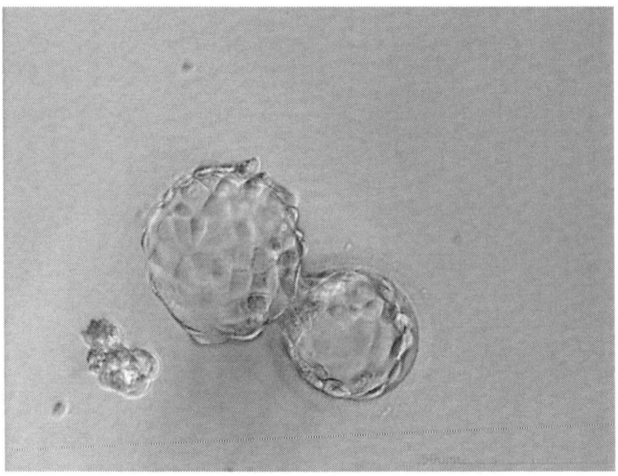

Figure 18.18 Hatching has advanced. Most of the embryo has come out of the zona pellucida (author's own archive).

Key performance indicators for blastocyst embryos in the embryology laboratory are defined as blastocyst development rate, good quality blastocyst growth rate, and good quality blastocyst transfer rate on day 5. The rate of development of blastocysts is the ratio of the number of zygotes with 2PN to the total number of blastocysts formed on the 5th and 6th days. The rate of good-quality blastocyst development is the ratio of the number of zygotes with 2PN to the number of good-quality blastocysts formed on the 5th day. A good quality blastocyst transfer rate can vary depending on conditions such as freezing or PGD (Alpha & ESHRE, 2017).

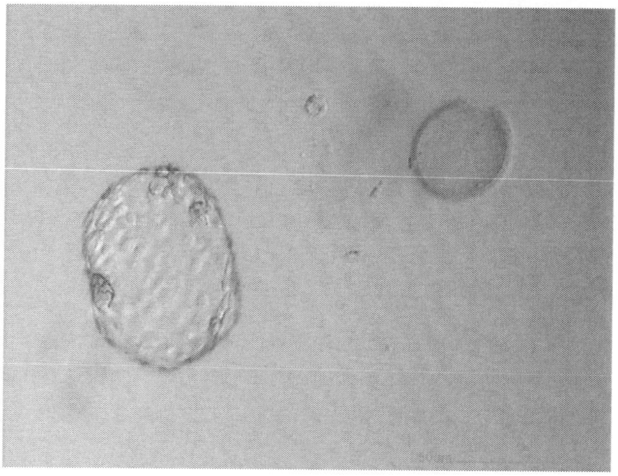

Figure 18.19 Hatching has completed and the embryo has completely emerged (on the left) from the zona pellucida (on the right) (author's own archive).

Embryo Imaging Systems

Since embryo development is a dynamic process, the morphological appearance and scoring of embryos may differ even within a few hours. Conventional morphological evaluations are performed each day in a very limited and specified time in many laboratories after removing the embryos from the incubator. As gas concentrations and temperature values are severely decreased when routinely used incubators are opened, it will take some time for the incubator to regain its normal values. In addition, no matter how fast the embryo is evaluated under the microscope; the embryo will be exposed to completely different atmospheric conditions. In addition, it may not be possible to detect the cleavage times and characteristics of embryos and the structural changes observed in the cells during conventional evaluations. Because most embryo development continues on time when it is not observed in the conventional incubators (Racowsky et al., 2015). Sequential embryo scoring increases both the amount of data obtained, the exposure time of the embryo to inappropriate environmental conditions, and the time for the incubators to reach the desired gas concentration again. Therefore, isolated culture systems, in which each patient's embryo is followed individually, have been used recently instead of large single-lid incubators. Embryo follow-ups made with standard culture systems provide immobile and a very short moment image for each embryo, while important indicators in the embryo development process can be captured by time-lapse imaging systems (Meseguer et al., 2011).

These systems consist of an incubator with a special camera system with a connected computer. The embryo cultured in time-lapse systems is monitored with a special digital invert microscope and captured photographs at predetermined intervals (5-20 minutes) without being taken out of the incubator and these images are transferred to the computer to follow the development of the embryos. Due to a special software, a video sequence is created that consists of these photos. Since embryos can be continuously monitored in full time with these systems, dynamic stages that are desired to be detected in embryo development can be easily observed. Embryo images recorded with time lapse systems repeatedly and sequential observations can be made. In this way, more detailed and complete follow-ups of the embryo are made by using morphokinetic parameters in different time periods. Since embryos are never taken out of the incubator during evaluation, negative effects of environmental conditions (temperature and gas changes, direct exposure to light, etc.) can be prevented, and a more stable culture environment is provided (Kovacs, 2014; Lundin & Park, 2020).

With the use of these systems, morphological criteria such as cell division time intervals, pronuclear and nuclear formations, cleavage and fragmentation can be evaluated in detail. In this way, the selection of the best embryo for transfer can be decided earlier.

The Embryology laboratory has Embryo Scope (FertiliTech), Primo Vision (Vitrolife) and EEVA (Early Embryo Viability Assessment) (Progyny/Merck Serono) time-lapse systems nowadays. Embryo Scope is a self-contained system with a fixed camera. The maximum quality of the resolution makes it advantageous compared to other systems. Time-lapse devices utilize visible light imaging, which is thought to be less damaging than ultraviolet, infrared, or fluorescent. The maximum quality of the resolution of Embryo Scope makes it advantageous compared to other systems. The constant movement of the surface holding the culture dishes to bring the embryo into the view area may have the potential for adverse effects. In the Primo Vision system, 16 embryos can be evaluated simultaneously without moving. Since embryos are viewed simultaneously in this system, adverse effects of light, electrical, and electromagnetic are minimized according to Embryo Scope. The resolutions of the images obtained in Primo Vision are lower than those of Embryo Scope. Embryo Scope and Primo Vision systems use bright-field technology. In the EEVA system, images are taken through a special microscope in the incubator using bright field technology, where the cell membrane can be observed better than in other systems. When they compared the exposure time of embryos to light during evaluations in conventional incubators with the light exposure used in imaging systems, they did not observe a negative effect of exposure in time-lapse systems on embryo development (Meseguer et al., 2011). In a meta-analysis conducted in 2019, no significant differences in embryo development and selection were observed between conventional culture systems and time-lapse culture systems (Armstrong et al., 2019). Although the superiority of time lapse systems over conventional incubators is not clear yet in scientific studies; the algorithms created as a result of the standardization and detailed analysis of the data groups used in the these systems will be able to replace the routine conventional systems in the future. They provide clear information about morphokinetic parameters that cannot be monitored in routine follow-ups of conventional systems. Today, this technology is used as a noninvasive technique to predict the emergence and disappearance of pronuclei, early cleavage monitoring, determination of the cleavage pattern and timing, blastulation and blastocyst expansion onset times, and estimation of euploid or aneuploid embryos based on morphokinetic data (Kovacs, 2014; Lemmen et al., 2008). Still, additional data are needed to support the safety and superiority of time-lapse technology.

These systems also have disadvantages. One of these is the limitation in obtaining the desired image, as the system does not allow rotation of the embryos. Another limitation of use is that the algorithms used in embryo selection are determined with sharp limits. One of the disadvantages of this system is the initial setup and the consumable usage costs of the system (Findikli & Oral, 2014). The decrease in production costs over time with developing technology may enable these systems to be used routinely in an IVF laboratory. The quantitative evaluation of embryo development stages, namely morphokinetic parameters, has come to the fore with the use of time-lapse systems. Various algorithms have been developed in many studies to be used in the selection of embryos with the highest implantation potential. In some cases, where dynamic imaging systems are used, there may be cases where the system selects more than one embryo with the determined algorithms and the final decision is left to the embryologist (Cruz et al., 2011; Storr et al., 2018).

Metabolomics

The researchers began investigating the measurements of glucose, lactate, pyruvate or amino acid levels in the culture medium, the oxygen evaluation of the embryo, the genomic and proteomic profile, and finally the analytical examination of the embryonic metabolome in order to better understand the cell function of embryo (Brison et al., 2004; Conaghan et al., 1993). Proteomic research includes the analysis of the protein content and protein profile of the embryo. Examining the protein profiles of different embryos can provide information on the effects of methods such as IVF or cryopreservation. Since proteomic analysis requires cell lysis, it is not possible to apply this method prior to transfer. For this reason, proteins secreted into IVF culture media, namely secretomics, have begun to be studied. The reproductive success rate was investigated by evaluating the secretion profiles of embryos (Katz-Jaffe et al., 2006). Recently, researchers have focused on the metabolites that are released in the culture environment to evaluate embryo viability and implantation potential because it is a noninvasive technique (Seli et al., 2007).

Metabolomics is a branch of biotechnology that enables the determination, quantification, and identification of small molecule metabolites, which are the products of lipids, carbohydrates, vitamins, and hormones, and cell component profiles in biological fluids with the help of high efficiency technology (Dettmer & Hammock, 2004). Metabolomics is used in many fields of science; it has also started to be used in the field of IVF, and research on this field continues. The embryo interacts with the culture medium during its development. While the embryo takes the molecules it needs from the media, it releases the waste molecules back into the environment. Metabolomics analysis includes the profiling of biomarkers released as a result of the oxidative and energy metabolism of embryos surrounding the culture medium. The composition of the culture fluid is examined with different techniques and the culture fluid is mapped according to the metabolism of each embryo, and this graph is associated with the development and pregnancy capacity of the embryo (Gardner et al., 2001). Since these changes in the metabolome reflect the physiological and metabolic state of the embryo, the composition of the culture media differs for each embryo. In metabolomics studies, it has been shown that embryo metabolism does not always morphologically indicate the embryo with the highest gestational capacity. Sometimes, it can also provide data independent of the morphology of the embryo (Seli et al., 2007).

As a result of metabolomics studies, the profiles of implanted and nonimplanted embryos can be compared, and markers that give information about reproductive potential can be determined. It can be helpful in identifying aneuploid embryos. Since aneuploid embryos show different amino acid turnover in vitro compared to genetically normal embryos, amino acid profiling can provide information on the genetic health of the embryo (Picton et al., 2010). In single embryo transfer, metabolomics evaluation of embryo quality in addition to the conventional morphological classification can be used to predict the one embryo with higher implantation potential between two embryos with the same scoring. In this way, more precise methods can be developed to determine which embryo will be transferred in IVF cycles. Studies have shown that the selection of embryo after coevaluation of embryo morphology and metabolomics profile increases the rate of implantation (Seli et al., 2007; Seli et al., 2008).

Conclusion

The selection and transfer of a good quality embryo together with a successful culture environment and laboratory-managed standards are the basic principles of increasing IVF success. The mediums used in IVF today are largely standardized, and the necessary performance criteria are clearly defined. Since embryo development is a dynamic process, in order to select the best quality embryo, it is necessary to evaluate the morphological parameters that determine the viability and quality of embryos. These evaluations begin with the embryo zygote development and cleavage stage and continue until the embryo transfer process. At these stages, many features of the embryo, such as cell number, cell symmetry, nuclear structures, and fragmentation rates, are evaluated. The purpose of the evaluations is to find the best quality embryo for pregnancy. These steps are done with conventional incubators in many laboratories. Recently, in addition to conventional culture systems, imaging and culture techniques called time-lapse system have started to take place of routine incubator in some IVF centers. The difference of these systems from conventional incubators is that embryo selection and evaluation can be made by determining certain morphokinetic parameters by images taken without the need to remove the embryo from the incubator devices. These systems are used for both embryo follow-up and choosing the best quality embryo by looking at morphokinetic parameters. In addition to these developments, metabolomic investigations, as a noninvasive method, have started to evaluate embryo viability created by examining the ratios of substances called metabolomes that released into the medium by the embryo. Research on this subject is still ongoing.

References

Ahlström, A., Westin, C., Reismer, E., Wikland, M., & Hardarson, T. (2011). Trophectoderm morphology: An important parameter for predicting live birth after single blastocyst transfer. *Human Reproduction, 26*(12), 3289-96. https://doi.org/10.1093/humrep/der325

Alikani, M. (2005). Epithelial cadherin distribution in abnormal human pre-implantation embryos. *Human Reproduction*, 20(12), 3369-75. https://doi.org/10.1093/humrep/dei242

Alikani, M., Cohen, J., Tomkin, G., Garrisi, G. J., Mack, C., & Scott, R. T. (1999). Human embryo fragmentation in vitro and its implications for pregnancy and implantation. *Fertility and Sterility,* 71(5), 836-42. https://doi.org/10.1016/S0015-0282(99)00092-8

Alpha & ESHRE. (2011). Alpha Scientists in Reproductive Medicine and ESHRE Special Interest Group of Embryology. The Istanbul consensus workshop on embryo assessment: Proceedings of an expert meeting. *Human Reproduction*, 26(6), 1270-83. https://doi.org/10.1093/humrep/der037

Armstrong, S., Bhide, P., Jordan, V., Pacey, A., Marjoribanks, J., & Farquhar, C. (2019). Time-lapse systems for embryo incubation and assessment in assisted reproduction. *Cochrane Database of Systematic Reviews,* 5(5), CD011320. https://doi.org/10.1002/14651858.cd011320.pub4

Balaban, B., Yakin, K., & Urman, B. (2006). Randomized comparison of two different blastocyst grading systems. *Fertility and Sterility*, 85(3), 559-63. https://doi.org /10.1016/j.fertnstert.2005.11.013

Biggers, J. D., & Racowsky, C. (2002). The development of fertilized human ova to the blastocyst stage in KSOM(AA) medium: is a two-step protocol necessary? *Reproductive Biomedicine Online*, 5(2), 133-40. https://doi.org/10.1016/S1472 -6483(10)61615-X

Borini, A., Lagalla, C., Cattoli, M., Sereni, E., Sciajno, R., Flamigni, C., & Coticchio, G. (2005). Predictive factors for embryo implantation potential. *Reproductive BioMedicine Online,* 10(5), 653-68. https://doi.org/10.1016/S1472 -6483(10)61675-6

Brison, D. R., Houghton, F. D., Falconer, D., Roberts, S. A., Hawkhead, J., Humpherson, P. G., Lieberman, B. A., & Leese, H. J. (2004). Identification of viable embryos in IVF by non-invasive measurement of amino acid turnover. *Human Reproduction*, 19(10), 2319-24. https://doi.org/10.1093/humrep/deh409

Bungum, M., Bungum, L., Humaidan, P., & Andersen, C. Y. (2003). Day 3 versus day 5 embryo transfer: A prospective randomized study. *Reproductive BioMedicine Online*, 7(1), 98-104. https://doi.org/10.1016/S1472-6483(10)61736-1

Cauffman, G., De Rycke, M., Sermon, K., Liebaers, I., & Van De Velde, H. (2009). Markers that define stemness in ESC are unable to identify the totipotent cells in human preimplantation embryos. *Human Reproduction*, 24(1), 63-70 https:// doi.org/10.1093/humrep/den351

Chavez, S. L., Loewke, K. E., Han, J., Moussavi, F., Colls, P., Munne, S., Behr, B., & Reijo Pera, R. A. (2012). Dynamic blastomere behaviour reflects human embryo ploidy by the four-cell stage. *Nature Communications*, 3, 1251. https://doi.org/10 .1038/ncomms2249

Cheng-He, Y., Ruo-Peng, Z., Juan, L., & Zhou-Cun, A. (2018). A predictive model for high-quality blastocyst based on blastomere number, fragmentation, and symmetry. *Journal of Assisted Reproduction and Genetics,* 35(5), 809-816. https://doi.org/10.1007/s10815-018-1132-6

Conaghan, J., Hardy, K., Handyside, A. H., Winston, R. M. L., & Leese, H. J. (1993). Selection criteria for human embryo transfer: A comparison of pyruvate uptake and morphology. *Journal of Assisted Reproduction and Genetics,* 10(1), 21-30. https://doi.org/10.1007/BF01204436

Cruz, M., Gadea, B., Garrido, N., Pedersen, K. S., Martínez, M., Pérez-Cano, I., Muñoz, M., & Meseguer, M. (2011). Embryo quality, blastocyst and ongoing pregnancy rates in oocyte donation patients whose embryos were monitored by time-lapse imaging. *Journal of Assisted Reproduction and Genetics*, 28(7), 569-73. https://doi.org/10.1007/s10815-011-9549-1

Dawson, K. J., Conaghan, J., Ostera, G. R., Winston, R. M. L., & Hardy, K. (1995). Delaying transfer to the third day post-insemination, to select non-arrested embryos, increases development to the fetal heart stage. *Human Reproduction*, 10(1), 177-82. https://doi.org/10.1093/humrep/10.1.177

Dennis, S. J., Thomas, M. A., Williams, D. B., & Robins, J. C. (2006). Embryo morphology score on day 3 is predictive of implantation and live birth rates. *Journal of Assisted Reproduction and Genetics*, 23(4), 171-5. https://doi.org/10.1007/s10815-006-9027-3

Desai, N. N., Goldstein, J., Rowland, D. Y., & Goldfarb, J. M. (2000). Morphological evaluation of human embryos and derivation of an embryo quality scoring system specific for day 3 embryos: A preliminary study. *Human Reproduction*, 15(10), 2190-6. https://doi.org/10.1093/humrep/15.10.2190

Desch, L., Bruno, C., Luu, M., Barberet, J., Choux, C., Lamotte, M., Schmutz, E., Sagot, P., & Fauque, P. (2017). Embryo multinucleation at the two-cell stage is an independent predictor of intracytoplasmic sperm injection outcomes. *Fertility and Sterility*, 107(1), 97-103. https://doi.org/10.1016/j.fertnstert.2016.09.022

Dettmer, K., & Hammock, B. D. (2004). Metabolomics - A new exciting field within the "omics" sciences. *Environmental Health Perspectives*, 112(7), A396-7. https://doi.org/10.1289/ehp.112-1241997

Ebner, T., Moser, M., Sommergruber, M., Gaiswinkler, U., Shebl, O., Jesacher, K., & Tews, G. (2005). Occurrence and developmental consequences of vacuoles throughout preimplantation development. *Fertility and Sterility*, 83(6), 1635-40. https://doi.org/10.1016/j.fertnstert.2005.02.009

Ebner, T., Moser, M., Sommergruber, M., & Tews, G. (2003). Selection based on morphological assessment of oocytes and embryos at different stages of preimplantation development: A review. *Human Reproduction Update,* 9(3), 251-62. https://doi.org/10.1093/humupd/dmg021

Ebner, T., Yaman, C., Moser, M., Sommergruber, M., Pölz, W., & Tews, G. (2001). Embryo fragmentation in vitro and its impact on treatment and pregnancy outcome. *Fertility and Sterility*, 76(2), 281-5. https://doi.org/10.1016/S0015-0282(01)01904-5

Edwards, R. G., Purdy, J. M., Steptoe, P. C., & Walters, D. E. (1981). The growth of human preimplantation embryos in vitro. *American Journal of Obstetrics and Gynecology*, 141(4), 108-16. https://doi.org/10.1016/0002-9378(81)90603-7

Edwards, Robert G., & Beard, H. K. (1997). Oocyte polarity and cell determination in early mammalian embryos. *Molecular Human Reproduction*, 3(10), 863-905. https://doi.org/10.1093/molehr/3.10.863

Edwards, Robert G., & Hansis, C. (2005). Initial differentiation of blastomeres in 4-cell human embryos and its significance for early embryogenesis and implantation. *Reproductive BioMedicine Online,* 11(2), 206-18. https://doi.org/10.1016/s1472-6483(10)60960-1

Findikli, N., & Oral, E. (2014). Time-lapse embryo imaging technology: Does it improve the clinical results? *Current Opinion in Obstetrics and Gynecology*, 26(3), 138-44. https://doi.org/10.1097/GCO.0000000000000072

Fujimoto, V. Y., Browne, R. W., Bloom, M. S., Sakkas, D., & Alikani, M. (2011). Pathogenesis, developmental consequences, and clinical correlations of human embryo fragmentation. *Fertility and Sterility*, 95(4), 1197-204. https://doi.org/10.1016/j.fertnstert.2010.11.033

Gardner, D. K., & Balaban, B. (2016). Assessment of human embryo development using morphological criteria in an era of time-lapse, algorithms and "OMICS": Is looking good still important? *Molecular Human Reproduction*, 22(10), 704-718. https://doi.org/10.1093/molehr/gaw057

Gardner, D. K., Lane, M., Stevens, J., & Schoolcraft, W. B. (2001). Noninvasive assessment of human embryo nutrient consumption as a measure of developmental potential. *Fertility and Sterility*, 76(6), 1175-80. https://doi.org /10.1016/S0015-0282(01)02888-6

Gardner, D. K., & Schoolcraft, W. B. (1999). Culture and transfer of human blastocysts. *Current Opinion in Obstetrics and Gynecology*, 11(3), 307-11. https://doi.org/10 .1097/00001703-199906000-00013

Giorgetti, C., Hans, E., Terriou, P., Salzmann, J., Barry, B., Chabert-Orsini, V., Chinchole, J. M., Franquebalme, J. P., Glowaczower, E., Sitri, M. C., Thibault, M. C., & Roulier, R. (2007). Early cleavage: An additional predictor of high implantation rate following elective single embryo transfer. *Reproductive BioMedicine Online*, 14(1), 85-91. https://doi.org/10.1016/ S1472- 6483(10)60768-7

Giorgetti, C., Terriou, P., Auquier, P., Hans, E., Spach, J. L., Salzmann, J., & Roulier, R. (1995). Implantation: Embryo score to predict implantation after in-vitro fertilization: Based on 957 single embryo transfers. *Human Reproduction*, 10(9), 2427-31. https://doi.org/10.1093/oxfordjournals.humrep.a136312

Gray, D., Plusa, B., Piotrowska, K., Na, J., Tom, B., Glover, D. M., & Zernicka-Goetz, M. (2004). First cleavage of the mouse embryo responds to change in egg shape at fertilization. *Current Biology*, 14(5), 397-405. https://doi.org/10.1016/j.cub .2004.02.031

Guerif, F., Le Gouge, A., Giraudeau, B., Poindron, J., Bidault, R., Gasnier, O., & Royere, D. (2007). Limited value of morphological assessment at days 1 and 2 to predict blastocyst development potential: A prospective study based on 4042 embryos. *Human Reproduction*, 22(7), 1973-81. https://doi.org/10.1093/ humrep/dem100

Gulyas, B. J. (1975). A reexamination of cleavage patterns in eutherian mammalian eggs: Rotation of blastomere pairs during second cleavage in the rabbit. *Journal of Experimental Zoology*, 193(2), 235-48. https://doi.org/10.1002/jez.1401930212

Hardarson, T., Hanson, C., Sjögren, A., & Lundin, K. (2001). Human embryos with unevenly sized blastomeres have lower pregnancy and implantation rates: Indications for aneuploidy and multinucleation. *Human Reproduction*, 16(2), 313-8. https://doi.org/10.1093/humrep/16.2.313

Hardarson, T., Löfman, C., Coull, G., Sjögren, A., Hamberger, L., & Edwards, R. G. (2002). Internalization of cellular fragments in a human embryo: time-lapse recordings. *Reproductive Biomedicine Online*, 5(1), 36-8. https://doi.org/10 .1016/S1472-6483(10)61594-5

Hardarson, T., Selleskog, U., Reismer, E., Wigander, A., Wennerström, S., Westin, C., Ahlström, A., Hanson, C. (2006). Zygotes cleaving directly into more than two cells after 25–27 h in culture are predominantly chromosomally abnormal. In *Human Reproduction* (Vol 21, p. i102). Oxford University Press: Oxford.

Hardarson, T., Van Landuyt, L., & Jones, G. (2012). The blastocyst. *Human Reproduction*, 27(1), 72–91. https://doi.org/10.1093/humrep/des230

Hardy, K. (1999). Apoptosis in the human embryo. *Reviews of Reproduction*, 4(3), 125-34. https://doi.org/10.1530/ror.0.0040125

Hartshorne, G. (2000). The embryo. *Human Reproduction*, 15(4), 31–41. https://doi .org/10.1093/humrep/15.suppl_4.31

Hill, G. A., Freeman, M., Bastias, M. C., Rogers, B. J., Herbert, C. M., Osteen, K. G., & Wentz, A. C. (1989). The influence of oocyte maturity and embryo quality on pregnancy rate in a program for in vitro fertilization-embryo transfer. *Fertility and Sterility*, 52(5), 801-6. https://doi.org/10.1016/s0015-0282(16)61034-8

Hnida, C., Engenheiro, E., & Ziebe, S. (2004). Computer-controlled, multilevel, morphometric analysis of blastomere size as biomarket of fragmentation and multinuclearity in human embryos. *Human Reproduction*, 19(2), 288-93. https:// doi.org/10.1093/humrep/deh070

Holte, J., Berglund, L., Milton, K., Garello, C., Gennarelli, G., Revelli, A., & Bergh, T. (2007). Construction of an evidence-based integrated morphology cleavage embryo score for implantation potential of embryos scored and transferred on day 2 after oocyte retrieval. *Human Reproduction*, 22(2), 548-57. https://doi.org /10.1093/humrep/del403

Hossain, A., Phelps, J., Agarwal, A., Sanz, E., & Mahadevan, M. (2016). A review of the society for assisted reproductive technology embryo grading system and proposed modification. *International Journal of Fertility and Sterility*, 10(2), 141-7. https://doi.org/10.22074/ijfs.2016.4956.

Jackson, K. V., Ginsburg, E. S., Hornstein, M. D., Rein, M. S., & Clarke, R. N. (1998). Multinucleation in normally fertilized embryos is associated with an accelerated ovulation induction response and lower implantation and pregnancy rates in vitro fertilization-embryo transfer cycles. *Fertility and Sterility*, 70(1), 60-6. https://doi.org/10.1016/S0015-0282(98)00100-9

Johansson, M., Hardarson, T., & Lundin, K. (2003). There is a cutoff limit in diameter between a blastomere and a small anucleate fragment. *Journal of Assisted Reproduction and Genetics*, 20(8), 309-13. https://doi.org/10.1023/A :1024805407058

Katz-Jaffe, M. G., Gardner, D. K., & Schoolcraft, W. B. (2006). Proteomic analysis of individual human embryos to identify novel biomarkers of development and viability. Fertility and Sterility, 85(1), 101-7. https://doi.org/10.1016/j.fertnstert .2005.09.011 101-7

Keltz, M. D., Skorupski, J. C., Bradley, K., & Stein, D. (2006). Predictors of embryo fragmentation and outcome after fragment removal in in vitro fertilization. *Fertility and Sterility*, 86(2), 321-4. https://doi.org/10.1016/j.fertnstert.2006.01.048

Kovacs, P. (2014). Embryo selection: The role of time-lapse monitoring. *Reproductive Biology and Endocrinology*, 12(1), 124. https://doi.org/10.1186/1477-7827-12-124

Le Cruguel, S., Ferré-L'Hôtellier, V., Morinière, C., Lemerle, S., Reynier, P., Descamps, P., & May-Panloup, P. (2013). Early compaction at day 3 may be a useful additional criterion for embryo transfer. *Journal of Assisted Reproduction and Genetics*, 30(5), 683-90. https://doi.org/10.1007/s10815-013-9983-3

Lee, M. J., Lee, R. K. K., Lin, M. H., & Hwu, Y. M. (2012). Cleavage speed and implantation potential of early-cleavage embryos in IVF or ICSI cycles. *Journal of Assisted Reproduction and Genetics*, 29(8), 745-50. https://doi.org/10.1007/ s10815-012-9777-z

Lemmen, J. G., Agerholm, I., & Ziebe, S. (2008). Kinetic markers of human embryo quality using time-lapse recordings of IVF/ICSI-fertilized oocytes. *Reproductive BioMedicine Online*, 17(3), 385-91. https://doi.org/10.1016/S1472-6483(10)60222-2

Liu, Y., Chapple, V., Roberts, P., & Matson, P. (2014). Prevalence, consequence, and significance of reverse cleavage by human embryos viewed with the use of the Embryoscope time-lapse video system. *Fertility and Sterility*, 102(5), 1295-1300. https://doi.org/10.1016/j.fertnstert.2014.07.1235

Lundin, K., & Park, H. (2020). Time-lapse technology for embryo culture and selection. *Upsala Journal of Medical Sciences*, 125(2):77-84. https://doi.org/10.1080/03009734.2020.1728444

MacHtinger, R., & Racowsky, C. (2013). Morphological systems of human embryo assessment and clinical evidence. *Reproductive BioMedicine Online*, 26(3), 210-21. https://doi.org/10.1016/j.rbmo.2012.10.021

Magli, M. C., Gianaroli, L., & Ferraretti, A. P. (2001). Chromosomal abnormalities in embryos. *Molecular and Cellular Endocrinology*, 183(1), 29-34. https://doi.org/10.1016/S0303-7207(01)00574-3

Magli, M. Cristina, Gianaroli, L., Ferraretti, A. P., Lappi, M., Ruberti, A., & Farfalli, V. (2007). Embryo morphology and development are dependent on the chromosomal complement. *Fertility and Sterility*, 87(3), 534-41. https://doi.org/10.1016/j.fertnstert.2006.07.1512

Marhuenda-Egea, F. C., Martínez-Sabater, E., Gonsálvez-Álvarez, R., Lledó, B., Ten, J., & Bernabeu, R. (2010). A crucial step in assisted reproduction technology: human embryo selection using metabolomic evaluation. *Fertility and Sterility*, 94(2), 772-4. https://doi.org/10.1016/j.fertnstert.2009.10.013

Maxwell, S. M., Melzer-Ross, K., McCulloh, D. H., & Grifo, J. A. (2015). A comparison of pregnancy outcomes between day 3 and day 5/6 embryo transfers: does day of embryo transfer really make a difference? *Journal of Assisted Reproduction and Genetics*, 32(2), 249-54. https://doi.org/10.1007/s10815-014-0404-z

Meseguer, M., Herrero, J., Tejera, A., Hilligsøe, K. M., Ramsing, N. B., & Remoh, J. (2011). The use of morphokinetics as a predictor of embryo implantation. *Human Reproduction,* 26(10), 2658-71. https://doi.org/10.1093/humrep/der256

Milewski, R., Kuć, P., Kuczyńska, A., Stankiewicz, B., Łukaszuk, K., & Kuczyński, W. (2015). A predictive model for blastocyst formation based on morphokinetic parameters in time-lapse monitoring of embryo development. *Journal of Assisted Reproduction and Genetics*, 32(4), 571-9. https://doi.org/10.1007/s10815-015-0440-3

Munné, S., Grifo, J., Cohen, J., & Weier, H. U. G. (1994). Chromosome abnormalities in human arrested preimplantation embryos: A multiple-probe FISH study. *American Journal of Human Genetics*, 55(1), 150-9.

Munné, S. C. J. (1998). Chromosome abnormalities in human embryos. *Human Reproduction Update,* 4(6), 842–855. https://doi.org/10.1093/humupd/4.6.842.

Nel-Themaat, L., & Nagy, Z. P. (2011). A review of the promises and pitfalls of oocyte and embryo metabolomics. *Placenta*, 32(SUPPL. 3). https://doi.org/10.1016/j.placenta.2011.05.011

Paternot, G., Debrock, S., D'Hooghe, T., & Spiessens, C. (2011). Computer-assisted embryo selection: A benefit in the evaluation of embryo quality? *Reproductive BioMedicine Online*, 23(3), 347-54. https://doi.org/10.1016/j.rbmo.2011.05.007

Pickering, S. J., Taylor, A., Johnson, M. H., & Braude, P. R. (1995). An analysis of multinucleated blastomere formation in human embryos. *Human Reproduction*, 10(7), 1912-22. https://doi.org/10.1093/oxfordjournals.humrep.a136206

Picton, H. M., Elder, K., Houghton, F. D., Hawkhead, J. A., Rutherford, A. J., Hogg, J. E., Leese, H. J., & Harris, S. E. (2010). Association between amino acid turnover and chromosome aneuploidy during human preimplantation embryo development in vitro. *Molecular Human Reproduction*, 16(8), 557-69 https://doi.org/10.1093/molehr/gaq040

Plusa, B., Hadjantonakis, A. K., Gray, D., Piotrowska-Nitsche, K., Jedrusik, A., Papaioannou, V. E., Glover, D. M., & Zernicka-Goetz, M. (2005). The first cleavage of the mouse zygote predicts the blastocyst axis. *Nature*, 434(7031), 391-5. https://doi.org/10.1038/nature03388

Prados, F. J., Debrock, S., Lemmen, J. G., & Agerholm, I. (2012). The cleavage stage embryo. *Human Reproduction*, 27(1), 50-71. https://doi.org/10.1093/humrep/des224

Racowsky, C., Kovacs, P., & Martins, W. P. (2015). A critical appraisal of time-lapse imaging for embryo selection: where are we and where do we need to go? *Journal of Assisted Reproduction and Genetics,* 32(7), 1025-30. https://doi.org/10.1007/s10815-015-0510-6

Racowsky, C., Vernon, M., Mayer, J., Ball, G. D., Behr, B., Pomeroy, K. O., Wininger, D., Gibbons, W., Conaghan, J., & Stern, J. E. (2010). Standardization of grading embryo morphology. *Journal of Assisted Reproduction and Genetics,* 27(8), 437-9. https://doi.org/10.1007/s10815-010-9443-2

Richter, K. S., Harris, D. C., Daneshmand, S. T., & Shapiro, B. S. (2001). Quantitative grading of a human blastocyst: Optimal inner cell mass size and shape. *Fertility and Sterility*, 76(6), 1157-67. https://doi.org/10.1016/S0015-0282(01)02870-9

Rienzi, L., Ubaldi, F., Giulia Minasi, M., Iacobelli, M., Martinez, F., Tesarik, J., & Greco, E. (2003). Blastomere cytoplasmic granularity is unrelated to developmental potential of day 3 human embryos. *Journal of Assisted Reproduction and Genetics*, 20(8), 314-7. https://doi.org/10.1023/A:1024857523896

Rienzi, L., Ubaldi, F., Iacobelli, M., Romano, S., Minasi, M. G., Ferrero, S., Sapienza, F., Baroni, E., & Greco, E. (2005). Significance of morphological attributes of the early embryo. *Reproductive BioMedicine Online*, 10(5), 669-8. https://doi.org/10.1016/S1472-6483(10)61676-8

Roux, C., Joanne, C., Agnani, G., Fromm, M., Clavequin, M. C., & Bresson, J. L. (1995). Fertilization and early embryology: Morphometric parameters of living human in-vitro fertilization embryos; importance of the asynchronous division process. *Human Reproduction*, 10(5), 1201-7. https://doi.org/10.1093/oxfordjournals.humrep.a136119

Rubio, I., Kuhlmann, R., Agerholm, I., Kirk, J., Herrero, J., Escribá, M. J., Bellver, J., & Meseguer, M. (2012). Limited implantation success of direct-cleaved human zygotes: A time-lapse study. *Fertility and Sterility*, 98(6), 1458-63. https://doi.org/10.1016/j.fertnstert.2012.07.1135

Sela, R., Samuelov, L., Almog, B., Schwartz, T., Cohen, T., Amit, A., Azem, F., & Ben-Yosef, D. (2012). An embryo cleavage pattern based on the relative blastomere size as a function of cell number for predicting implantation outcome. *Fertility and Sterility*, 98(3), 650-656. https://doi.org/10.1016/j.fertnstert.2012.05.041

Seli, E., Botros, L., Sakkas, D., & Burns, D. H. (2008). Noninvasive metabolomic profiling of embryo culture media using proton nuclear magnetic resonance correlates with reproductive potential of embryos in women undergoing in vitro fertilization. *Fertility and Sterility*, 90(6), 2183-9 https://doi.org/10.1016/j.fertnstert.2008.07.1739

Seli, E., Sakkas, D., Scott, R., Kwok, S. C., Rosendahl, S. M., & Burns, D. H. (2007). Noninvasive metabolomic profiling of embryo culture media using Raman and near-infrared spectroscopy correlates with reproductive potential of embryos in women undergoing in vitro fertilization. *Fertility and Sterility*, 88(5), 1350-7. https://doi.org/10.1016/j.fertnstert.2007.07.1390

Special Interest Group of Embryology, E., & Scientists in Reproductive Medicine, A. (2017). The Vienna consensus: report of an expert meeting on the development of ART laboratory performance indicators ESHRE Special Interest Group of Embryology and Alpha Scientists in Reproductive Medicine. Nova Baran Center, 4.

Staessen, C., Camus, M., Bollen, N., Devroey, P., & Van Steirteghem, A. C. (1992). The relationship between embryo quality and the occurrence of multiple pregnancies. *Fertility and Sterility*, 57(3), 626-30. https://doi.org/10.1016/s0015-0282(16)54911-5

Stephenson, E. L., Braude, P. R., Mason, C., & Rowland, K. (2007). International community consensus standard for reporting derivation of human embryonic stem cell lines. *Regenerative Medicine*, 2(4), 349-62. https://doi.org/10.2217/17460751.2.4.349

Storr, A., Venetis, C., Cooke, S., Kilani, S., & Ledger, W. (2018). Time-lapse algorithms and morphological selection of day-5 embryos for transfer: a preclinical validation study. *Fertility and Sterility*, 109(2), 276-283. https://doi.org/10.1016/j.fertnstert.2017.10.036

Thurin, A., Hardarson, T., Hausken, J., Jablonowska, B., Lundin, K., Pinborg, A., & Bergh, C. (2005). Predictors of ongoing implantation in IVF in a good prognosis group of patients. *Human Reproduction*, 20(7), 1876-80. https://doi.org/10.1093/humrep/deh872

Van Blerkom, J. (1990). Occurrence and developmental consequences of aberrant cellular organization in meiotically mature human oocytes after exogenous ovarian hyperstimulation. *Journal of Electron Microscopy Technique*, 16(4), 324-46. https://doi.org/10.1002/jemt.1060160405

Van Montfoort, A. P. A., Dumoulin, J. C. M., Kester, A. D. M., & Evers, J. L. H. (2004). Early cleavage is a valuable addition to existing embryo selection parameters: A study using single embryo transfers. *Human Reproduction*, 19(9), 2103-8. https://doi.org/10.1093/humrep/deh385

Van Royen, E., Mangelschots, K., De Neubourg, D., Laureys, I., Ryckaert, G., & Gerris, J. (2001). Calculating the implantation potential of day 3 embryos in women younger than 38 years of age: A new model. *Human Reproduction*, 162), 326-32. https://doi.org/10.1093/humrep/16.2.326

Veeck, L. (1999). Preembryo grading and degree of cytoplasmic fragmentation. In An Atlas of Human Gametes and Conceptuses: An Illustrated Reference for Assisted Reproductive Technology (p. 49–51). New York, USA: Parthenon Publishing. https://doi.org/10.1201/9780367803001

Vergouw, C. G., Al Nofal, M., Kostelijk, E. H., Rooth, H., Hompes, P. G. A., Schats, R., & Lambalk, C. B. (2013). The association of the blastomere volume index (BVI), the blastomere symmetry index (BSI) and the mean ovality (MO) with ongoing implantation after single embryo transfer. *Journal of Assisted Reproduction and Genetics*, 30(4), 587-92. https://doi.org/10.1007/s10815-013-9970-8

Ziebe, S., Petersen, K., Lindenberg, S., Andersen, A. G., Gabrielsen, A., & Andersen, A. N. (1997). Embryo morphology or cleavage stage: How to select the best embryos for transfer after in-vitro fertilization. *Human Reproduction*, 12(7), 1545-9. https://doi.org/10.1093/humrep/12.7.1545

Chapter 19

Embryo Culture Systems

Fatma Nur Karakuş, MD*
Department of Histology and Embryology, Eskişehir Yunus Emre State Hospital, Eskişehir, Türkiye

Abstract

In IVF, there are many factors that affect success, such as patient age and lifestyle, indication of treatment, controlled ovarian stimulation protocol, and endometrial receptivity. Factors belonging to the IVF laboratory affect the treatment outcome at least as much as other factors. In particular, suboptimal culture conditions have prevented expected responses in IVF treatment. Today, optimizing culture conditions has become even more important, due to the single embryo transfer targeted to prevent multiple pregnancies and other complications. Fertilization, embryo development, and implantation are highly complex processes. The ability to carry out these complex processes in vitro and obtain pregnancies resulting in live births depends on many components gathered under the title of "embryo culture system".

Key Words: IVF success, Embryo, Culture conditions, Culture system

Introduction

In the last four decades since 1978, when the first live birth was achieved with assisted reproductive technology (ART) treatment, significant progress has been made in the field of ART, through many question marks about reproductive physiology and embryo metabolism have been resolved. In IVF

---

* Corresponding Author's E-mail: fatmanur.karakus1@saglik.gov.tr

In: Holistic Approach to Assisted Reproductive Technology
Editor: Kenan Demir and Rümeysa Yılmaz Göç
ISBN: 979-8-89113-017-3
© 2023 Nova Science Publishers, Inc.

laboratories, embryos are created under in vitro conditions and developed until the day of transfer to the expectant mother. Gametes and embryos are sensitive to the slightest changes in the culture environment such as medium content, pH, osmolality, and laboratory conditions such as temperature, light, air quality. Therefore, the aim of clinical embryologists should be to standardize all variables and to provide a stable and stress-free culture environment for gamets and embryos to achieve healthy developing embryos and high live birth rates. The main components of culture media and the environmental factors required for an optimal culture environment are the subject of this chapter.

Components of Culture Media

Ions and Osmolality

Along with amino acids, inorganic ions in embryo culture mediums are the main determinants of osmolality. In addition to being an osmolyte, ions maintain cell membrane potential and low Na^+ and Cl^- and high K^+ concentrations in the cell through Na^+K^+ATPase (Kaplan, 2002). Ions play a role in many physiological processes, such as the regulation of intracellular pH, through transmembrane ion gradients (Hediger et al., 2004). The ionic content of the currently available embryo culture mediums is based on Krebs-Ringer Bicarbonate (KRB) solution and mainly Na^+, K^+, Cl^-, Ca^{2+}, Mg^{2+}, SO_4^{2-}, HCO_3^- and PO_4^{2-}ions constitute this content.

Whitten first performed a successful mouse embryo culture using a medium prepared by adding glucose and bovine serum albumin to KRB (Whitten, 1956). Until the 1980s, various mediums such as M16, Earle's, Ham's F10, Quinn's HTF, etc. were developed with minor modifications to Whitten's medium, but none of them was able to overcome the developmental blocks observed in various mammalian species, including humans (Baltz, 2012). The mentioned blocks were able to be overcome with KSOM (K^+-Simplex Optimization Medium) and CZB media. The main difference between these media (KSOM, CZB) from previous media is their low osmolality. Interestingly, although mammalian genital tract fluid is characterized by high osmolality (>360 mOsmol), successful results can be achieved with low osmolality (Borland et al., 1980). The osmolality of the media used for human embryos is also in the range of 249-290 mOsmol (Baltz, 2012). The main explanation for this situation is the interaction between ions and other media components such as amino acids, carbohydrates, etc. For example, a "2-cell block" was observed when phosphate was added to simple salt solutions containing glucose, such as HTF, but this effect of phosphate was not observed in the presence of amino acids (Gardner & Simón, 2017). In the presence of organic osmolytes such as glycine, taurine, hypotaurine, betaine, β-alanine and proline, embryo development can continue even at high osmolality.

The effects of ions on the development of human preimplantation embryos are still unknown, and an optimal osmolality has yet to be determined. In addition to studies reporting that high K+ concentrations support embryo development and sperm capacitation, there are also studies reporting negative effects. Calcium is known to be necessary for compaction. Oocytes do not have efficient transport systems and are protected from ionic stress by cumulus cells. Therefore, the denudation process should be delayed as much as possible (Gardner & Simón, 2017).

Energy Metabolism and Carbohydrates

The development of the preimplantation embryo, which has complex multicellular organization, from gametes is a very dynamic process. This process, which begins in the female fallopian tubes with fertilization, ends with implantation in the uterus. During this journey, the microenvironment of embryo constantly changes and a healthy embryo continues its development by keeping up with these changes with some physiological, biochemical, and metabolic changes. The major stages of embryo development such as cleavage, rapid increase in cell number, embryonic genome activation (EGA), formation of morula with compaction, differentiation of blastomeres into inner cell mass and trophectoderm, formation of blastocoele, development of homeostatic regulatory mechanisms are energy dependent (Smith & Sturmey, 2013). As in other cells, the embryo uses the basic pathways of energy metabolism to produce energy, intermediates for macromolecule synthesis, and substrates for various cellular processes (acetylation, methylation, etc.) (Figure 19.1) (Gardner & Wale, 2013; Zander-Fox & Lane, 2012). Each substrate in these pathways interacts with each other, and alteration of any of them affects all pathways. Therefore, the metabolic equilibrium of the embryo is associated with increased viability, implantation, and live birth rates. Leese et al. defined this situation as the "Silent Embryo Hypothesis" and observed that there is a balanced, controlled, and low metabolic activity in embryos with high development potential (Leese, 2002). Disruption of the balance between metabolic pathways, and uncontrolled high metabolism is associated with a decrease in the energy production capacity of the embryo and even loss of viabilility (Lane & Gardner, 2005a; Zander-Fox & Lane, 2012).

Carbohydrates are one of the main energy sources. The developing embryo encounters different levels of carbohydrate on its journey from the female genital tract to the uterus (Gardner et al., 1996). Pyruvate and lactate concentrations are high in the oviduct, while glucose levels are high in the uterus. This

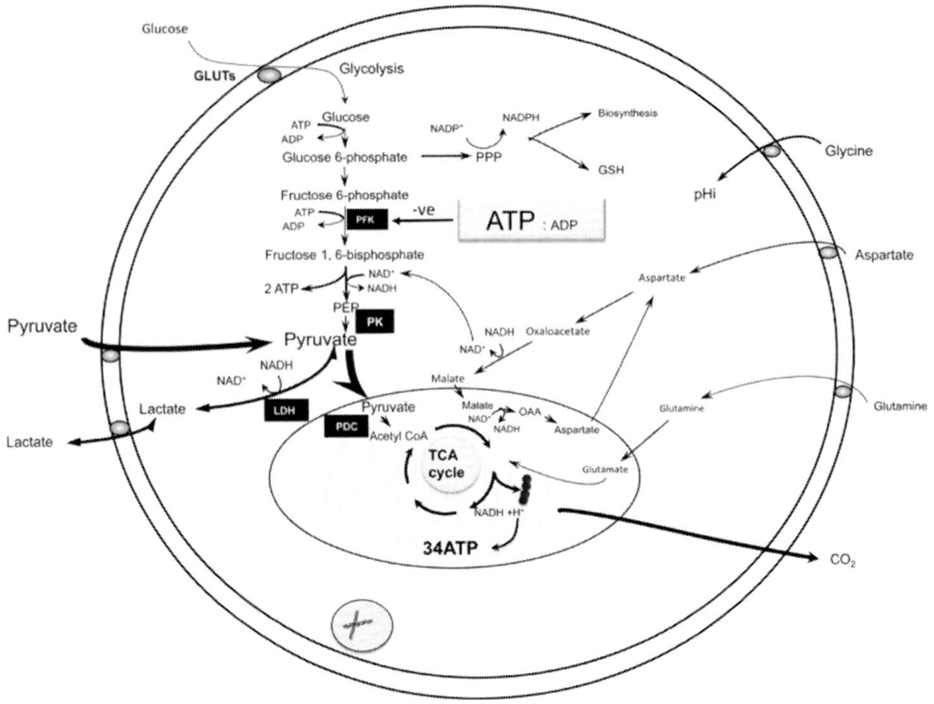

Figure 19.1 Metabolic pathways (Gardner & Wale, 2013).

situation is compatible with the carbohydrate requirement of the developing embryo. There is low metabolic activity and therefore high ATP levels during the process from fertilization to EGA. High ATP level inhibits glycolysis (Barbehenn et al., 1974a; Biggers et al., 2021). Early cleavage embryos have limited capacity to use nutrients, so the main energy source is pyruvate. Before compaction, 85-90% of ATP is produced by oxidative phosphorylation. After EGA, the increased energy requirement results in an approximately six-fold increase in metabolic activity compared to early cleavage embryos (Leese, 1991). In the blastocyst stage, the main energy source is glucose, ATP is rapidly consumed, and AMP levels increase. Despite the presence of oxygen in the environment, abundant lactate is produced from glucose through "aerobic glycolysis". This phenomenon observed in rapidly dividing cells, such as cancer cells, is called the "Warburg effect" (Smith & Sturmey, 2013).

Adding pyruvate to the media prevents "2-cell block". EGA occurs in the presence of nuclear pyruvate dehydrogenase (Nagaraj et al., 2017). When pyruvate was removed from embryo culture fluids, approximately 84% of human embryos had early cleavage arrest (Conaghan et al., 1993). The dependence of pyruvate in embryo development can be overcome with pyruvate precursors such as arginine and α-ketoglutarate, or with the activity of malate-aspartate shuttle in the presence of aspartate and lactate (Lane & Gardner, 2005b). Lactate can be used as an energy source in the 2-cell stage and is also a signaling molecule that influences immune and vascular responses in the endometrium. Lactate causes the pH value of the environment to decrease and facilitates the degradation of uterine tissue. Through these effects, lactate supports trophoblast invasion and thus implantation. Aerobic glycolysis and increased lactate production observed in blastocysts also coincide with the contribution of lactate to implantation. Lactate and pyruvate act synergistically and both must be present in the culture medium for optimal embryo development (Cross & Brinster, 1973). The pyruvate/lactate ratio is an important parameter for the developmental competence of the embryo. There is still no consensus on the ideal lactate concentration to be added to the culture medium. However, high lactate concentration affects pyruvate oxidation rate and ATP production, redox potential through its action on NAD+ and NADH, and regulation of gene expression through its action on sirtuin activity and ADP ribosylation (Gardner, 2015; Wales & Whittingham, 1973). Lactate can reduce the intracellular pH value (pHi). Although only the L-isomer is the biologically active isomer of lactate, the D-isomer is also effective on pHi. Therefore, sodium lactate salt should be preferred instead of 50:50 sodium DL lactate syrup to reduce the amount of D-isomer that does not have biological activity in culture media (Gardner & Simón, 2017).

Although it has been known that early cleavage embryos do not prefer glucose as an energy substrate and that glucose in the presence of phosphate in the culture fluids causes a developmental delay or arrest, the culture fluids used at every stage of embryo development contain glucose at various levels. The negative effect of glucose on embryo development in the presence of phosphate was prevented by adding EDTA, various amino acids, and vitamins to the medium (Gardner & Simón, 2017). Glucose is added to the culture media of early cleavage-stage embryos because of its roles other than as an energy substrate. First of all, sperm needs glucose during fertilization; cumulus cells produce pyruvate and lactate from glucose (Gardner et al., 1996; Leese & Barton, 1985). Glucose plays a role in many biosynthetic pathways. The metabolism of glucose through the pentose-phosphate pathway produces ribose fragments required for the synthesis of nucleic acid and triacylglycerol and NADPH required for the synthesis of lipids / membranes (Gardner & Harvey, 2015). The expression of various nutrient transporters (such as MCT1 and MCT4) that play a role in the response to oxidative stress and the regulation of the pHi value in the blastocyst stage depends on the presence of glucose in the microenvironment of the early cleavage stage embryo (Jansen et al., 2006; Leese, 1991). The reason why the blastocyst prefers glycolysis may be that the uterine microenvironment is partially anoxic (Rogers et al.,

1982). If the glucose in the culture medium is insufficient, the glucose stores of the embryo are depleted and therefore the implantation capacity is reduced (Gardner & Simón, 2017). Metabolomic studies show a relationship between glucose consumption and embryo quality, viability, and implantation potential. For example, it has been observed that embryos that are parthenogenetic, polyspermic, or have poor morphology have lower glucose consumption than high-quality embryos (Gardner et al., 2001; Hardy et al., 1989).

Amino Acids

Large-scale studies on human embryos have some limitations. Therefore, there are still no definitive data on which amino acids should be used in what amounts for human embryo culture. However, amino acids are routinely added to human embryo culture media in light of information obtained from animal experiments.

Amino acids are classified as essential, nonessential, and conditionally essential amino acids. The embryo is indiscriminately exposed to all amino acids found in the female reproductive tract and uterus, so a classification of essential and nonessential amino acids makes no sense for embryo development. Classifications such as "cleavage stage amino acids" and "blastocyst stage amino acids" seem more plausible (Gardner & Simón, 2017).

Amino acids have important physiological roles in embryo development. In addition to being mainly an energy substrate and used in protein synthesis, they are also intracellular organic osmolytes (especially glycine), pH buffers (especially nonessential amino acids), chelators, and antioxidants (Dawson et al., 1998; Edwards et al., 1998; Gardner, 2008; Li & Foote, 1995; Van Winkle et al., 1990). The fact that arginine is the precursor of the signal molecule nitric oxide (NO), which plays an important role in embryo development, and that leucine regulates trophoblast invasion through the mammalian target of rapamycin protein complex (mTOR) pathway; are examples of amino acids' roles in signaling in embryo development (Manser et al., 2004; Martin et al., 2003; Martin & Sutherland, 2001).

While there were no amino acids in embryo culture media in the initial studies, the high amino acid content in the female genital tract and the presence of various amino acid transport systems in the oocyte and embryos led to the idea of adding amino acids to the media (Harris et al., 2005; Menezo, 1975; Miller & Schultz, 1987; Van Winkle, 1988). An increase in the rate of blastocyst development was observed in many mammalian species, such as mice, hamsters, sheep, and cows, with culture media supplemented with amino acids (Gardner & Simón, 2017). Thanks to the culture media with Eagle's non-essential amino acids and glutamine, which do not support somatic cell culture; alleviation of the "2 cell block", and an increase in cleavage, blastocyst formation, hatching, viability, implantation, and fetal development rates were observed (Gardner & Simón, 2017; Mehta & Kiessling, 1990; Zhang & Armstrong, 1990). There is a similarity between Eagle's nonessential amino acids and amino acids such as alanine, aspartate, glutamate, glycine, and serine, which are found at high levels in the female genital tract (Eagle, 1959). As with carbohydrates, the amino acids that must be present in the medium for optimal embryo development differ according to the stage of embryo development. While non-essential amino acids and glutamine are required for early embryonic development, essential amino acids are needed after the 8-cell stage (Lane & Gardner, 1997). While the the essential amino acids, which were low levels in the female genital tract, inhibited embryo development until the 8-cell stage, they lead to an increase in cleavage, inner cell mass, and blastocoel formation, and viability rates after the 8-cell stage (Lane & Gardner, 1997). The content of the currently available sequential culture media has also been determined by considering these changes in amino acid requirement.

The level of amino acid consumption has the potential to be a noninvasive tool for measuring the developmental potential of embryos and selecting the best embryo to be transferred (Houghton et al., 2002). Houghton et al. observed that the total amino acid consumption level of embryos that could reach the blastocyst stage was lower than that of embryos that arrest, although their morphological characteristics were similar (Houghton et al., 2002). These data also support the "silent embryo hypothesis". Brison et al. found that the live birth rates of ICSI embryos were correlated with their leucine, asparagine, and glycine consumption (Brison et al., 2004).

An important handicap of the presence of amino acids in embryo culture fluids is the formation of ammonium. Ammonium, which is formed as a result of spontaneous degradation of amino acids in culture fluids at 37°C and embryo metabolism, is almost absent in the female genital tract (Casslén, 1987; Lane & Gardner, 1995). Ammonium has negative effects on preimplantation embryo development, implantation, and fetal development. In embryos exposed to ammonium, changes in metabolism and gene expression and fetal developmental abnormalities such as exencephaly are observed (Lane & Gardner, 1994; Zander et al., 2006). Atmospheric oxygen has been reported to increase the negative effects of ammonium on embryo development (Wale & Gardner, 2013). Ammonium amounts can be reduced by using more stable amino acids such as alanyl-glutamine or glycyl-glycine instead of glutamine, which is the most labile amino acid in culture fluids, and by changing the medium every 48 hours. In single-step culture media and time-lapse culture system without medium change, amino acids should be used at the lowest concentrations at which they are effective (Hardarson et al., 2015).

Vitamins

Ascorbic acid (vitamin C) has promoted the development of human embryos through its antioxidant activity when added to slow freezing medium (Lane et al., 2002). Ascorbic acid has also shown a positive effect on mouse embryos (Wang et al., 2002). However, the antioxidant activity of vitamin C carries the risk of evolution into pro-oxidant depending on its cellular localization, exposure time, and concentration changes (Osiecki et al., 2010). Vitamin E also has antioxidant activity and although it is not used for human embryo culture, there are many animal studies reporting its positive effects. Increased blastocyst rates were obtained with vitamin E supplementation in studies on mouse, bovine, pig, and buffalo embryos (Combelles & Hennet, 2012; Wang et al., 2002). As with vitamin C, vitamin E has a pro-oxidant effect under certain conditions, for example in the presence of iron (Osiecki et al., 2010; Yamamoto & Niki, 1988). When both vitamin E and C were added to the medium, increased apoptosis was observed in bovine embryos and increased DNA damage in human sperm cells (Donnelly et al., 1999; Jeong et al., 2006). B vitamins play an important role in amino acid and carbohydrate metabolism, and there are various combinations of B vitamins in current embryo culture fluids (Combelles & Hennet, 2012; Gardner & Simón, 2017). Folic acid (B9), panthothenate (B5), and pyridoxine (B6) have antioxidant activity (Stocker et al., 2003). No positive effects of B6 on animal embryos have been observed (Kane, 1988). Folic acid is essential for in vivo embryo development; however, it has not promoted in vitro embryo development in rabbits, hamsters, and mice (Kane & Bavister, 1988; Kane, 1988; O'Neill, 1998). In in vitro conditions, the embryo does not need exogenous folic acid, when the endogenous folic acid pool is sufficient (O'Neill, 1998). B5 has increased the blastocyst development and live birth rates of hamster embryos, when used alone or in a cocktail with other B vitamins. A similar effect has not been achieved with B vitamins other than B5 and vitamin B cocktails without B5 (McKiernan & Bavister, 2000). Water-soluble vitamins, especially Nicotinamide (B3) and cobalamin (B12), have inhibited blastocyst development and decreased viability (Kane & Bavister, 1988; Tsai & Gardner, 1994). In the presence of amino acids in the medium, the same vitamins did not have a negative effect on embryo development (Gardner & Sakkas, 1993). Human embryos can complete their development under vitamin-free culture conditions (Hardy, 1993) and the effects of vitamins on embryos developing in vitro and their interactions with other culture components have not been fully elucidated yet. Therefore, further research is required to add information, such as the type, dose, and stage of development of the vitamins they should be used in, to the culture fluids.

Antioxidants and Chelators

It is known that nontoxic doses of reactive oxygen species (ROS) are necessary for cells and support embryo development (Morales et al., 1999; Thomas et al., 1997). High ROS levels are one of the main stressors for the embryo. ROS are commonly found in the female genital tract and various antioxidant systems are present in oocytes, embryos, and fluids of the genital tract (Agarwal et al., 2012; Dumoulin et al., 1992; Premkumar & Agarwal, 2012). High amounts of ROS that cannot be balanced with various antioxidant systems; lead to lipid peroxidation, so cell and organelle membrane damage, mitochondrial damage, aggregation of endoplasmic reticulum and cytoskeleton components, inactivation of various enzymes, DNA fragmentation, and apoptosis (Combelles & Hennet, 2012). Embryos exposed to high ROS levels show a slow cleavage rate, uneven blastomeres, increased cytoplasmic fragmentation due to increased apoptosis, and developmental arrest (Aguilar & Reyley, 2005; Barbehenn et al., 1974b).

During in vitro culture, embryos are exposed to ROS levels higher than those developed in the female genital tract (Bedaiwy et al., 2004). While the metabolic activity of the embryo is the source of endogenous ROS; leukocytes, dead spermatozoa, cell debris, metal ions, exposure of some photosensitive components in medium and oil to visible light, high glucose level, atmospheric oxygen concentration (21%), and insufficient medium content are the sources of exogenous ROS (Combelles & Hennet, 2012). Various antioxidants and chelators are used in embryo culture systems to combat ROS and its possible effects. Antioxidants act as enzymes such as superoxide dismutase (SOD), catalase, glutathione peroxidase (GPx), or non-enzymatically such as ascorbic acid, pyruvate, taurine, hypotaurine, cysteamine (CSH), glutathione (GSH), thioredoxin, etc. Chelators, whose name is derived from the Greek word "chele" meaning claw, form complexes with positively charged metal ions through their negative charges (Figure 19.2) (Combelles & Hennet, 2012). All amino acids in culture media also have chelator effects to varying degrees. Ethylenediaminetetraacetic acid (EDTA), ethylenediaminediacetate (EDDA), ethyleneglycolbistetraacetate (EGTA), diethylenetriaminepentaacetic acid (DTPA), desferrioxamine (DFO), transferrin, and citrate are examples of other molecules used as chelators, in addition to amino acids (Combelles & Hennet, 2012).

Despite many studies on human and animal embryos, there is no consensus on ideal antioxidants and chelators, suitable combinations of antioxidants and chelators, exposure time, and dose to be added to culture fluids. Even in different studies with the same antioxidant or chelator, conflicting data are presented. Differences in animal species, culture fluids, and oxygen concentration used in

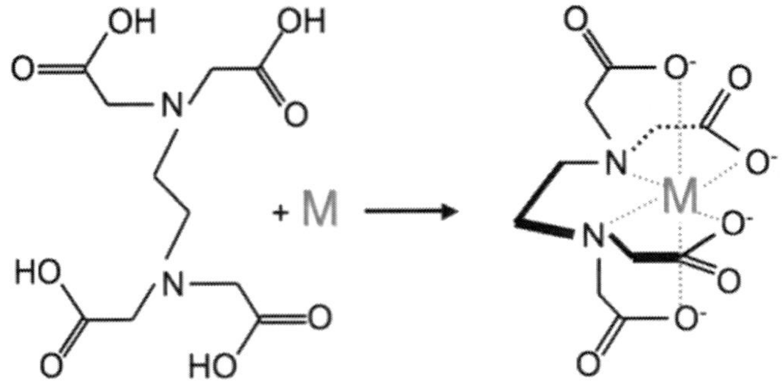

Figure 19.2 Structures of EDTA and EDTA-metal complex (Combelles & Hennet, 2012).

the experiments affected the results. For example, in mouse strains sensitive to the "2-cell block", embryos were able to reach the blastocyst stage as a result of SOD supplementation; however, no effects were observed in other studies in different mouse species, cattle and rabbits (Chun et al., 1994; Lindenau & Fischer, 1994; Noda et al., 1991; Payne et al., 1992). A high glucose concentration is associated with higher ROS levels, and Karja NW et al. reported that the antioxidant effect of SOD was masked when glucose concentration increased in culture media (Karja et al., 2006). Another problem with antioxidants and chelators is that these substances are highly labile in solution. Ascorbic acid added to the slow-freezing medium and GSH, which is highly effective in female genital tract fluids, supports embryo development (Lane et al., 2002; Legge & Sellens, 1991). However, both ascorbate and GSH are not stable in solution (Gardner & Simón, 2017). The half-life of cysteine, the precursor of GSH, in culture media is only ten minutes (Guérin et al., 2001). Studies generally focused on only one antioxidant. However, the functions of antioxidants in vivo are intertwined (Figure 19.3) (Combelles & Hennet, 2012). Troung et al. observed that α-lipoic acid, acetyl-l-cysteine and acetyl-l-carnitine were more effective when used in a group (Truong et al., 2016). The results of the studies also vary according to the stage of development of the embryo. For example, taurine, which is found in high concentrations in female genital tract fluids, has antioxidant and chelator activity and is especially effective in fertilization and the 2-cell stage (Bavister, 1995). Today, the G1 and P1 mediums contain taurine (Gardner & Simón, 2017). Another example that shows varying effects depending on the developmental stage of the embryo is pyruvate, which is present in all culture fluids, especially as a nutritional supplement. Pyruvate has strong antioxidant activity (Andrae et al., 1985). In bovine embryos, the protective effect of pyruvate against H_2O_2 damage was sufficient in zygotes but insufficient in the blastocyst stage (Morales et al., 1999). Supplementation with EDTA has been reported to support embryo development in the early cleavage

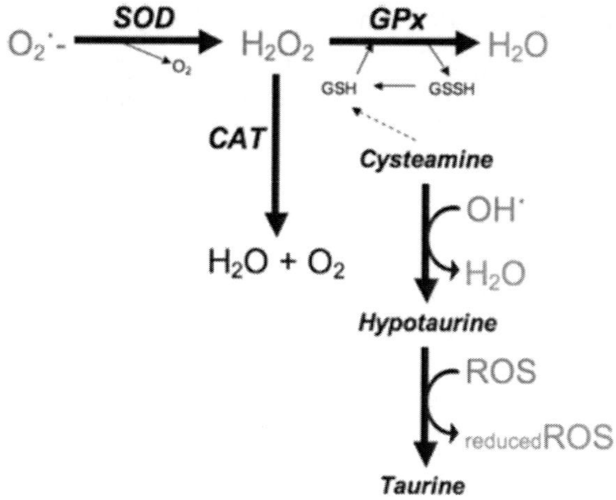

Figure 19.3 The example of antioxidant cooperation (Combelles & Hennet, 2012).

stage similar to taurine and may even affect negatively after compaction. There is no consensus on the optimal dose of EDTA. Both 10 μM and 100 μM doses of EDTA have reduced glycolytic 3-phosphoglycerate kinase enzyme activity, so supplementation with EDTA in culture media should be avoided in the blastocyst stage, where glycolysis is the main energy source (Lane & Gardner, 2001). Transferrin, not yet used in human embryo culture media, has promoted embryo development in mouse strains sensitive to the "2-cell block" (Nasr-esfahani et al., 1990; Nasr-Esfahani & Johnson, 1992). However, no beneficial effect was observed when human transferrin was used instead of bovine transferrin in the same experiment, and embryotoxic effects were observed at some doses (Nasr-esfahani et al., 1990). It has been reported that the presence or absence of transferrin does not cause any change in embryo development, in the presence of glutamine, nonessential amino acids, and EDTA in the culture medium (Gardner & Lane, 1996).

ROS plays a role in embryo development through its effects on cell signaling. Therefore, when supplementing culture fluids with antioxidants and chelators, the aim should be to keep ROS within a safe range rather than eliminate it. The interactions of the antioxidant and chelator molecules with each other and other components of the culture medium, as well as the developmental stage and oxygen concentration at which they are effective should be considered.

Antibiotics

Through improved sterile working conditions in IVF laboratories, antibiotics (especially gentamicin, penicillin, streptomycin) are routinely added to culture fluids, although the risk of contamination has decreased, except in cases such as infected seminal plasma. Penicillin and streptomycin cause developmental arrest in hamster embryos (Zhou et al., 2000). With the removal of both antibiotics from the media, increased cleavage rates in humans, increased chromatin integrity, and decreased apoptosis in mouse embryos were observed (Liu et al., 2011; Magli et al., 1996). Gentamicin, the most common antibiotic in commercially available culture fluids, has no known embryotoxic effect (Cohen & Rieger, 2012). Although the use of antibiotic-free culture fluids seems to be a better option because the embryo developing under physiological conditions is not exposed to antibiotics and the possible embryotoxic effects of antibiotics, it is not recommended due to the risk of contamination (Cohen & Rieger, 2012). The need for antibiotics in the media used for sperm preparation is indisputable (Gardner & Simón, 2017).

Proteins and Other Macromolecules

In the first years of human IVF studies, somatic cell culture fluids with added serum obtained from various sources (fetal bovine, calf, human fetal cord, fertile donor, maternal serum) were used as culture medium. The insufficiency of somatic cell media and simple salt solutions to support embryo development led to the idea of supplementing these fluids with serum. Embryo coculture was very popular in the 1990s, and coculture studies were performed with various cells such as oviduct, vero, ampulla, fetal bovine uterine cells (Bongso et al., 1990; Killian et al., 2001; Ménézo et al., 1995; Rieger et al., 1995; Wiemer et al., 1989). The purpose of preserving the viability of the cells mentioned above has made it essential to supplement the culture fluids with serum.

Although serum has the capacity to support simple culture media with its energy sources such as amino acids, glucose, intermediate metabolites, growth factors and hormones, and to function as a chelator and pH buffer in more complex culture media, it also brings many negatives (Gardner & Simón, 2017).

The preparation of the serum is a very time-consuming and costly process. In addition to major components such as albumin and transferrin, serum also contains many minor components such as energy sources, lipids, hormones, growth factors and minerals, whose concentrations and effects on the embryo will never be known. It is not possible to ensure the consistency of the sources from which the serum is obtained, hence the standardization of the serum content. Even from the same source, conditions such as menstrual cycle day, fasting, satiety, and illness cause changes in serum content (Gardner & Simón,

2017). Sera belonging to some patient groups such as unexplained infertility, polycystic ovary syndrome, and endometriosis showed embryotoxic effects (Damewood et al., 1990; Deaton et al., 1996; Dokras et al., 1993). The serum may be contaminated with prions or viruses (such as HIV and hepatitis B) and may infect the embryo, patient, and laboratory staff. Hepatitis B infection has been developed in 79 women after transfer of embryos cultured with serum contaminated with hepatitis B (Alberda et al., 1989). Serum supplemented embryo culture has resulted in fetal macrosomia (large baby syndrome), post-natal malformations, increased neonatal mortality, and abortion rates in sheep and cattle (Thompson, 2000). In mice, excephalopathy, increased postnatal organ weight, and low birth weight were observed (Fernández-Gonzalez et al., 2004; Khosla et al., 2001; Lawrence & Moley, 2008). Large baby syndrome resulting from serum supplementation has been associated with decreased M6P/IGF-IIR gene expression, which plays a role in fetal organogenesis and humans do not have this locus (Killian et al., 2001; Young et al., 2001). Therefore, it is not surprising that large-baby syndrome has not been observed after serum supplementation in human studies. Ultrastructural changes such as abnormal folding of mitochondrial crystae and trophectoderm vesiculation have also been observed with serum supplementation (Dorland, 1994; Gardner & Simón, 2017).

In addition to the negative effects mentioned, serum utilization is not physiological for embryo culture. Embryos that develop in vivo are exposed to specialized female genital tract fluids for embryo development rather than pathological serum transudates resulting from platelet activity (Gardner et al., 1996; Leese, 1988; Menezo et al., 1984). As a result of these data from the literature, current embryo culture fluids are not supplemented with serum.

Macromolecules facilitate in vitro manipulation by preventing gametes and embryos from adhering to each other or to their contact surfaces. Nowadays, albumin solutions enriched with α and β globulin such as Human Serum Albumin (HSA), Plasmatein®, Plasmanate® and Synthetic Serum Substitute (SSS®); recombinant albumin, hyaluronic acid; and synthetic polymers such as polyvinyl alcohol (PVA) and polyvinylpyrrolidone (PVP) are used as an alternative to serum. Proteins, especially HSA, are an essential nutritional source for embryos and other macromolecules such as hyaluronic acid, PVA, and PVP cannot perform this function (Pemble & Kaye, 1986). Albumin maintains cell membrane stabilization and osmotic pressure, neutralizes toxins accumulated in the culture medium, carries embryotrophic products such as growth factors, amino acids, fatty acids, vitamins, and hormones, and has a pH buffering effect (Meintjes, 2012).

α and β globulins increased blastocyst development and hatching rates in mouse embryos (Tanikawa et al., 1999). In the study by Meintjes M et al., higher live birth rates were found in the HSA+SSS group compared to the HSA group (Meintjes et al., 2009). Interestingly, there were no differences in embryo morphology and pregnancy rates between the two groups. Live birth rates for the HSA and HSA+SSS groups are similar on day 2 or day 3 embryo transfer. The positive effect of SSS was observed after EGA and was associated with possible growth factors. In the same study, the male / female sex ratio was found to increase significantly in the HSA group. It is thought that HSA may cause selective loss of female embryos after the 8-cell stage (Chang et al., 2009). Thus, the increase in live birth rates observed in the HSA+SSS group may be a direct result of the increased viability of female embryos (Meintjes, 2012).

Embryo developing in vivo is exposed to many autocrine and paracrine molecules and has the capacity to respond to these substances according to its requirements. Currently used protein supplements contain also heavy metals, fatty acids and other small molecules, hormones, growth factors, and many compounds that have not been fully characterized. In addition to contaminants, HSA solutions also contain stabilizers such as sodium caprylate and sodium acetyl tryptophanate. Various growth factors and hormones such as VEGF, IGF-II, FSH, TSH, progesterone, hCG, DHEA-S and insulin have been detected in SSS solutions (Meintjes, 2012). In protein supplements even produced by the same company, there are differences from batch to batch. The standardization problem as with serum also exists for alternative protein sources, and the effect of contaminants such as hormones and growth factors in protein solutions on embryos is not fully known. Endotoxin contamination is another risk found in protein supplements. In embryos exposed to endotoxin, delayed development, increased fragmentation, and decreased live birth rates were observed (Fishel et al., 1988; Nagata & Shirakawa, 1996).

Recombinant albumin is a better macromolecule option because it does not have the risks mentioned in HSA and other serum extracts, it can be standardized, and its effectiveness has been clinically proven (Bungum et al., 2002). Recombinant albumin has been associated with increased cryotolerance, as well as its equivalent success with HSA in embryo development and pregnancy rates under in vitro conditions (Murakami et al., 2014).

Hyaluronic acid is a member of glycosaminoglycans, and both endometrium and embryo have hyaluronate receptors (Behzad et al., 1994). In a study in mice an increase in endometrial hyaluronate concentration during implantation has been observed (Zorn et al., 1995). Increased blastocyst development, implantation, and fetal development rates were observed with the addition of hyaluronic acid to culture media. Like recombinant albumin, hyaluronic acid also increased cryotolerance (Stojkovic et al., 2002). Hyaluronate supplementation, especially to embryo transfer medium, supports pregnancy and live birth (Bontekoe et al., 2014).

Growth Factors

Currently available culture fluids do not contain growth factors except granulocyte-macrophage colony stimulating factor (GM-CSF). However, oocytes and embryos interact with many growth factors in the female genital tract and uterine fluids through their receptors. Growth factors are expressed with hCG stimulation in corpus luteum (vascular endothelial growth factor [VEGF] and inhibin) and granulosa cells (insulin-like growth factor-2 [IGF-2], inhibin, VEGF and activin A). Various growth factors such as IGF-1, IGF-2, macrophage colony stimulating factor (MCSF), and fibroblast growth factor (FGF)) were detected in follicular fluids obtained during the oocyte pick up. In addition to the growth factors found in the in vivo microenvironment, many growth factors are expressed in embryos. All this knowledge supports the role of growth factors in embryo development. In experiments with human and various mammal embryos, growth factors have been shown to support embryo development. Increased pregnancy rates in humans have been obtained with GM-CSF, platelet activating factor (PAF), and leukemia inhibitory factor (LIF). Increased blastocyst formation and hatching with heparin-binding epidermal growth factor (HB-EGF) and GM-CSF; increased blastocyst formation and decreased apoptosis were observed with IGF-1. Although current culture fluids are not fully optimized yet, healthy embryos can be developed and live births can be obtained with these fluids. Although growth factors interact with each other in the in vivo microenvironment, each growth factor was used in isolation in the experiments. Today's technologies are insufficient to obtain data on the concentrations of growth factors in female genital tract fluids. High levels of growth factors can cause developmental abnormalities, and long-term follow-up is required if there is exposure to any growth factor during in vitro culture. Further studies are needed on the combinations and amounts of growth factors that should be added to embryo culture fluids (Hegde & Behr, 2012).

pH and Buffer Systems

pH is another important parameter that needs to be regulated for optimal embryo development and to reduce the stress that the embryo will be exposed to in culture medium. Currently, the pH value of embryo culture media (pHe) is mainly balanced by the bicarbonate buffer system. According to the Henderson-Hasselbalch Equation ($CO_2+H_2O \rightleftharpoons H_2CO_3 \rightleftharpoons HCO_3^-+H^+$), the concentration of H^+ ions balanced with HCO_3^- in the environment, hence pHe, is affected by changes in CO_2 concentration (Michelle Lane et al., 2000). To maintain the physiological pH range (7.2-7.4), 25 mM HCO_3^- and 5-6% CO_2

concentration are used in culture systems. Besides the effect of CO_2 gas on pH value, it has also been observed that it is incorporated into nucleic acids and proteins of mouse preimplantation embryos (Graves & Biggers, 1970).

pH values of the female genital tract have been reported to vary according to the stage of the menstrual cycle and are lower in the uterus than in the oviduct (Dale et al., 1998a; Maas et al., 1977). In studies conducted with various mammalian embryos, it has been found that the CO_2 concentration in the uterus is 10% and that in vitro embryo development is also better than at a concentration of 5% CO_2 (Carney & Bavister, 1987; Garris, 1984; Hallden et al., 1992). Although a 5-6% CO_2 concentration is used for human embryos, the optimal CO_2 concentration has not yet been determined (Gardner & Simón, 2017).

Although the pHe value in embryo culture systems is tried to be adjusted in the range of 7,2-7,4, pH is a very dynamic variable. Depending on the type of commercial culture medium used; the differences in some components (especially ions such as Na^+, K^+, Mg^{2+}, Cl^-, amino acids such as glycine, which acts as a zwitterionic buffer, lactate, and pyruvate), the interactions of these components with each other, the temperature, and even the altitude of the laboratory affect the pH value. Even if the same culture medium and the same CO_2 concentration are used, the pH value that needs to be adjusted may vary from laboratory to laboratory and incubator to incubator (Edwards et al., 1998; Swain, 2012; Swain & Pool, 2009).

The intracellular pH value (pHi) of the embryo is at least as important as pHe for development and is affected by changes in pHe (Edwards et al., 1998). When the pHe value is not optimal, the embryo needs to consume more energy to maintain the pHi value. The pHi value has many functions in the maintenance of intracellular homeostasis and in the regulation of embryo development. Deviations in pHi impair the developmental competence of mouse embryos by causing disruption in the cytoplasmic localization of organelles, metabolic changes such as decreased oxidative phosphorylation, and increased glycolysis (Edwards et al., 1998; Lane et al., 2000; Squirrell et al., 2001; Zander-Fox et al., 2010). The pHi value of human oocytes and embryos is approximately 7.1. The reason for keeping the pHe value of culture systems in the range of 7.2-7.4 is that this value decreases as a result of embryo metabolism (Swain, 2012). In addition to the short-acting buffering capacity of the cytoplasm, the embryo regulates pHi through various transport systems such as HCO_3^- / Cl^- exchanger, Na^+/H^+ antiporter, monocarboxylate transporter (MCT). However, oocytes and early clevage embryos lack transport systems, thus the capacity to regulate pHi and are more sensitive to changes in pHe (Swain, 2012). Cumulus cells are known to regulate pHi, and fluctuations in pH values should especially be avoided in processes after denudation (such as ICSI, IVM) (Gardner & Simón, 2017). Morula and blastocyst stage embryos are more competent to regulate pHi through their intercellular tight junctions (Edwards et al., 1998). The pH regulation capacity that varied according to the stage of development and the increase in the binding of sperm to the zona pellucida at higher pH values revealed the model of "high-low-high" (Dale et al., 1998b). According to this model, some centers prefer to use a high pH during fertilization, a lower pH for the culture of embryos in the cleavage stage, and again a high pH for the culture of the morula and blastocyst.

When culture plates are removed from the incubator for various procedures such as oocyte pick up, ICSI, cryopreservation, embryo transfer, the HCO_3^- buffer system is insufficient. A rapid increase in pH occurs as a result of the low concentration of CO_2 in the air and, therefore, the rapid decrease in the concentration of CO_2 in the culture medium. Although precautions are taken to delay this increase, such as supplementing culture media with amino acids with pH buffering function, the use of incubators with lids in each compartment and oil overlay, more effective solutions are required. Today, N-2-hydroxyethylpiperazine-N′-2-ethanesulfonic acid (HEPES) and 4-morpholinepropanesulfonic acid (MOPS) buffer systems are used for this purpose. Among the zwitterionic buffers, these buffers, which have the closest pKa value (7.2) to the pHi value of 7.1, are very successful in pH regulation. It has also been reported that HEPES can function as a heavy metal chelator and support embryo development in the presence of optimal culture conditions (Mash et al., 2002).

Environmental Factors

Temperature

Today, it is accepted that the optimal temperature value required for embryo development is 37°C. Decreased cleavage and blastocyst development rates were observed in mouse and rabbit embryos exposed to room temperature, while meiotic spindle disruption was observed in human oocytes. Meiotic spindle damage was also observed at temperatures of 38°C and above (Sun et al., 2004). Although such data are not available for humans, in many species the temperature of the female genital tract is lower than that of the rest of the body. (Simopoulou et al., 2018). Leese et al. also reported that 37°C may not be optimal for embryo development (Leese et al., 2008). Although this view is not supported in human embryo studies, it is an indication that the optimum culture environment is still not reached in current IVF practice and each parameter should be questioned until the best embryo is reached.

The aim in IVF laboratories is to maintain the optimal temperature value and to prevent temperature fluctuations that will adversely affect embryo development. Incubators, tube warmers, and hot plates should be routinely checked and calibrated as needed. Procedures outside the incubator should be kept as short as possible, and patient planning should be done in such a way that the incubator doors are opened the least. To prevent evaporation, the use of a heating work surface should be avoided during the preparation of the culture plates and medium the day before the procedures.

Oxygen

Embryo culture for many years has been performed at an atmospheric oxygen concentration. However, in many mammalian species, it has been observed that the oxygen concentration in the oviduct is in the range of 5-8.7%, and this rate drops to 1.5-2% in the uterus (Fischer & Bavister, 1993).

High oxygen concentration can cause toxicity by increasing the amount of ROS in the culture medium (Kovačič, 2012). Atmospheric oxygen has detrimental effects on the epigenome, proteome, and metabolism of the embryo. Hypoxia-inducible factors (HIFs), which are DNA-binding proteins and are stable only at low oxygen concentrations, activate the transcription of genes that regulate embryo development and metabolism. At a 21% oxygen concentration, dysregulation of the expression of various genes associated with cell growth and gastrulation has been observed (Rinaudo et al., 2006). Harvey AJ et al. observed an increase in ICM formation and the expression of genes related to glucose metabolism in bovine embryos at a 2% oxygen concentration (Harvey et al., 2007). Low oxygen concentration is also associated with increased expression of antioxidant enzymes (Otsuki et al., 2007). Atmospheric oxygen increases the susceptibility of the embryo to various stress factors in the culture medium, as is the case with increasing the negative effects of ammonium on embryo development (Otsuki et al., 2007; Wale & Gardner, 2013).

When the oxygen concentration is reduced to 5%; increased fertilization, cleavage rate, blastocyst development, embryo quality, hatching, implantation, and live birth rates, and decreased apoptosis and incidence of mosaicism were observed (Bean et al., 2002; Gardner & Lane, 2003; Meintjes et al., 2009; Waldenström et al., 2009; Wale & Gardner, 2010; Yuan et al., 2003).

Although the optimal oxygen concentration for human embryo culture is still unknown, the need for a low oxygen concentration is obvious. Embryos that develop in vivo are exposed to a decrease in oxygen concentration from the oviduct to the uterus, coinciding with a shift in embryo metabolism from oxidative phosphorylation to glycolysis (Leese, 1995). In vitro culture at varying oxygen concentrations according to the embryo development stage may be the subject of future studies.

Incubators

Incubators are one of the most important pieces of equipment in IVF laboratories. Optimal conditions required for embryo development (such as pH and temperature) are provided through incubators. The most important feature sought in incubators is the ability to quickly recover the lowered temperature and gas concentration values after opening the lid. Embryo quality increases markedly when the incubator opening frequency decreases (Gardner & Lane, 1996). Conventional-type large incubators and bench-top mini-incubators are the two main types of incubators. In conventional incubators, models with inner lids for each compartment in addition to the outer lid should be preferred. Bench-top incubators have separate compartments with their own lids, and recovery time is shorter than conventional incubators. Another advantage of bench-top incubators is that they are compatible with time-lapse technology. However, heat loss is faster in bench-top types. The recovery rate of CO_2 concentration in incubators with infrared CO_2 sensors is faster than in incubators with thermal conductive CO_2 sensors (Gardner & Simón, 2017). Water jacketed incubators are superior to air jacketed in temperature fluctuations (Coward & Wells, 2013). There are incubator types that use only CO_2, CO_2, and N_2 and premix gas (CO_2, O_2, and N_2) cylinders as gas source. Incubators that are gassed only with CO_2 should not be preferred, as they have an atmospheric O_2 concentration. During the setup of the IVF laboratory, a mix of different types of incubator should be adopted rather than relying on just one type of incubator that does not have a clear advantage over the other (Swain, 2014). There should be a sufficient number of incubators according to the patient density of the center. Separate incubators can be used for embryo culture and equilibration to reduce the frequency of opening the lid.

Light

Visible light is a stress factor for mammalian embryos (Hirao & Yanagimachi, 1978; Ottosen et al., 2007). With low lighting conditions; increased rates of cleavage and blastocyst development were observed in rabbits and hamsters, and increased rates of blastocyst development, pregnancy rates, and live birth weights were observed in humans (Noda et al., 1994; Schumacher & Fischer, 1988; Umaoka et al., 1992). Prolonged exposure to visible light causes degradation in culture fluids and peroxidation in paraffin oil (Kovačič, 2012). Procedures such as oocyte collection and embryo manipulation in IVF laboratories should be performed under low lighting conditions, procedures under the microscope should be kept as short as possible, and the culture fluids and paraffin oil used should be stored in the dark.

"Back to Nature" or "Let the Embryo Choose"

As mentioned above, both the fluid content of the female genital tracts and the requirements of the embryo change during the process from fertilization to implantation. These changes are especially evident after EGA and compaction. In sequential culture systems that adopt the "back to nature" principle, two different media with different contents are used for the early cleavage and late blastocyst stages, similar to in vivo conditions (Lane & Gardner, 2007; Leese, 1998). In the "let the embryo choose" principle, all possible requirements of the embryo are collected in a single medium at tolerable concentrations. The opinion is that the embryo determines which component and how much it will consume at which stage (Biggers, 2001).

Embryos can be developed and live birth can be obtained in both culture systems, and there are not enough clinical data to prove that one of the two culture systems is superior to the other (Dieamant et al., 2017; Sfontouris et al., 2016). However, today there is a trend towards single-step culture systems for the following reasons:

- Affordable than the sequential culture system
- Less workload
- Reduced removal from incubator→ more stable culture conditions (pH, temperature, etc.)
- Less handling of embryo→ reduced risk of possible embryo damage/loss
- Providing the continuity of the microenvironment formed by the embryo→accumulation of embryotrophic molecules such as endogenous growth factors
- Suitable for Time-Lapse culture systems→improved embryo selection (Swain, 2019).

Incubation Volume and Group Culture

The aim in human IVF practices is to select the best-developed embryo and to transfer a single embryo. Therefore, group culture is not common. However, there are studies reporting that group culture supports embryo development in many mammalian species (O'Neill, 2008). With group culture; increased cell number, blastocyst development, and viability have been observed in cattle, mice, and sheep embryos (Ahern & Gardner, 1998; Gardner et al., 1997; Gardner et al., 1994; Salahuddin et al., 1995). In humans, by adding a good quality embryo to the medium, an improvement in development and pregnancy rates was observed in embryos with delayed development (Lightman et al., 1997). T. Ebner et al. have reported that group culture was associated with increased blastocyst development, implantation, and live birth rates in human embryos (Ebner et al., 2010). However, stronger evidence is needed that group culture is definitively beneficial in human embryos (Rijnders & Jansen, 1999).

Embryos that develop in vivo are exposed to very low volumes of female genital tract fluids, and the beneficial effects of group culture on embryo development also become more prominent when the volume of microdrops was reduced. Embryos produce a variety of autocrine and paracrine embryotrophic factors, and these factors are diluted in high-media volumes. Microdrops with a volume of 20-50 μl, which are widely used in today's IVF laboratories, are large enough to dilute and inactivate embryotrophic factors. In addition to embryotrophic factors; ROS, metabolic wastes, and cellular toxins accumulate in culture fluids, which may be one reason why the use of small-volume microdrops is avoided. Another drawback is the increased risk of osmolality and pH fluctuations that will develop as a result of evaporation of low volumes, despite oil overlay, and the possibility of being denatured more easily as a result of being closer to the surface of fat-soluble embryotrophic factors (Reed, 2012). An increase in embryo development has been observed with ultramicrodrop systems using volumes as low as 0.5-1 μl in cattle and mice and 1.5-2 μl in humans (Vajta et al., 2010). Today, culture plates suitable for both group culture and the evaluation of each embryo separately have been developed (Vajta et al., 2000). As a result of this information, the traditional culture system (20-50 μl volume/1-4 embryos) should be reviewed, and the beneficial effects of group culture on human embryos should be evaluated by making appropriate modifications to culture plates (Vajta et al., 2010).

Conclusion

Infertility is an important health problem, and there are approximately 48 million infertile couples worldwide (The Lancet Global Health, 2022). In the last four decades, significant advances have been made in the treatment of infertility and more than 8 million children have been born with ART treatments (Fauser, 2019). One of the most important factors that played a role in this success is the "embryo culture systems", the main members of which are examined in this chapter.

Studies in the laboratory phase of infertility treatment have especially focused on determining the optimal culture conditions required for gametes and embryos. There are many interrelated conditions that need to be optimized from the consumable used to the culture media, from the incubator to the laboratory temperature. There are certain standards in current human IVF practice, and embryos can be developed successfully. However, the 'optimal' conditions identified are based mostly on animal experiments because of the limitations of large-scale human studies. The "optimum" has not yet been reached for each parameter that makes up the embryo culture systems. Many more questions continue to be discussed, such as sequential or single-stage culture, which culture medium component, in which developmental stage, in what quantity, and which incubator. A multidisciplinary approach is required for system optimization, and many disciplines such as biology, medicine, chemistry, genetics, and mechanics should work together. Time-lapse technology, which can eliminate stress factors that will develop due to removal from the incubator, is a good example of this multidisciplinary approach. Nowadays, various microfluidic tools such as microwells, microchannels, etc., dynamic culture systems (shaking, rotation, tilting, etc.), and specialized culture surfaces such as agarose and matrigel, etc. are being developed for in vitro embryo culture (Swain & Smith, 2011). However, further studies are required on the effects on human embryos for the routine use of the mentioned tools in human ART practices.

As seen, each parameter that makes up the "embryo culture system" is open to being questioned and developed. However, it is not possible to determine a single optimal system for each IVF laboratory. Therefore, clinical embryologists should establish an "optimal" system based on individual laboratory performance and key components that have been proven superior in the literature, such as low oxygen culture. Finally, the physiology, metabolism and requirements of gametes and embryos should be sufficiently known and understood. In case of unsuccessful results, the parameters of the system should be questioned, possible solutions should be known, and innovation should be open.

References

Agarwal, A., Aponte-Mellado, A., Premkumar, B. J., Shaman, A., & Gupta, S. (2012). The effects of oxidative stress on female reproduction: A review. In *Reproductive Biology and Endocrinology* (Vol. 10). Reprod Biol Endocrinol. https://doi.org/10.1186/1477-7827-10-49

Aguilar, J., & Reyley, M. (2005). The uterine tubal fluid : secretion , composition and biological effects. *Animal Reproduction Science*, *2*(2), 91–105.

Ahern, T., & Gardner, D. K. (1998). Culturing bovine embryos in groups stimulates blastocyst development and cell allocation to the inner cell mass. *Theriogenology*, *49*(1), 194. https://doi.org/10.1016/s0093-691x(98)90547-7

Alberda, A. T., Van Os, H. C., & Zeilmaker, G. H. (1989). Hepatitis Bvirusinfectie bij Vrouwen behandeld met in-vitro fertilisatie [Hepatitis B virus infection in women treated with in vitro fertilization]. *Nederlands Tijdschrift Voor Gieneeskunde*, *133*, 20–25.

Andrae, U., Singh, J., & Ziegler-Skylakakis, K. (1985). Pyruvate and related α-ketoacids protect mammalian cells in culture against hydrogen peroxide-induced cytotoxicity. *Toxicology Letters*, *28*(2–3), 93–98. https://doi.org/10.1016/0378-4274(85)90015-3

Baltz, J. M. (2012). Media composition: Salts and osmolality. *Methods in Molecular Biology*, *912*, 61–80. https://doi.org/10.1007/978-1-61779-971-6_5

Barbehenn, E. K., Wales, R. G., & Lowry, O. H. (1974a). The explanation for the blockade of glycolysis in early mouse embryos. *Proceedings of the National Academy of Sciences of the United States of America*, *71*(4), 1056–1060. https://doi.org/10.1073/pnas.71.4.1056

Barbehenn, E. K., Wales, R. G., & Lowry, O. H. (1974b). The explanation for the blockade of glycolysis in early mouse embryos. *Proceedings of the National Academy of Sciences of the United States of America*, *71*(4), 1056–1060. https://doi.org/10.1073/pnas.71.4.1056

Bavister, B. D. (1995). Culture of preimplantation embryos: Facts and artifacts. *Human Reproduction Update*, *1*(2), 91–148. https://doi.org/10.1093/humupd/1.2.91

Bean, C. J., Hassold, T. J., Judis, L. A., & Hunt, P. A. (2002). Fertilization in vitro increases non-disjunction during early cleavage divisions in a mouse model system. *Human Reproduction*, *17*(9), 2362–2367. https://doi.org/10.1093/humrep/17.9.2362

Bedaiwy, M. A., Falcone, T., Mohamed, M. S., Aleem, A. A. N., Sharma, R. K., Worley, S. E., Thornton, J., & Agarwal, A. (2004). Differential growth of human embryos in vitro: Role of reactive oxygen species. *Fertility and Sterility*, *82*(3), 593–600. https://doi.org/10.1016/j.fertnstert.2004.02.121

Behzad, F., Seif, M. W., Campbell, S., & Aplin, J. D. (1994). Expression of two isoforms of CD44 in human endometrium. *Biology of Reproduction*, *51*(4), 739–747. https://doi.org/10.1095/biolreprod51.4.739

Biggers, J. D., Gardner, D. K., & Leese, H. J. (2021). Control of Carbohydrate Metabolism in Preimplantation Mammalian Embryos. In *Growth Factors in Mammalian Development* (pp. 19–32). CRC Press. https://doi.org/10.1201/9781003210351-2

Biggers, John D. (2001). Thoughts on embryo culture conditions. *Reproductive BioMedicine Online*, *4*(June), 30–38. https://doi.org/10.1016/S1472-6483(12)60009-1

Bongso, A., Ng, S. C., & Ratnam, S. (1990). Co-cultures: their relevance to assisted reproduction. *Human Reproduction (Oxford, England)*, *5*(8), 893–900. https://doi.org/10.1093/OXFORDJOURNALS.HUMREP.A137216

Bontekoe, S., Heineman, M. J., Johnson, N., & Blake, D. (2014). Adherence compounds in embryo transfer media for assisted reproductive technologies. In *Cochrane*

Database of Systematic Reviews (Vol. 2014, Issue 2, pp. CD007421–CD007421). John Wiley and Sons Ltd. https://doi.org/10.1002/14651858.CD007421.pub3

Borland, R. M., Biggers, J. D., Lechene, C. P., & Taymor, M. L. (1980). Elemental composition of fluid in the human Fallopian tube. *Journal of Reproduction and Fertility*, *58*(2), 479–482. https://doi.org/10.1530/jrf.0.0580479

Brison, D. R., Houghton, F. D., Falconer, D., Roberts, S. A., Hawkhead, J., Humpherson, P. G., Lieberman, B. A., & Leese, H. J. (2004). Identification of viable embryos in IVF by non-invasive measurement of amino acid turnover. *Human Reproduction (Oxford, England)*, *19*(10), 2319–2324. https://doi.org/10.1093/HUMREP/DEH409

Bungum, M., Humaidan, P., & Bungum, L. (2002). Recombinant human albumin as protein source in culture media used for IVF: a prospective randomized study. *Reproductive Biomedicine Online*, *4*(3), 233–236. https://doi.org/10.1016/S1472-6483(10)61811-1

Carney, E. W., & Bavister, B. D. (1987). Regulation of hamster embryo development in vitro by carbon dioxide. *Biology of Reproduction*, *36*(5), 1155–1163. https://doi.org/10.1095/biolreprod36.5.1155

Casslén, B. G. (1987). Free amino acids in human uterine fluid. Possible role of high taurine concentration. *The Journal of Reproductive Medicine*, *32*(3), 181–184.

Chang, H. J., Lee, J. R., Jee, B. C., Suh, C. S., & Kim, S. H. (2009). Impact of blastocyst transfer on offspring sex ratio and the monozygotic twinning rate: a systematic review and meta-analysis. *Fertility and Sterility*, *91*(6), 2381–2390. https://doi.org/10.1016/j.fertnstert.2008.03.066

Chun, Y. S., Kim, J. H., Lee, H. T., & Chung, K. S. (1994). Effect of superoxide dismutase on the development of preimplantation mouse embryos. *Theriogenology*, *41*(2), 511–520. https://doi.org/10.1016/0093-691X(94)90087-Y

Cohen, J., & Rieger, D. (2012). Historical background of gamete and embryo culture. *Methods in Molecular Biology*, *912*, 1–18. https://doi.org/10.1007/978-1-61779-971-6_1

Combelles, C. M. H., & Hennet, M. L. (2012). Media composition: Antioxidants/chelators and cellular function. *Methods in Molecular Biology*, *912*, 129–159. https://doi.org/10.1007/978-1-61779-971-6_9

Conaghan, J., Handyside, A. H., Winston, R. M. L., & Leese, H. J. (1993). Effects of pyruvate and glucose on the development of human preimplantation embryos in vitro. *Journal of Reproduction and Fertility*, *99*(1), 87–95. https://doi.org/10.1530/jrf.0.0990087

Coward, K., & Wells, D. (2013). Textbook of clinical embryology. In *Textbook of Clinical Embryology*. https://doi.org/10.1017/CBO9781139192736

Cross, P. C., & Brinster, R. L. (1973). The sensitivity of one-cell mouse embryos to pyruvate and lactate. *Experimental Cell Research*, *77*(1–2), 57–62. https://doi.org/10.1016/0014-4827(73)90552-1

Dale, B., Menezo, Y., Cohen, J., Dimatteo, L., & Wilding, M. (1998a). Intracellular pH regulation in the human oocyte. *Human Reproduction (Oxford, England)*, *13*(4), 964–970. https://doi.org/10.1093/HUMREP/13.4.964

Dale, B., Menezo, Y., Cohen, J., Dimatteo, L., & Wilding, M. (1998b). Intracellular pH regulation in the human oocyte. *Human Reproduction*, *13*(4), 964–970. https://doi.org/10.1093/humrep/13.4.964

Damewood, M. D., Hesla, J. S., Schlaff, W. D., Hubbard, M., Gearhart, J. D., & Rock, J. A. (1990). Effect of serum from patients with minimal to mild endometriosis on mouse embryo development in vitro. *Fertility and Sterility*, *54*(5), 917–920. https://doi.org/10.1016/s0015-0282(16)53956-9

Dawson, K. M., Collins, J. L., & Baltz, J. M. (1998). Osmolarity-dependent glycine accumulation indicates a role for glycine as an organic osmolyte in early preimplantation mouse embryos. *Biology of Reproduction*, *59*(2), 225–232. https://doi.org/10.1095/BIOLREPROD59.2.225

Deaton, J. L., Dempsey, R. A., & Miller, K. A. (1996). Serum from women with polycystic ovary syndrome inhibits fertilization and embryonic development in the murine in vitro fertilization model. *Fertility and Sterility*, *65*(6), 1224–1228. https://doi.org/10.1016/S0015-0282(16)58343-5

Dieamant, F., Petersen, C. G., Mauri, A. L., Comar, V., Mattila, M., Vagnini, L. D., Renzi, A., Petersen, B., Ricci, J., Oliveira, J. B. A., Baruffi, R. L. R., & Franco, J. G. (2017). Single versus sequential culture medium: Which is better at improving ongoing pregnancy rates? a systematic review and meta-analysis. In *Jornal Brasileiro de Reproducao Assistida* (Vol. 21, Issue 3, pp. 240–246). https://doi.org/10.5935/1518-0557.20170045

Dokras, A., Sargent, I. L., Redman, C. W. G., & Barlow, D. H. (1993). Sera from women with unexplained infertility inhibit both mouse and human embryo growth in vitro. *Fertility and Sterility*, *60*(2), 285–292. https://doi.org/10.1016/S0015-0282(16)56099-3

Donnelly, E. T., McClure, N., & Lewis, S. E. M. (1999). The effect of ascorbate and α-tocopherol supplementation in vitro on DNA integrity and hydrogen peroxide-induced DNA damage in human spermatozoa. *Mutagenesis*, *14*(5), 505–511. https://doi.org/10.1093/mutage/14.5.505

Dorland, & M. (1994). Serum in synthetic oviduct fluid causes mitochondrial degeneration in ovine embryos. *J. Reprod. Fertil.*, *13*, 25.

Dumoulin, J. C. M., Evers, J. L. H., Bakker, J. A., Bras, M., Pieters, M. H. E. C., & Geraedts, J. P. M. (1992). Temporal effects of taurine on mouse preimplantation development in vitro. *Human Reproduction*, *7*(3), 403–407. https://doi.org/10.1093/oxfordjournals.humrep.a137658

Eagle, H. (1959). Amino acid metabolism in mammalian cell cultures. *Science (New York, N.Y.)*, *130*(3373), 432–437. https://doi.org/10.1126/SCIENCE.130.3373.432

Ebner, T., Shebl, O., Moser, M., Mayer, R. B., Arzt, W., & Tews, G. (2010). Group culture of human zygotes is superior to individual culture in terms of blastulation, implantation and life birth. *Reproductive Biomedicine Online*, *21*(6), 762–768. https://doi.org/10.1016/J.RBMO.2010.06.038

Edwards, L. J., Williams, D. A., & Gardner, D. K. (1998). Intracellular pH of the mouse preimplantation embryo: Amino acids act as buffers of intracellular pH. *Human Reproduction*, *13*(12), 3441–3448. https://doi.org/10.1093/humrep/13.12.3441

Fauser, B. C. (2019). Towards the global coverage of a unified registry of IVF outcomes. In *Reproductive BioMedicine Online* (Vol. 38, Issue 2, pp. 133–137). https://doi.org/10.1016/j.rbmo.2018.12.001

Houghton, F. D., Hawkhead, J. A., Humpherson, P. G., Hogg, J. E., Balen, A. H., Rutherford, A. J., & Leese, H. J. (2002). Non-invasive amino acid turnover predicts human embryo developmental capacity. *Human Reproduction (Oxford, England)*, *17*(4), 999–1005. https://doi.org/10.1093/HUMREP/17.4.999

Fernández-Gonzalez, R., Moreira, P., Bilbao, A., Jiménez, A., Pérez-Crespo, M., Ramírez, M. A., De Fonseca, F. R., Pintado, B., & Gutiérrez-Adán, A. (2004). Long-term effect of in vitro culture of mouse embryos with serum on mRNA expression of imprinting genes, development, and behavior. *Proceedings of the National Academy of Sciences of the United States of America*, *101*(16), 5880–5885. https://doi.org/10.1073/PNAS.0308560101

Fischer, B., & Bavister, B. D. (1993). Oxygen tension in the oviduct and uterus of rhesus monkeys, hamsters and rabbits. *Journal of Reproduction and Fertility*, *99*(2), 673–679. https://doi.org/10.1530/JRF.0.0990673

Fishel, S., Jackson, P., Webster, J., & Faratian, B. (1988). Endotoxins in culture medium for human in vitro fertilization. *Fertility and Sterility*, *49*(1), 108–111. https://doi.org/10.1016/S0015-0282(16)59659-9

Gardner, D. K., Lane, M., Calderon, I., & Leeton, J. (1996). Environment of the preimplantation human embryo in vivo: metabolite analysis of oviduct and uterine fluids and metabolism of cumulus cells. *Fertility and Sterility*, *65*(2), 349–353. https://doi.org/10.1016/S0015-0282(16)58097-2

Gardner, D. K., Lane, M., Spitzer, A., & Batt, P. A. (1994). Enhanced rates of cleavage and development for sheep zygotes cultured to the blastocyst stage in vitro in the absence of serum and somatic cells: Amino acids, vitamins, and culturing embryos in groups stimulate development. *Biology of Reproduction*, *50*(2), 390–400. https://doi.org/10.1095/biolreprod50.2.390

Gardner, D., Lane, M., & Lane, M. (1997). Development of the inner cell mass in mouse blastocysts is stimulated by reducing the embryo:incubation volume ratio. *Human Reproduction*, *12*(Suppl_2), 182–183. https://doi.org/10.1093/humrep/12.suppl_2.182-a

Gardner, D. K. (2008). Dissection of culture media for embryos: the most important and less important components and characteristics. *Reproduction, Fertility, and Development*, *20*(1), 9–18. https://doi.org/10.1071/RD07160

Gardner, D. K. (2015). Lactate production by the mammalian blastocyst: Manipulating the microenvironment for uterine implantation and invasion? *BioEssays*, *37*(4), 364–371. https://doi.org/10.1002/bies.201400155

Gardner, D. K., & Harvey, A. J. (2015). Blastocyst metabolism. In *Reproduction, Fertility and Development* (Vol. 27, Issue 4, pp. 638–654). https://doi.org/10.1071/RD14421

Gardner, D. K., & Lane, M. (1996). Alleviation of the "2-cell block" and development to the blastocyst of CF1 mouse embryos: Role of amino acids, EDTA and physical parameters. *Human Reproduction*, *11*(12), 2703–2712. https://doi.org/10.1093/oxfordjournals.humrep.a019195

Gardner, D. K., & Lane, M. (2003). Towards a single embryo transfer. In *Reproductive BioMedicine Online* (Vol. 6, Issue 4, pp. 470–481). https://doi.org/10.1016/s1472-6483(10)62170-0

Gardner, D. K., Lane, M., Stevens, J., & Schoolcraft, W. B. (2001). Noninvasive assessment of human embryo nutrient consumption as a measure of developmental potential. *Fertility and Sterility*, *76*(6), 1175–1180. https://doi.org/10.1016/S0015-0282(01)02888-6

Gardner, D. K., & Sakkas, D. (1993). Mouse embryo cleavage, metabolism and viability: Role of medium composition. *Human Reproduction*, *8*(2), 288–295. https://doi.org/10.1093/oxfordjournals.humrep.a138039

Gardner, D. K., & Simón, C. (2017). Handbook of In Vitro Fertilization: Fourth Edition. In *Handbook of in Vitro Fertilization, Fourth Edition*. https://doi.org/10.1201/9781315157269

Gardner, D. K., & Wale, P. L. (2013). Analysis of metabolism to select viable human embryos for transfer. *Fertility and Sterility*, *99*(4), 1062–1072. https://doi.org/10.1016/j.fertnstert.2012.12.004

Garris, D. R. (1984). Uterine blood flow, pH, and pCO2 during nidation in the guinea pig: Ovarian regulation. *Endocrinology*, *114*(4), 1219–1224. https://doi.org/10.1210/endo-114-4-1219

Graves, C. N., & Biggers, J. D. (1970). Carbon dioxide fixation by mouse embryos prior to implantation. *Science (New York, N.Y.)*, *167*(3924), 1506–1508. https://doi.org/10.1126/SCIENCE.167.3924.1506

Guérin, P., El Mouatassim, S., & Ménézo, Y. (2001). Oxidative stress and protection against reactive oxygen species in the pre-implantation embryo and its surroundings. *Human Reproduction Update*, *7*(2), 175–189. https://doi.org/10.1093/HUMUPD/7.2.175

Hallden, K., Li, J., Carney, E. W., & Foote, R. H. (1992). Increasing carbon dioxide from five percent to ten percent improves rabbit blastocyst development from cultured zygotes. *Molecular Reproduction and Development*, *33*(3), 276–280. https://doi.org/10.1002/MRD.1080330307

Hardarson, T., Bungum, M., Conaghan, J., Meintjes, M., Chantilis, S. J., Molnar, L., Gunnarsson, K., & Wikland, M. (2015). Noninferiority, randomized, controlled trial comparing embryo development using media developed for sequential or undisturbed culture in a time-lapse setup. *Fertility and Sterility*, *104*(6), 1452-1459.e4. https://doi.org/10.1016/J.FERTNSTERT.2015.08.037

Hardy, K, Hooper, M. A. K., Handyside, A. H., Rutherford, A. J., Winston, R. M. L., & Leese, H. J. (1989). Non-invasive measurement of glucose and pyrovate uptake by individual human oocytes and preimplantation embryos. In *Human Reproduction* (Vol. 4, Issue 3, p. 348). https://doi.org/10.1093/oxfordjournals.humrep.a136905

Hardy, Kate. (1993). Development of Human Blastocysts In Vitro. In *Preimplantation Embryo Development* (pp. 184–199). Springer, New York, NY. https://doi.org/10.1007/978-1-4613-9317-7_14

Harris, S. E., Gopichandran, N., Picton, H. M., Leese, H. J., & Orsi, N. M. (2005). Nutrient concentrations in murine follicular fluid and the female reproductive tract. *Theriogenology*, *64*(4), 992–1006. https://doi.org/10.1016/J.THERIOGENOLOGY.2005.01.004

Harvey, A. J., Kind, K. L., & Thompson, J. G. (2007). Regulation of gene expression in bovine blastocysts in response to oxygen and the iron chelator desferrioxamine. *Biology of Reproduction*, *77*(1), 93–101. https://doi.org/10.1095/BIOLREPROD.106.058826

Hediger, M. A., Romero, M. F., Peng, J. Bin, Rolfs, A., Takanaga, H., & Bruford, E. A. (2004). The ABCs of solute carriers: Physiological, pathological and therapeutic implications of human membrane transport proteins. In *Pflugers*

Archiv European Journal of Physiology (Vol. 447, Issue 5, pp. 465–468). Pflugers Arch. https://doi.org/10.1007/s00424-003-1192-y

Hegde, A., & Behr, B. (2012). Media composition: Growth factors. *Methods in Molecular Biology*, *912*, 177–198. https://doi.org/10.1007/978-1-61779-971-6_11

Hirao, Y., & Yanagimachi, R. (1978). Detrimental effect of visible light on meiosis of mammalian eggs in vitro. *Journal of Experimental Zoology*, *206*(3), 365–369. https://doi.org/10.1002/jez.1402060308

Jansen, S., Esmaeilpour, T., Pantaleon, M., & Kaye, P. L. (2006). Glucose affects monocarboxylate cotransporter (MCT) 1 expression during mouse preimplantation development. *Reproduction*, *131*(3), 469–479. https://doi.org/10.1530/rep.1.00953

Jeong, Y. W., Park, S. W., Hossein, M. S., Kim, S., Kim, J. H., Lee, S. H., Kang, S. K., Lee, B. C., & Hwang, W. S. (2006). Antiapoptotic and embryotrophic effects of α-tocopherol and l-ascorbic acid on porcine embryos derived from in vitro fertilization and somatic cell nuclear transfer. *Theriogenology*, *66*(9), 2104–2112. https://doi.org/10.1016/j.theriogenology.2006.06.007

Kane, M. T., & Bavister, B. D. (1988). Vitamin requirements for development of eight-cell hamster embryos to hatching blastocysts in vitro. *Biology of Reproduction*, *39*(5), 1137–1143. https://doi.org/10.1095/biolreprod39.5.1137

Kane, Michael T. (1988). The effects of water-soluble vitamins on the expansion of rabbit blastocysts in vitro. *Journal of Experimental Zoology*, *245*(2), 220–223. https://doi.org/10.1002/jez.1402450211

Kaplan, J. H. (2002). Biochemistry of Na,K-ATPase. In *Annual Review of Biochemistry* (Vol. 71, pp. 511–535). Annu Rev Biochem. https://doi.org/10.1146/annurev.biochem.71.102201.141218

Karja, N. W. K., Kikuchi, K., Fahrudin, M., Ozawa, M., Somfai, T., Ohnuma, K., Noguchi, J., Kaneko, H., & Nagai, T. (2006). Development to the blastocyst stage, the oxidative state, and the quality of early developmental stage of porcine embryos cultured in alteration of glucose concentrations in vitro under different oxygen tensions. *Reproductive Biology and Endocrinology*, *4*, 54. https://doi.org/10.1186/1477-7827-4-54

Khosla, S., Dean, W., Brown, D., Reik, W., & Feil, R. (2001). Culture of preimplantation mouse embryos affects fetal development and the expression of imprinted genes. *Biology of Reproduction*, *64*(3), 918–926. https://doi.org/10.1095/biolreprod64.3.918

Killian, J. K., Nolan, C. M., Wylie, A. A., Li, T., Vu, T. H., Hoffman, A. R., & Jirtle, R. L. (2001). Divergent evolution in M6P/IGF2R imprinting from the Jurassic to the Quaternary. *Human Molecular Genetics*, *10*(17), 1721–1728. https://doi.org/10.1093/hmg/10.17.1721

Kovačič, B. (2012). Culture systems: Low-oxygen culture. *Methods in Molecular Biology*, *912*, 249–272. https://doi.org/10.1007/978-1-61779-971-6_15

Lane, M., & Gardner, D. K. (1994). Increase in postimplantation development of cultured mouse embryos by amino acids and induction of fetal retardation and exencephaly by ammonium ions. *Journal of Reproduction and Fertility*, *102*(2), 305–312. https://doi.org/10.1530/JRF.0.1020305

Lane, M., & Gardner, D. K. (1997). Differential regulation of mouse embryo development and viability by amino acids. *Journal of Reproduction and Fertility*, *109*(1), 153–164. https://doi.org/10.1530/JRF.0.1090153

Lane, M., & Gardner, D. K. (1995). Removal of embryo-toxic ammonium from the culture medium by in situ enzymatic conversion to glutamate. *The Journal of Experimental Zoology*, *271*(5), 356–363. https://doi.org/10.1002/JEZ.1402710505

Lane, M., & Gardner, D. K. (2001). Inhibiting 3-phosphoglycerate kinase by EDTA stimulates the development of the cleavage stage mouse embryo. *Molecular Reproduction and Development*, *60*(2), 233–240. https://doi.org/10.1002/mrd.1083

Lane, M., & Gardner, D. K. (2005a). Understanding cellular disruptions during early embryo development that perturb viability and fetal development. *Reproduction, Fertility, and Development*, *17*(3), 371–378. https://doi.org/10.1071/RD04102

Lane, M., & Gardner, D. K. (2005b). Mitochondrial malate-aspartate shuttle regulates mouse embryo nutrient consumption. *Journal of Biological Chemistry*, *280*(18), 18361–18367. https://doi.org/10.1074/jbc.M500174200

Lane, M., & Gardner, D. K. (2007). Embryo culture medium: which is the best? *Best Practice and Research: Clinical Obstetrics and Gynaecology*, *21*(1), 83–100. https://doi.org/10.1016/j.bpobgyn.2006.09.009

Lane, M., Lyons, E. A., & Bavister, B. D. (2000). Cryopreservation reduces the ability of hamster 2-cell embryos to regulate intracellular pH. *Human Reproduction (Oxford, England)*, *15*(2), 389–394. https://doi.org/10.1093/HUMREP/15.2.389

Lane, M., Maybach, J. M., & Gardner, D. K. (2002). Addition of ascorbate during cryopreservation stimulates subsequent embryo development. *Human Reproduction*, *17*(10), 2686–2693. https://doi.org/10.1093/humrep/17.10.2686

Lawrence, L. T., & Moley, K. H. (2008). Epigenetics and assisted reproductive technologies: Human imprinting syndromes. *Seminars in Reproductive Medicine*, *26*(2), 143–152. https://doi.org/10.1055/S-2008-1042953

Leese, H. J. (1988). The formation and function of oviduct fluid. *Journal of Reproduction and Fertility*, *82*(2), 843–856. https://doi.org/10.1530/JRF.0.0820843

Leese, H. J. (1991). Metabolism of the preimplantation mammalian embryo. In *Oxford reviews of reproductive biology* (Vol. 13, pp. 35–72).

Leese, H. J. (1995). Metabolic control during preimplantation mammalian development. *Human Reproduction Update*, *1*(1), 63–72. https://doi.org/10.1093/humupd/1.1.63

Leese, H. J. (1998). Human embryo culture: Back to nature. In *Journal of Assisted Reproduction and Genetics* (Vol. 15, Issue 8, pp. 466–468). Springer. https://doi.org/10.1023/A:1022526219202

Leese, H. J. (2002). Quiet please, do not disturb: a hypothesis of embryo metabolism and viability. *BioEssays : News and Reviews in Molecular, Cellular and Developmental Biology*, *24*(9), 845–849. https://doi.org/10.1002/BIES.10137

Leese, H. J., & Barton, A. M. (1985). Production of pyruvate by isolated mouse cumulus cells. *Journal of Experimental Zoology*, *234*(2), 231–236. https://doi.org/10.1002/jez.1402340208

Leese, H. J., Baumann, C. G., Brison, D. R., McEvoy, T. G., & Sturmey, R. G. (2008). Metabolism of the viable mammalian embryo: Quietness revisited. In *Molecular Human Reproduction* (Vol. 14, Issue 12, pp. 667–672). Oxford University Press. https://doi.org/10.1093/molehr/gan065

Legge, M., & Sellens, M. H. (1991). Free radical scavengers ameliorate the 2-cell block in mouse embryo culture. *Human Reproduction*, *6*(6), 867–871. https://doi.org/10.1093/oxfordjournals.humrep.a137442

Li, J., & Foote, R. H. (1995). Effect of inositol and glycine with increasing sodium chloride and constant osmolality on development of rabbit embryos. *Journal of Assisted Reproduction and Genetics, 12*(2), 141–146. https://doi.org/10.1007/BF02211384

Lightman, A., Vertman, D., Shahar, K., Manor, D., Wayner, V., & Itskovitz-Eldor, J. (1997). The presence of a sponsoring embryo in a batch of poor quality thawed embryos significantly increases pregnancy and implantation rate. *Fertility and Sterility, 67*(4), 711–716. https://doi.org/10.1016/S0015-0282(97)81371-4

Lindenau, A., & Fischer, B. (1994). Effect of oxygen concentration in the incubator's gas phase on the development of cultured preimplantation rabbit embryos. *Theriogenology, 41*(4), 889–898. https://doi.org/10.1016/0093-691X(94)90504-C

Liu, J., Tang, S., Xu, W., Wang, Y., Yin, B., & Zhang, Y. (2011). Detrimental effects of antibiotics on mouse embryos in chromatin integrity, apoptosis and expression of zygotically activated genes. *Zygote, 19*(2), 137–145. https://doi.org/10.1017/S0967199410000249

Maas, D. H. A., Storey, B. T., & Mastroianni, L. (1977). Hydrogen ion and carbon dioxide content of the oviductal fluid of the rhesus monkey (Macaca mulatta). *Fertility and Sterility, 28*(9), 981–985. https://doi.org/10.1016/s0015-0282(16)42801-3

Magli, M. C., Gianaroli, L., Fiorentino, A., Ferraretti, A. P., Fortini, D., & Panzella, S. (1996). Improved cleavage rate of human embryos cultured in antibiotic-free medium. *Human Reproduction, 11*(7), 1520–1524. https://doi.org/10.1093/oxfordjournals.humrep.a019430

Manser, R. C., Leese, H. J., & Houghton, F. D. (2004). Effect of Inhibiting Nitric Oxide Production on Mouse Preimplantation Embryo Development and Metabolism. *Biology of Reproduction, 71*(2), 528–533. https://doi.org/10.1095/BIOLREPROD.103.025742

Martin, P. M., & Sutherland, A. E. (2001). Exogenous amino acids regulate trophectoderm differentiation in the mouse blastocyst through an mTOR-dependent pathway. *Developmental Biology, 240*(1), 182–193. https://doi.org/10.1006/DBIO.2001.0461

Martin, P. M., Sutherland, A. E., & Van Winkle, L. J. (2003). Amino acid transport regulates blastocyst implantation. *Biology of Reproduction, 69*(4), 1101–1108. https://doi.org/10.1095/BIOLREPROD.103.018010

Mash, H. E., Chin, Y. P., Sigg, L., Hari, R., & Xue, H. (2002). Complexation of Copper by Zwitterionic Aminosulfonic (Good) Buffers. *Analytical Chemistry, 75*(3), 671–677. https://doi.org/10.1021/AC0261101

McKiernan, S. H., & Bavister, B. D. (2000). Culture of one-cell hamster embryos with water soluble vitamins: Pantothenate stimulates blastocyst production. *Human Reproduction, 15*(1), 157–164. https://doi.org/10.1093/humrep/15.1.157

Mehta, T. S., & Kiessling, A. A. (1990). Development potential of mouse embryos conceived in vitro and cultured in ethylenediaminetetraacetic acid with or without amino acids or serum. *Biology of Reproduction, 43*(4), 600–606. https://doi.org/10.1095/BIOLREPROD43.4.600

Meintjes, M. (2012). Media composition: Macromolecules and embryo growth. *Methods in Molecular Biology, 912*, 107–127. https://doi.org/10.1007/978-1-61779-971-6_8

Meintjes, M., Chantilis, S. J., Douglas, J. D., Rodriguez, A. J., Guerami, A. R., Bookout, D. M., Barnett, B. D., & Madden, J. D. (2009). A controlled randomized trial evaluating the effect of lowered incubator oxygen tension on live births in a predominantly blastocyst transfer program. *Human Reproduction*, *24*(2), 300–307. https://doi.org/10.1093/humrep/den368

Menezo, Y. J. R. (1975). Amino constituents of tubal and uterine fluids of the estrous ewe: comparison with blood serum and ram seminal fluid. In *The biology of spermatozoa* (pp. 174–181). Karger Publishers.

Ménézo, Y. J. R., Sakkas, D., & Janny, L. (1995). Co-culture of the early human embryo: factors affecting human blastocyst formation in vitro. *Microscopy Research and Technique*, *32*(1), 50–56. https://doi.org/10.1002/JEMT.1070320105

Menezo, Y., Testart, J., & Perrone, D. (1984). Serum is not necessary in human in vitro fertilization, early embryo culture, and transfer. *Fertility and Sterility*, *42*(5), 750–755. https://doi.org/10.1016/S0015-0282(16)48202-6

Miller, J. G., & Schultz, G. A. (1987). Amino acid content of preimplantation rabbit embryos and fluids of the reproductive tract. *Biology of Reproduction*, *36*(1), 125–129. https://doi.org/10.1095/BIOLREPROD36.1.125

Morales, H., Tilquin, P., Rees, J. F., Massip, A., Dessy, F., & Van Langendonckt, A. (1999). Pyruvate prevents peroxide-induced injury of in vitro preimplantation bovine embryos. *Molecular Reproduction and Development*, *52*(2), 149–157. https://doi.org/10.1002/(SICI)1098-2795(199902)52:2<149::AID-MRD5>3.0.CO;2-4

Murakami, M., Egashira, A., Tanaka, K., Mine, C., Otsubo, H., & Kuramoto, T. (2014). Perinatal outcomes for transfer of blastocysts vitrified and warmed in defined solutions with recombinant human albumin: 374 babies born after 898 embryo transfers. *Journal of Assisted Reproduction and Genetics*, *31*(12), 1605–1610. https://doi.org/10.1007/s10815-014-0343-8

Nagaraj, R., Sharpley, M. S., Chi, F., Braas, D., Zhou, Y., Kim, R., Clark, A. T., & Banerjee, U. (2017). Nuclear Localization of Mitochondrial TCA Cycle Enzymes as a Critical Step in Mammalian Zygotic Genome Activation. *Cell*, *168*(1–2), 210-223.e11. https://doi.org/10.1016/J.CELL.2016.12.026

Nagata, Y., & Shirakawa, K. (1996). Setting standards for the levels of endotoxin in the embryo culture media of human in vitro fertilization and embryo transfer. *Fertility and Sterility*, *65*(3), 614–619. https://doi.org/10.1016/s0015-0282(16)58164-3

Nasr-Esfahani, M. H., & Johnson, M. H. (1992). How does transferrin overcome the in vitro block to development of the mouse preimplantation embryo? *Journal of Reproduction and Fertility*, *96*(1), 41–48. https://doi.org/10.1530/jrf.0.0960041

Nasr-Esfahani, M., Johnson, M. H., & Aitken, R. J. (1990). The effect of iron and iron chelators on the in-vitro block to development of the mouse preimplantation embryo: BAT6 a new medium for improved culture of mouse embryos in vitro. *Human Reproduction*, *5*(8), 997–1003. https://doi.org/10.1093/oxfordjournals.humrep.a137235

Noda, Y, Goto, Y., Umaoka, Y., Shiotani, M., Nakayama, T., & Mori, T. (1994). Culture of human embryos in alpha modification of eagle's medium under low oxygen tension and low illumination. *Fertility and Sterility*, *62*(5), 1022–1027. https://doi.org/10.1016/s0015-0282(16)57068-x

Noda, Yoichi, Matsumoto, H., Umaoka, Y., Tatsumi, K., Kishi, J., & Mori, T. (1991). Involvement of superoxide radicals in the mouse two-cell block. *Molecular Reproduction and Development*, *28*(4), 356–360. https://doi.org/10.1002/MRD.1080280408

O'Neill, C. (1998). Endogenous folic acid is essential for normal development of preimplantation embryos. *Human Reproduction*, *13*(5), 1312–1316. https://doi.org/10.1093/humrep/13.5.1312

O'Neill, Chris. (2008). The potential roles for embryotrophic ligands in preimplantation embryo development. *Human Reproduction Update*, *14*(3), 275–288. https://doi.org/10.1093/humupd/dmn002

Osiecki, M., Ghanavi, P., Atkinson, K., Nielsen, L. K., & Doran, M. R. (2010). The ascorbic acid paradox. *Biochemical and Biophysical Research Communications*, *400*(4), 466–470. https://doi.org/10.1016/j.bbrc.2010.08.052

Otsuki, J., Nagai, Y., & Chiba, K. (2007). Peroxidation of mineral oil used in droplet culture is detrimental to fertilization and embryo development. *Fertility and Sterility*, *88*(3), 741–743. https://doi.org/10.1016/J.FERTNSTERT.2006.11.144

Ottosen, L. D. M., Hindkjær, J., & Ingerslev, J. (2007). Light exposure of the ovum and preimplantation embryo during ART procedures. *Journal of Assisted Reproduction and Genetics*, *24*(2–3), 99–103. https://doi.org/10.1007/s10815-006-9081-x

Payne, S. R., Munday, R., & Thompson, J. G. (1992). Addition of superoxide dismutase and catalase does not necessarily overcome developmental retardation of one-cell mouse embryos during in-vitro culture. *Reproduction, Fertility and Development*, *4*(2), 147–167. https://doi.org/10.1071/RD9920167

Pemble, L. B., & Kaye, P. L. (1986). Whole protein uptake and metabolism by mouse blastocysts. *Journal of Reproduction and Fertility*, *78*(1), 149–157. https://doi.org/10.1530/jrf.0.0780149

Premkumar, B. J., & Agarwal, A. (2012). Female Infertility and Assisted Reproduction: Impact of Oxidative Stress-- An Update. *Current Women's Health Reviews*, *8*(3), 183–207. https://doi.org/10.2174/157340412803760711

Reed, M. L. (2012). Culture systems: Embryo density. *Methods in Molecular Biology*, *912*, 273–312. https://doi.org/10.1007/978-1-61779-971-6_16

Rieger, D., Grisart, B., Semple, E., Van Langendonckt, A., Betteridge, K. J., & Dessy, F. (1995). Comparison of the effects of oviductal cell co-culture and oviductal cell-conditioned medium on the development and metabolic activity of cattle embryos. *Journal of Reproduction and Fertility*, *105*(1), 91–98. https://doi.org/10.1530/JRF.0.1050091

Rijnders, P. M., & Jansen, C. A. M. (1999). Influence of group culture and culture volume on the formation of human blastocysts: A prospective randomized study. *Human Reproduction*, *14*(9), 2333–2337. https://doi.org/10.1093/humrep/14.9.2333

Rinaudo, P. F., Giritharan, G., Talbi, S., Dobson, A. T., & Schultz, R. M. (2006). Effects of oxygen tension on gene expression in preimplantation mouse embryos. *Fertility and Sterility*, *86*(4 Suppl), 1265.e1-1265.e36. https://doi.org/10.1016/J.FERTNSTERT.2006.05.017

Rogers, P. A. W., C.R., & Gannon, B. J. (1982). Changes in the spatial organization of the uterine vasculature during implantation in the rat. *Journal of Reproduction and Fertility*, *65*(1), 211–214. https://doi.org/10.1530/jrf.0.0650211

Salahuddin, S., Ookutsu, S., Goto, K., Nakanishi, Y., & Nagata, Y. (1995). Fertilization and early embryology: Effects of embryo density and co-culture of unfertilized oocytes on embryonic development of in-vitro fertilized mouse embryos. *Human Reproduction*, *10*(9), 2382–2385. https://doi.org/10.1093/oxfordjournals.humrep.a136303

Schumacher, A., & Fischer, B. (1988). Influence of visible light and room temperature on cell proliferation in preimplantation rabbit embryos. *Journal of Reproduction and Fertility*, *84*(1), 197–204. https://doi.org/10.1530/jrf.0.0840197

Sfontouris, I. A., Martins, W. P., Nastri, C. O., Viana, I. G. R., Navarro, P. A., Raine-Fenning, N., van der Poel, S., Rienzi, L., & Racowsky, C. (2016). Blastocyst culture using single versus sequential media in clinical IVF: a systematic review and meta-analysis of randomized controlled trials. In *Journal of Assisted Reproduction and Genetics* (Vol. 33, Issue 10, pp. 1261–1272). Springer New York LLC. https://doi.org/10.1007/s10815-016-0774-5

Simopoulou, M., Sfakianoudis, K., Rapani, A., Giannelou, P., Anifandis, G., Bolaris, S., Pantou, A., Lambropoulou, M., Pappas, A., Deligeoroglou, E., Pantos, K., & Koutsilieris, M. (2018). Considerations regarding embryo culture conditions: From media to epigenetics. In *In Vivo* (Vol. 32, Issue 3, pp. 451–460). https://doi.org/10.21873/invivo.11261

Smith, D. G., & Sturmey, R. G. (2013). Parallels between embryo and cancer cell metabolism. *Biochemical Society Transactions*, *41*(2), 664–669. https://doi.org/10.1042/BST20120352

Squirrell, J. M., Lane, M., & Bavister, B. D. (2001). Altering intracellular pH disrupts development and cellular organization in preimplantation hamster embryos. *Biology of Reproduction*, *64*(6), 1845–1854. https://doi.org/10.1095/biolreprod64.6.1845

Stocker, P., Lesgards, J. F., Vidal, N., Chalier, F., & Prost, M. (2003). ESR study of a biological assay on whole blood: Antioxidant efficiency of various vitamins. *Biochimica et Biophysica Acta - General Subjects*, *1621*(1), 1–8. https://doi.org/10.1016/S0304-4165(03)00008-4

Stojkovic, M., Kölle, S., Peinl, S., Stojkovic, P., Zakhartchenko, V., Thompson, J. G., Wenigerkind, H., Reichenbach, H.-D., Sinowatz, F., & Wolf, E. (2002). Effects of high concentrations of hyaluronan in culture medium on development and survival rates of fresh and frozen-thawed bovine embryos produced in vitro. *Reproduction (Cambridge, England)*, *124*(1), 141–153.

Sun, X. F., Wang, W. H., & Keefe, D. L. (2004). Overheating is detrimental to meiotic spindles within in vitro matured human oocytes. *Zygote*, *12*(1), 65–70. https://doi.org/10.1017/S0967199404002631

Swain, J. E., & Smith, G. D. (2011). Advances in embryo culture platforms: Novel approaches to improve preimplantation embryo development through modifications of the microenvironment. *Human Reproduction Update*, *17*(4), 541–557. https://doi.org/10.1093/humupd/dmr006

Swain, J. E. (2012). Media composition: pH and buffers. *Methods in Molecular Biology (Clifton, N.J.)*, *912*, 161–175. https://doi.org/10.1007/978-1-61779-971-6_10

Swain, J. E. (2014). Decisions for the IVF laboratory: Comparative analysis of embryo culture incubators. *Reproductive BioMedicine Online*, *28*(5), 535–547. https://doi.org/10.1016/j.rbmo.2014.01.004

Swain, Jason E., & Pool, T. B. (2009). New pH-buffering system for media utilized during gamete and embryo manipulations for assisted reproduction. *Reproductive Biomedicine Online*, *18*(6), 799–810. https://doi.org/10.1016/S1472-6483(10)60029-6

Tanikawa, M., Harada, T., Ito, M., Yoshida, S., Iwabe, T., & Terakawa, N. (1999). Globulins in protein supplements promote the development of preimplantation embryos. *Journal of Assisted Reproduction and Genetics*, *16*(10), 555–557. https://doi.org/10.1023/A:1020557422982

The Lancet Global Health. (2022). Infertility—why the silence? In *The Lancet Global Health* (Vol. 10, Issue 6, p. e773). Elsevier Ltd. https://doi.org/10.1016/S2214-109X(22)00215-7

Thomas, M., Jain, S., Kumar, G. P., & Laloraya, M. (1997). A programmed oxyradical burst causes hatching of mouse blastocysts. *Journal of Cell Science*, *110*(14), 1597–1602. https://doi.org/10.1242/jcs.110.14.1597

Thompson, J. G. (2000). In vitro culture and embryo metabolism of cattle and sheep embryos - A decade of achievement. *Animal Reproduction Science*, *60–61*, 263–275. https://doi.org/10.1016/S0378-4320(00)00096-8

Truong, T. T., Soh, Y. M., & Gardner, D. K. (2016). Antioxidants improve mouse preimplantation embryo development and viability. *Human Reproduction*, *31*(7), 1445–1454. https://doi.org/10.1093/humrep/dew098

Tsai, F. C. H., & Gardner, D. K. (1994). Nicotinamide, a component of complex culture media, inhibits mouse embryo development in vitro and reduces subsequent developmental potential after transfer. *Fertility and Sterility*, *61*(2), 376–382. https://doi.org/10.1016/s0015-0282(16)56534-0

Umaoka, Y., Noda, Y., Nakayama, T., Narimoto, K., Mori, T., & Iritani, A. (1992). Effect of visual light on in vitro embryonic development in the hamster. *Theriogenology*, *38*(6), 1043–1054. https://doi.org/10.1016/0093-691X(92)90118-B

Vajta, G., Peura, T. T., Holm, P., Páldi, A., Greve, T., Trounson, A. O., & Callesen, H. (2000). New method for culture of zona-included or zona-free embryos: The Well of the Well (WOW) system. *Molecular Reproduction and Development*, *55*(3), 256–264. https://doi.org/10.1002/(SICI)1098-2795(200003)55:3<256::AID-MRD3>3.0.CO;2-7

Vajta, G., Rienzi, L., Cobo, A., & Yovich, J. (2010). Embryo culture: Can we perform better than nature? *Reproductive BioMedicine Online*, *20*(4), 453–469. https://doi.org/10.1016/j.rbmo.2009.12.018

Van Winkle, L. J. (1988). Amino acid transport in developing animal oocytes and early conceptuses. *Biochimica et Biophysica Acta*, *947*(1). https://doi.org/10.1016/0304-4157(88)90024-X

Van Winkle, L. J., Haghighat, N., & Campione, A. L. (1990). Glycine protects preimplantation mouse conceptuses from a detrimental effect on development of the inorganic ions in oviductal fluid. *The Journal of Experimental Zoology*, *253*(2), 215–219. https://doi.org/10.1002/JEZ.1402530211

Waldenström, U., Engström, A. B., Hellberg, D., & Nilsson, S. (2009). Low-oxygen compared with high-oxygen atmosphere in blastocyst culture, a prospective randomized study. *Fertility and Sterility*, *91*(6), 2461–2465. https://doi.org/10.1016/j.fertnstert.2008.03.051

Wale, P. L., & Gardner, D. K. (2010). Time-lapse analysis of mouse embryo development in oxygen gradients. *Reproductive Biomedicine Online*, *21*(3), 402–410. https://doi.org/10.1016/J.RBMO.2010.04.028

Wale, Petra L, & Gardner, D. K. (2013). Oxygen Affects the Ability of Mouse Blastocysts to Regulate Ammonium1. *Biology of Reproduction*, *89*(3), 1-10,75. https://doi.org/10.1095/biolreprod.113.109256

Wales, R. G., & Whittingham. (1973). The metabolism of specifically labelled lactate and pyruvate by two-cell mouse embryos. *Journal of Reproduction and Fertility*, *33*(2), 207–222. https://doi.org/10.1530/jrf.0.0330207

Wang, X., Falcone, T., Attaran, M., Goldberg, J. M., Agarwal, A., & Sharma, R. K. (2002). Vitamin C and vitamin E supplementation reduce oxidative stress-induced embryo toxicity and improve the blastocyst development rate. *Fertility and Sterility*, *78*(6), 1272–1277. https://doi.org/10.1016/S0015-0282(02)04236-X

Whitten, W. K. (1956). Culture of Tubal Mouse Ova. *Nature*, *177*(4498), 96. https://doi.org/10.1038/177096a0

Wiemer, K. E., Cohen, J., Amborskir, G. F., Wright, G., Wiker, S., Munyakazi, L., & Godke, R. A. (1989). In-vitro development and implantation of human embryos following culture on fetal bovine uterine fibroblast cells. *Human Reproduction (Oxford, England)*, *4*(5), 595–600. https://doi.org/10.1093/OXFORDJOURNALS.HUMREP.A136949

Yamamoto, K., & Niki, E. (1988). Interaction of α-tocopherol with iron: antioxidant and prooxidant effects of α-tocopherol in the oxidation of lipids in aqueous dispersions in the presence of iron. *Biochimica et Biophysica Acta (BBA)/ Lipids and Lipid Metabolism*, *958*(1), 19–23. https://doi.org/10.1016/0005-2760(88)90241-X

Young, L. E., Fernandes, K., McEvoy, T. G., Butterwith, S. C., Gutierrez, C. G., Carolan, C., Broadbent, P. J., Robinson, J. J., Wilmut, I., & Sinclair, K. D. (2001). Epigenetic change in IGF2R is associated with fetal overgrowth after sheep embryo culture. *Nature Genetics*, *27*(2), 153–154. https://doi.org/10.1038/84769

Yuan, Y. Q., Van Soom, A., Coopman, F. O. J., Mintiens, K., Boerjan, M. L., Van Zeveren, A., De Kruif, A., & Peelman, L. J. (2003). Influence of oxygen tension on apoptosis and hatching in bovine embryos cultured in vitro. *Theriogenology*, *59*(7), 1585–1596. https://doi.org/10.1016/S0093-691X(02)01204-9

Zander-Fox, D. L., Mitchell, M., Thompson, J. G., & Lane, M. (2010). Alterations in mouse embryo intracellular pH by DMO during culture impair implantation and fetal growth. *Reproductive BioMedicine Online*, *21*(2), 219–229. https://doi.org/10.1016/j.rbmo.2010.05.001

Zander-Fox, D., & Lane, M. (2012). Media composition: energy sources and metabolism. *Methods in Molecular Biology (Clifton, N.J.)*, *912*, 81–96. https://doi.org/10.1007/978-1-61779-971-6_6

Zander, D. L., Thompson, J. G., & Lane, M. (2006). Perturbations in mouse embryo development and viability caused by ammonium are more severe after exposure at the cleavage stages. *Biology of Reproduction*, *74*(2), 288–294. https://doi.org/10.1095/BIOLREPROD.105.046235

Zhang, X., & Armstrong, D. T. (1990). Presence of amino acids and insulin in a chemically defined medium improves development of 8-cell rat embryos in vitro and subsequent implantation in vivo. *Biology of Reproduction*, *42*(4), 662–668. https://doi.org/10.1095/BIOLREPROD42.4.662

Zhou, H., McKiernan, S. H., Ji, W., & Bavister, B. D. (2000). Effect of antibiotics on development in vitro of hamster pronucleate ova. *Theriogenology*, *54*(7), 999–1006. https://doi.org/10.1016/S0093-691X(00)00408-8

Zorn, T. M., Pinhal, M. A., Nader, H. B., Carvalho, J. J., Abrahamsohn, P. A., & Dietrich, C. P. (1995). Biosynthesis of glycosaminoglycans in the endometrium during the initial stages of pregnancy of the mouse. *Cellular and Molecular Biology (Noisy-Le-Grand, France)*, *41*(1), 97–106.

Chapter 20

Polar Body, Cleavage Stage and Trophectoderm Biopsy

Selin Kenan[1], MD* and Çiğdem Karaca[2], MD

[1]Department of Histology and Embryology, Cengiz Gökçek Obstetrics and Gynecology Hospital, Gaziantep, Turkiye

[2]Department of Histology and Embryology, İslam, Science and Technology University Faculty of Medicine, Gaziantep, Turkiye

Abstract

Embryo biopsy (EB) is the method used to analyze the chromosomal content of the embryo without damaging the integrity of the embryo prior to implantation. The sample taken by this method is obtained by biopsy of one or both polar bodies, blastomere biopsy in the cleavage stage, or trophectoderm biopsy after blastulation. Biopsy is preferred for the preimplantation genetic test (PGT) especially in couples who have advanced maternal age (AMA), recurrent implantation failure (RIF), recurrent miscarriage (RM), and severe male factor (SMF) problems. As a result of PGT, genetic causes such as structural chromosomal disorders or single gene diseases are analyzed before pregnancy occurs and couples are offered the opportunity to choose healthy embryos. Additionally, PGT is a method that increases the chance of pregnancy and eliminates unnecessary terminations due to numerical chromosomal anomalies by performing aneuploidy screening in couples who cannot have children in the normal way and who apply for assisted reproductive techniques (Audibert et al., 2009; Group et al., 2020; Handyside et al., 1990; von Wolff, 2019).

Key Words: Cleavage stage biopsy, Trophectoderm biopsy, Polar body biopsy, Preimplantation genetic testing

---

* Corresponding Author's E-mail: selinseymen@gmail.com

In: Holistic Approach to Assisted Reproductive Technology
Editor: Kenan Demir and Rümeysa Yılmaz Göç
ISBN: 979-8-89113-017-3
© 2023 Nova Science Publishers, Inc.

Introduction

Although the history of PGTs is not very long, the first trial was made in 1968 from a blastomere biopsy taken from a rabbit embryo. After almost 20 years, a blastomere biopsy was performed on mouse embryos at the stage with 4 blastomeres in 1989 and it was stated that this procedure did not affect embryo development and would allow genetic studies. After the success of these studies, it was thought that biopsy could be performed for clinical purposes in human embryos as well. EB started as an experimental procedure for sex selection and detection of monogenic diseases in humans with methods based on polymerase chain reaction (PCR) (Gardner et al., 2012). The first pregnancy after biopsy was reported in 1990 by Handyside et al. The first live birth was reported in 1992 by Grifo et al. (Edwards & Gardner, 1967; Grifo et al., 1992; Wilton & Trounson, 1989). Today, the primary purpose of EB is to remove a cell or genetic material in the preimplantation period without causing damage to the developing embryo as much as possible. It is important that the diagnosis is made correctly and in a way that represents the whole embryo when performing this procedure. The biopsy techniques used and the experience of the personnel performing the procedure constitute the most important stage in terms of both embryo development and test reliability. Different methods are used in different laboratories for PGT. The main biopsy methods and preparation stages for biopsy are presented in detail below.

Cleavage-Stage Biopsy

Cleavage stage biopsy involves the removal of a single cell from the embryo with at least 6 blastomeres and less than 30% fragmentation on day 3, as recommended by the ESCHRE and ASRM guidelines. Depending on the number of blastomeres, 2 cells can also be removed (1 cell in embryos with 6-7 cells, 2 cells in embryos with ≥8 cells) (Goossens et al., 2008). Although cleavage stage biopsy is more invasive, it is preferred more than polar body biopsy and has been used as the most preferred method for many years because blastomeres provide information about both maternal and paternal genomes. Biopsies performed on day 3 have been reported to significantly reduce embryonic reproductive potential, whereas trophectoderm biopsy is a more reliable method for embryo biopsy (Scott et al., 2013a). Furthermore, late morphokinetic events in the morula and blastocyst stages were found to occur significantly earlier in biopsied embryos than in nonbiopsied control embryos (Lammers et al., 2021), while another study showed that embryos that were aneuploid in the cleavage stage after biopsy may be euploid in the blastocyst stage (Kalma et al., 2018). After biopsy, the embryo can be frozen and stored, or it can be cultured and transferred to the blastocyst stage. Therefore, centers that do not want to perform cryopreservation are also preferred (Gardner & Simón, 2017).

Advantages

- Provide information about both the maternal and paternal genomes.
- Access to more resources on the reliability and effectiveness of the application method, as it is a method that has been used for a long time.

Disadvantages

- It is the most invasive biopsy method in which the largest part of the embryonic mass is removed.
- High margin of error
- Allele dropout risk

Stages of biopsy

- First, the preparation of the containers to be biopsied is done. Drops are prepared using 10 nl of Ca^{2+} / Mg^{2+} free culture broth or HEPES/MOPS buffered culture solution for each embryo. A drop of PVP (polyvinylpyrrolidone) is also added to any part of the culture vessel and covered with oil.
- Embryos are added to numbered drops and placed under an inverted microscope for biopsy.
- A small amount of PVP is drawn into the biopsy pipette.
- After the ZP is punctured with one of the 3 methods used, the blastomere to be biopsied is brought to the 3 o'clock direction, aspirated into the biopsy pipette, and slowly pulled out of the embryo. It is transferred to the labeled biopsy cup or PCR (polymerase chain reaction) tube and sent to the genetics laboratory for analysis.
- After the biopsy procedure, the embryo is thoroughly washed in the washing drops in the culture solution, cleared of the HEPES/MOPS solution, and incubated.

Polar Body (PB) Biopsy

PB biopsy has been developed as an alternative to the blastomere biopsy procedure, as it is thought to have less impact on the further development of the embryo. PBs are structures that degenerate and disappear over time during the embryo development process. It is the only option in countries with legal restrictions for biopsy procedures and is still actively used, but the chance of success is very low (Montag & Morbeck, 2017). Since PBs are waste products of maternal meiosis, they do not provide information about the paternal genome; therefore, it is preferred in the detection of single gene diseases of maternal origin, balanced translocations, and aneuploidies with age-related increase. Furthermore, since not every oocyte that is biopsied can continue to develop, performing a biopsy on all oocytes is very costly and increases the workload (Capalbo et al., 2013).

While the first polar body is formed after the completion of the 1st meiosis in oogenesis; the second polar body is formed after the completion of the second meiotic division initiated by the sperm (after fertilization). A biopsy can only be performed on day 0 or on day 1 after fertilization. If a simultaneous biopsy is performed (day 1), the optimal time interval is 6-10 hours after microinjection. If sequential, 4-10 hours after microinjection for the first polar body; 8-16 hours for the second polar body. In any case, both PBs are necessary for a correct diagnosis and must be reliably distinguished. Simultaneous biopsy is less time consuming but more complex than sequential biopsies because differentiation of PB1 and PB2 can be difficult, especially in the case of PB fragmentation.

Stages of biopsy

- Zona pellucida is opened with one of the 3 preferred methods.
- A small amount of PVP is drawn into the biopsy pipette. (To prevent the biopsy material from sticking to the pipette)
- By slowly inserting the biopsy pipette into the perivitelline space through the opening created in the ZP, the polar bodies are aspirated in sequence.
- The biopsy piece taken is left as far away from the oocyte/zygote as possible in the drop, and the oocyte/zygote is put back into the culture dish and removed to the incubator.
- The same steps are repeated for each oocyte; The pieces taken are placed in biopsy cups or PCR tubes that are clearly labeled on the top and side and sent to the genetic laboratory for analysis.

Advantages

- Does not affect embryo development because it is less invasive
- Allow a large amount of time for genetic analysis due to the early period
- Good information on the maternal genome
- Not being affected by legal limitations

Disadvantages

- Not providing information about the paternal genome and the postzygotic period.
- Necessity of biopsy of both polar bodies for correct diagnosis, thus requiring technical experience.

Trophectoderm (TE) Biopsy

TE biopsy was first reported in a study conducted in the marmoset monkey in 1988 and it was shown that the in vivo development of these embryos was normal after biopsy (Summers et al., 1988). The first clinical application in human blastocysts was achieved in 2004, and the first pregnancy was achieved in 2005 (De Boer et al., 2004; Kokkali et al., 2005). Since cryopreservation is required after TE biopsy, laboratories must have an effective cryopreservation program. Today, TE biopsy has become more preferable because vitrification procedures are so advanced. In addition, since only embryos that can continue to develop until the 5th day are biopsied, it saves laboratories from serious cost, labor, and time loss.

In the study by Scott et al. in 2013, the biopsy procedure performed at the cleavage stage and the trophectoderm biopsy were compared and the embryo implantation rate leading to permanent implantation was found to be significantly higher in the trophectoderm biopsy. Additionally, a significantly lower mosaicism rate in the blastocyst stage has also been shown to be a reason for preference (Scott et al., 2013b).

There are 3 different methods for TE biopsy; in the first, a hole is made in the zona pellucida (ZP) on the 3rd day and the culture is continued until the 5th day, and TE cells are expected to come out of this opening. In the second method, the embryo is cultured until it reaches the expanded blastocyst stage, the ZP is examined, and a laser shot is made from the farthest point to the inner cell mass; 5-10 TE cells are removed. The third method is the method developed to avoid the disadvantages of the second method. In the enlarged blastocyst stage, a laser shot is made to a point far from the inner cell mass and incubated again for 1-2 hours, and a biopsy is performed from the protruding TE cells (Capalbo. et al., 2014; McArthur et al., 2005).

Stages of biopsy

- The dishes for the biopsy are prepared. For blastocysts, a 10 µl culture solution containing 4-5 drops of HEPES / MOPS and two 10 µl wash solutions are prepared in biopsy dishes. Additionally, PVP is added to a 5 µl HEPES/MOPS drop of HEPES / MOPS during biopsy. The droplets are covered with oil.
- The holding and biopsy pipettes are attached to the inverted microscope.
- The blastocysts to be biopsied are controlled and placed in the drops.
- After some PVP is filled into the biopsy pipette, the trophectoderm cells that have come out of the zona pellucida are aspirated into the pipette.
- A laser pulse is applied to release the cells drawn into the pipette.
- The biopsy piece is placed away from the blastocyst. The biopsy piece is placed in the PCR tube and the blastocyst is removed by placing it in the culture dish.
- The same steps are repeated by changing the biopsy pipette for each blastocyst.
- The biopsied blastocysts are frozen one by one using the vitrification method until the results of the genetic analysis are obtained.

Advantages

- Provide information on both the paternal and maternal genomes
- Proven and high reliability
- Low cost since it is made from embryos that can continue to develop up to the blastocyst stage

Disadvantages

- Requires manipulation skills due to technical difficulty
- Obligatory vitrification

Blastosol Fluid Aspiration

The purpose of blastocoel fluid aspiration is to think that the DNA fragments contained in the blastocoel fluid reflect the embryo and to perform DNA analysis without damaging the integrity of the embryo. However, it is still unclear whether this genetic material reflects the entire embryo.

The first report on the presence of embryonic DNA in blastocoel fluid was published in 2013 (Palini et al., 2013). Although one study found 93.5%, 94%, and 96.6% concordance rates per chromosome in polar bodies, blastomeres, and trophectoderm, respectively, compared to blastocoel fluid, another study found only concordance of 63% (Gianaroli et al., 2014; Tobler et al., 2015). Given these inconsistencies, blastocoel fluid analysis should still be considered experimental and further studies should be performed to prove its effectiveness.

Introduction to Biopsy and Specimen Collection

Biopsy Laboratory Infrastructure

The embryology laboratory design should include a dedicated area for biopsy. Whether the biopsy laboratory is a private space or a room, it must comply with all safety and environmental standards criteria (air quality, positive pressure, laboratory access, etc.) (De Los Santos et al., 2016).

Preliminary

Before biopsy, the surfaces and equipment to be worked with should be cleaned using proven disinfectants and this process should be repeated before each use. DNA decontamination solutions, 10% bleach, UV-C irradiation, or autoclaving (when applicable, for example, tube racks) are used for cleaning and DNA decontamination. Since it does not decontaminate DNA, 70% alcohol should not be used (ESHRE PGT Consortium Steering Committee et al., 2020).

To avoid contamination, all embryologists should wear personal protective equipment such as full surgical gowns (clean, non-sterile, and regularly changed), gloves, bonnets, masks (covering the nose and mouth), and special shoes/overshoes. Gloves should be changed frequently and should never be handled without gloves. These gloves should be powder-free (vinyl) and fit snugly to the body. Another procedure to be done before the biopsy is to provide genetic counseling to couples. To select embryos with normal genetic structure, the procedure should be explained in detail to couples (Harper et al., 2014).

Equipment and materials

- Laminar airflow (airflow cabinet)
- Inverted microscope
- Microinjection system
- Incubator system
- Laser system (1.48 mm diode laser)
- Hepes/mops buffered culture fluid
- PVP
- Biopsy container
- Holding pipette
- Culture vessels
- Micropipettes that vary in diameter depending on the biopsy stage (10-15μm, 30-35μm for the cleavage stage, 25-30μm for the trophectoderm biopsy) (De Los Santos et al., 2016; Zegers-Hochschild et al., 2017).

Training for biopsy

The biopsy procedure should be performed by experienced embryologists with basic skills in general embryology and micromanipulation. The embryologist must have undergone complementary biopsy training to be able to complete all the steps. The biopsy should be supervised by a clinical embryologist, preferably with the relevant certification for their country.

Stages of biopsy

- Opening of the Zona Pellucida (ZP) (mechanical, chemical or using a laser)
- Removal of Polar Bodies (PBs) or embryonic cells

Opening of the Zona Pellucida (ZP)

Mechanical ZP opening (partial zona dissection); This is the first method used to open the ZP, in which a slit is created in the zona with a sharp micropipette. It is still used by laboratories that do not have a laser system.

Chemical ZP opening; It involves puncturing the ZP with an acid thyroid, but is not preferred because the resulting patency cannot be standardized and the solution used has potentially harmful effects on the embryo.

Laser method; ZP opening using a diode laser is the most preferred method today. First of all, the ZP region, which is planned to be opened, is taken to the 3 o'clock position and held at the 9 o'clock position with the embryo holding pipette. By switching to the laser objective, a laser shot is thrown on the desired area and the diameter of the hole is adjusted according to the biopsy procedure to be performed (e.g., 20 mm for PB biopsy, 40 mm for blastomere biopsy).

Removal of Polar Bodies (PBs) or Embryonic Cells

Different methods are used in the biopsy procedure to obtain PB and cells. The most commonly used and preferred method is the removal of cell/cells or PBs by aspiration. The second method is to remove the cells by pulling them after they have been partially aspirated. In recent years, the most preferred method, especially in TE biopsies, has been excision of aspirated cells with the help of a laser. Alternatively, this method can be used in combination with the mechanical separation of TE cells, called flicking (Group et al., 2020).

Conclusion

Today, many genetic diseases can be diagnosed. However, although there is no treatment for many of them after birth, the treatment of those who do is very costly. Performing PGT with IVF in individuals with familial predisposition means that these diseases can be treated before implantation. In this way, many couples will be able to have healthy children by preventing genetic diseases that may occur.

References

Audibert, F., Wilson, R. D., Allen, V., Audibert, F., Blight, C., Brock, J. A., Désilets, V. A., Gagnon, A., Johnson, J. A., Langlois, S., & Wyatt, P. (2009). Preimplantation Genetic Testing. *Journal of Obstetrics and Gynaecology Canada, 31*(8), 761–767. https://doi.org/10.1016/S1701-2163(16)34284-0

Capalbo, A., Bono, S., Spizzichino, L., Biricik, A., Baldi, M., Colamaria, S., Ubaldi, F. M., Rienzi, L., & Fiorentino, F. (2013). Sequential comprehensive chromosome analysis on polar bodies, blastomeres and trophoblast: insights into female meiotic errors and chromosomal segregation in the preimplantation window of embryo development. *Human Reproduction*, *28*(2), 509–518. https://doi.org/10.1093/HUMREP/DES394

Capalbo, A., Rienzi, L., Cimadomo, D., Maggiulli, R., Elliott, T., Wright, G., Nagy, Z. P., & Ubaldi, F. M. (2014). Correlation between standard blastocyst morphology, euploidy and implantation: An observational study in two centers involving 956 screened blastocysts. *Human Reproduction*, *29*(6), 1173–1181. https://doi.org/10.1093/humrep/deu033

ESHRE PGT Consortium Steering Committee, Carvalho, F., Coonen, E., Goossens, V., Kokkali, G., Rubio, C., Meijer-Hoogeveen, M., Moutou, C., Vermeulen, N., & De Rycke, M. (2020). ESHRE PGT Consortium good practice recommendations for the organisation of PGT. *Human Reproduction Open*, *2020*(3).

De Boer, K. A., Catt, J. W., Jansen, R. P. S., Leigh, D., & McArthur, S. (2004). Moving to blastocyst biopsy for preimplantation genetic diagnosis and single embryo transfer at Sydney IVF. *Fertility and Sterility*, *82*(2), 295–298. https://doi.org/10.1016/j.fertnstert.2003.11.064

De Los Santos, M. J., Apter, S., Coticchio, G., Debrock, S., Lundin, K., Plancha, C. E., Prados, F., Rienzi, L., Verheyen, G., Woodward, B., & Vermeulen, N. (2016). Revised guidelines for good practice in IVF laboratories (2015). *Human Reproduction*, *31*(4), 685–686. https://doi.org/10.1093/HUMREP/DEW016

Edwards, R. G., & Gardner, R. L. (1967). Sexing of Live Rabbit Blastocysts. *Nature 1967 214:5088*, *214*(5088), 576–577. https://doi.org/10.1038/214576a0

Gardner, D. K., & Simón, C. (2017). Handbook of In Vitro Fertilization: Fourth Edition. *Handbook of in Vitro Fertilization, Fourth Edition*, 1–371. https://doi.org/10.1201/9781315157269

Gardner, D. K., Weissman, A., Howles, C. M., & Shoham, Z. (2012). *Textbook of assisted reproductive techniques fourth edition: volume 2: Clinical perspectives* (Vol. 2). CRC press.

Gianaroli, L., Magli, M. C., Pomante, A., Crivello, A. M., Cafueri, G., Valerio, M., & Ferraretti, A. P. (2014). Blastocentesis: a source of DNA for preimplantation genetic testing. Results from a pilot study. *Fertility and Sterility*, *102*(6), 1692-1699.e6. https://doi.org/10.1016/J.FERTNSTERT.2014.08.021

Goossens, V., De Rycke, M., De Vos, A., Staessen, C., Michiels, A., Verpoest, W., Van Steirteghem, A., Bertrand, C., Liebaers, I., Devroey, P., & Sermon, K. (2008). Diagnostic efficiency, embryonic development and clinical outcome after the biopsy of one or two blastomeres for preimplantation genetic diagnosis. *Human Reproduction*, *23*(3), 481–492. https://doi.org/10.1093/humrep/dem327

Grifo, J. A., Tang, Y. X., Cohen, J., Gilbert, F., Sanyal, M. K., & Rosenwaks, Z. (1992). Pregnancy After Embryo Biopsy and Coamplification of DNA From X and Y Chromosomes. *JAMA*, *268*(6), 727–729. https://doi.org/10.1001/JAMA.1992.03490060055016

Group, E. P. C. and S.-E. B. W., Kokkali, G., Coticchio, G., Bronet, F., Celebi, C., Cimadomo, D., Goossens, V., Liss, J., Nunes, S., Sfontouris, I., Vermeulen, N., Zakharova, E., & De Rycke, M. (2020). ESHRE PGT Consortium and SIG Embryology good practice recommendations for polar body and embryo biopsy for PGT. *Human Reproduction Open*, *2020*(3), 1–12. https://doi.org/10.1093/HROPEN/HOAA020

Group, E. P. G. T. C. and S.-E. B. W., Kokkali, G., Coticchio, G., Bronet, F., Celebi, C., Cimadomo, D., Goossens, V., Liss, J., Nunes, S., & Sfontouris, I. (2020). ESHRE PGT Consortium and SIG Embryology good practice recommendations for polar body and embryo biopsy for PGT. *Human Reproduction Open*, *2020*(3).

Handyside, A. H., Kontogianni, E. H., Hardy, K., & Winston, R. M. L. (1990). Pregnancies from biopsied human preimplantation embryos sexed by Y-specific DNA amplification. *Nature*, *344*(6268), 768–770. https://doi.org/10.1038/344768A0

Harper, J., Geraedts, J., Borry, P., Cornel, M. C., Dondorp, W. J., Gianaroli, L., Harton, G., Milachich, T., Kääriäinen, H., Liebaers, I., Morris, M., Sequeiros, J., Sermon, K., Shenfield, F., Skirton, H., Soini, S., Spits, C., Veiga, A., Vermeesch, J. R., Viville, S., de Wert, G., & Macek, M. (2014). Current issues in medically assisted reproduction and genetics in Europe: research, clinical practice, ethics, legal issues and policy. *Human Reproduction*, *29*(8), 1603–1609. https://doi.org/10.1093/HUMREP/DEU130

Kalma, Y., Bar-El, L., Asaf-Tisser, S., Malcov, M., Reches, A., Hasson, J., Amir, H., Azem, F., & Ben-Yosef, D. (2018). Optimal timing for blastomere biopsy of 8-cell embryos for preimplantation genetic diagnosis. *Human Reproduction*, *33*(1), 32–38. https://doi.org/10.1093/humrep/dex343

Kokkali, G., Vrettou, C., Traeger-Synodinos, J., Jones, G. M., Cram, D. S., Stavrou, D., Trounson, A. O., Kanavakis, E., & Pantos, K. (2005). Birth of a healthy infant following trophectoderm biopsy from blastocysts for PGD of beta-thalassaemia major. *Human Reproduction (Oxford, England)*, *20*(7), 1855–1859. https://doi.org/10.1093/HUMREP/DEH893

Lammers, J., Reignier, A., Loubersac, S., Chtourou, S., Lefebvre, T., Barrière, P., & Fréour, T. (2021). Modification of late human embryo development after blastomere removal on day 3 for preimplantation genetic testing. *Systems Biology in Reproductive Medicine*, *67*(2), 121–126. https://doi.org/10.1080/19396368.2020.1834008

McArthur, S. J., Leigh, D., Marshall, J. T., De Boer, K. A., & Jansen, R. P. S. (2005). Pregnancies and live births after trophectoderm biopsy and preimplantation genetic testing of human blastocysts. *Fertility and Sterility*, *84*(6), 1628–1636. https://doi.org/10.1016/j.fertnstert.2005.05.063

Montag, M., & Morbeck, D. (2017). Principles of IVF laboratory practice: Optimizing performance and outcomes. In *Principles of IVF Laboratory Practice: Optimizing Performance and Outcomes*. https://doi.org/10.1017/9781316569238

Palini, S., Galluzzi, L., De Stefani, S., Bianchi, M., Wells, D., Magnani, M., & Bulletti, C. (2013). Genomic DNA in human blastocoele fluid. *Reproductive BioMedicine Online*, *26*(6), 603–610. https://doi.org/10.1016/J.RBMO.2013.02.012

Scott, R. T., Upham, K. M., Forman, E. J., Zhao, T., & Treff, N. R. (2013a). Cleavage-stage biopsy significantly impairs human embryonic implantation potential while blastocyst biopsy does not: a randomized and paired clinical trial. *Fertility and Sterility*, *100*(3), 624–630. https://doi.org/10.1016/J.FERTNSTERT.2013.04.039

Scott, R. T., Upham, K. M., Forman, E. J., Zhao, T., & Treff, N. R. (2013b). Cleavage-stage biopsy significantly impairs human embryonic implantation potential while blastocyst biopsy does not: a randomized and paired clinical trial.

Fertility and Sterility, *100*(3), 624–630. https://doi.org/10.1016/J.FERTNSTERT.2013.04.039

Summers, P. M., Campbell, J. M., & Miller, M. W. (1988). Normal in-vivo development of marmoset monkey embryos after trophectoderm biopsy. *Human Reproduction (Oxford, England)*, *3*(3), 389–393. https://doi.org/10.1093/OXFORDJOURNALS.HUMREP.A136713

Tobler, K. J., Zhao, Y., Ross, R., Benner, A. T., Xu, X., Du, L., Broman, K., Thrift, K., Brezina, P. R., & Kearns, W. G. (2015). Blastocoel fluid from differentiated blastocysts harbors embryonic genomic material capable of a whole-genome deoxyribonucleic acid amplification and comprehensive chromosome microarray analysis. *Fertility and Sterility*, *104*(2), 418–425. https://doi.org/10.1016/J.FERTNSTERT.2015.04.028

von Wolff, M. (2019). The role of Natural Cycle IVF in assisted reproduction. *Best Practice & Research. Clinical Endocrinology & Metabolism*, *33*(1), 35–45. https://doi.org/10.1016/J.BEEM.2018.10.005

Wilton, L. J., & Trounson, A. O. (1989). Biopsy of preimplantation mouse embryos: development of micromanipulated embryos and proliferation of single blastomeres in vitro. *Biology of Reproduction*, *40*(1), 145–152. https://doi.org/10.1095/BIOLREPROD40.1.145

Zegers-Hochschild, F., Adamson, G. D., Dyer, S., Racowsky, C., de Mouzon, J., Sokol, R., Rienzi, L., Sunde, A., Schmidt, L., Cooke, I. D., Simpson, J. L., & van der Poel, S. (2017). The International Glossary on Infertility and Fertility Care, 2017. *Fertility and Sterility*, *108*(3), 393–406. https://doi.org/10.1016/J.FERTNSTERT.2017.06.005

Chapter 21

Pre-implantation Genetic Testing

Ozlem Sezer[1], MD* and Aslihan Kiraz[2], MD

[1]Department of Medical Genetics, Samsun University, Faculty of Medicine, Samsun, Turkiye

[2]Department of Medical Genetics, Erciyes University, Faculty of Medicine, Kayseri, Turkiye

Abstract

With the advancement of genetic science and the development of diagnostic and examination methods, the diagnostic rate of genetic diseases is increasing day by day. Today, early diagnosis of the disease in future generations and even the birth of healthy individuals with healthy embryos can be ensured with genetic counseling and advanced examination studies. The preimplantation genetic test (PGT) refers to any test that evaluates whether oocytes or embryos are healthy. These tests are divided mainly into three categories: PGT-A, which evaluates numerical chromosomal disorders, namely aneuploidies, PGT-M, which evaluates single gene diseases, and PGT-SR, which evaluates structural chromosomal abnormalities. This evaluation, which was originally performed using Fluorescence in Situ Hybridization (FISH), is now also performed using different techniques such as Comparative Genomic Hybridization (aCGH), Next Generation Sequencing (NGS), and Real-Time Quantitative Polymerase Chain Reaction (qPCR).

Key Words: Infertility, Genetics, Preimplantation, Testing

---

* Corresponding Author's Email: ozlemturkeli@yahoo.com

In: Holistic Approach to Assisted Reproductive Technology
Editor: Kenan Demir and Rümeysa Yılmaz Göç
ISBN: 979-8-89113-017-3
© 2023 Nova Science Publishers, Inc.

Introduction

The early diagnosis methods of genetic diseases can be evaluated in two groups, prenatal genetic diagnosis and preimplantation genetic diagnosis (PGD). Prenatal genetic diagnosis is the process of diagnosing genetic diseases while the embryo is still in the womb. Samples examined in the prenatal genetic diagnosis differ according to the examination period. The prenatal genetic diagnosis methods are briefly summarized below;

Chorionic villus sampling (CVS) is a genetic diagnosis method applied to chorionic villi at 11-14 weeks of gestation.

Amniocentesis (AS) is a genetic examination method performed with fetal cells in the amniotic fluid at 16-20 weeks of pregnancy.

Cordocentesis (CS) is a genetic examination method applied to cord blood at 20-24 weeks in the advanced stages of pregnancy.

The preimplantation genetic diagnosis is offered to families with known risk of hereditary disease as an alternative to prenatal diagnosis (Ingerslev et al., 2018). With PGD, at-risk couples have the opportunity to have healthy children without having to terminate their pregnancy. In its simplest definition, PGD is the process of genetic examination of the oocyte or zygote during the preimplantation period and the implant of the healthy one into the uterus. In this method, cell biopsy procedures are performed before pregnancy occurs. The cells are genetically examined, and the product of conception is obtained by selecting genetically healthy ones (Fesahat et al., 2020). Therefore, families with known genetic diseases are ensured to have healthy children. The indications for PGD indications are similar to the indications for prenatal diagnosis. However, an additional indication is the need for a Human Leukocyte Antigen (HLA) matching sibling for the child who needs bone marrow transplantation (Ingerslev et al., 2018).

The first treatment with PGD was introduced in 1989 by Handyside et al. (Handyside et al., 1989) with the selection of female embryos to prevent births with X-linked recessive disease (Handyside et al., 1990), in 1990, Verlinsky et al. applied the PGD method with polar cell biopsy from a heterozygous mother with alpha-1-antitrypsin deficiency and Storm et al., from a couple with cystic fibrosis (Verlinsky et al., 1990; Strom et al., 1990). With the development and use of in vitro fertilization (IVF) and PGD methods, it has become possible to detect many chromosomal damage in the preimplantation period, diagnose single-gene diseases, and provide HLA-matched siblings. The lack of a general formula for all mutations is the method's biggest technical problem.

To make an accurate diagnosis by PGD, in addition to preparing special individual designs, it is necessary to have fast result times, especially in fresh embryo transfer (Chen et al., 2018).

Three approaches are commonly used in PGD. The 3rd-day biopsy procedure is the most preferred method in PGD. The processes are performed on 1 or 2 blastomeres. Blastocyst biopsy is the other alternative. FISH (Fluorescent In Situ Hybridization) for cytogenetic diagnosis and PCR (Polymerase Chain Reaction) test for molecular genetic diagnosis are applied to biopsy materials. The study of polar bodies is used to examine the maternal genetic contribution. As a result of the examination, only healthy embryos are transferred to the uterus (Basille et al., 2009).

The sampling methods in PGD are polar body analysis, blastomere analysis, and trophectoderm analysis. In all three applications, cell removal is well tolerated and does not cause congenital anomalies.

Polar Body Examination (Prefertilized Period of Oocytes)

In this method, the status of the oocyte is determined after polar body examination. The presence of polar cells with the nonmutated gene indicates the normal oocyte. The embryo fertilized with this oocyte will not be affected by genetic disease. Technical limitations of this method are the misdiagnosis due to the cross-over occurring during meiosis. This limitation is less common with direct gene analysis and linkage markers. However, since polar body examination shows only maternal contribution to the embryo, it cannot distinguish between carrier and patient in recessive diseases. Only the normal oocyte should be processed to avoid this resulting problem.

Blastomere Examination (Day 3, 1-2 cells)

In this second approach, one or two blastomeres are removed by biopsy from the embryo of the 8-cell stage (day 3). By genetic examination of these blastomeres, genetically normal embryos are transferred to the uterus. Examination of a single cell in the blastomere biopsy can lead to incomplete or erroneous results due to insufficient amplification. However, conditions such as faulty amplification of sperm DNA in the zona pellucida or allele dropout can lead to a false negative result at the blastomere stage. After marker analysis and whole genome amplification, single nucleotide polymorphism (SNP) microarray applications can circumvent these issues.

Trophectoderm Examination (Day 5-7, 5-12 cells):

This is the examination of cells taken from the trophectoderm layer, which is the early placental form, at the blastocyst stage. While the ability to examine more cells is an advantage of the method, the long culture time is its disadvantage, since it is done in the advanced stages of fertilization. Therefore, genetic analyzes should be completed before 24 hours or blastocysts should be frozen during examination (Wapner et al., 2009).

In studies, there is no increased risk of congenital anomalies in babies who have undergone PGD, and all three approaches are safe (Wapner et al., 2009).

Preimplantation genetic screening (PGS) is a preimplantation genetic screening test that screens for aneuploidy combined with routine IVF. The European Society of Human Reproduction and Embryology (ESHRE) has divided PGS into two categories: high-risk PGS (PGT for chromosome structural rearrangements (PGT-SR) and PGT for single gene / monogenic disorders (PGT-M)) and low-risk PGS (PGT for aneuploidies (PGT-A)). PGD-A is an analysis that includes the selection of euploid embryos and improves fertility outcomes by providing genetic screening for aneuploidies in couples with infertility or spontaneous pregnancy loss (Brezina et al., 2016). PGD-A

Table 21.1 Sampling methods in PGD; biopsy methods and their advantages and disadvantages (Fesahat et al., 2020)

Source of DNA	Aim and methods	Advantages	Disadvantages
PB biopsy	Indirect analysis Day 0-1, one PB Day 1, both PBs	Non-invasive An alternative method (Prohibited) Fresh ET possibility	Only the maternal genome Time-consuming Single-cell analysis
Blastomere biopsy	Direct analysis Day 3, Biopsy of 1-2 blastomeres Depending on: embryo quality	Routine procedure Whole genome analysis of the embryo Well-matched with fresh ET	Low amplification rate Influence on developmental competence of embryo Single-cell analysis Weak diagnostic power
Trophectoderm	Direct analysis Day 5-7, 5 to 10 cell TE Depending on: the embryo development stage	Diagnostic power Cost-effectiveness No influence on embryo High amplification rate	The IVF center must be qualified Inadequate experience Limited time to fresh ET

Abbreviations: ET, embryo transfer; IVF, in vitro fertilization; PB, Polar body; TE, trophectoderm.

Table 21.2 Features of preimplantation genetic testing (Fesahat et al., 2020)

Types of preimplantation genetic testing	
PGT-A *Aneuploidies*	Today, it is used instead of PGS, PGD-AS, and CCS. Detection of numerical anomalies ● Recurrent pregnancy losses ● Recurrent IVF failure ● Couples with a previously affected child ● Women over 35 years of age of late reproductive age ● History of radiotherapy or chemotherapy ● Poor-quality embryos in IVF cycles ● Severe male-factored infertility, such as azoospermia or severe oligospermia
PGT-M *Single gene / monogenic disorders*	Detection of monogenic or single-gene diseases / PGD ● Carrier families of an identified hereditary genetic disease caused by mutations ● HLA compatible sibling
PGT-SR *Chromosome structural rearrangements*	Detection of chromosomal rearrangements / PGD ● Parents with Robertsonian translocations or inversions ● Uses FISH and NGS ● NGS allows all chromosomes to be studied and does not require preliminary PGD testing ● FISH can only be used for relevant chromosomes and requires a prior informative study ● In most cases, massive sequencing techniques are used ● The FISH technique is used in the presence of an unbalanced chromosomal abnormality of less than 20 Mb.
Combined PGT	PGD-M+ PGD-A It is used to simultaneously diagnose and screen embryos ● If both couples are carriers of the mutation ● If one of the couples is affected by a genetic disorder ● If there is more than one clinical indication for couples; one of the parents is a carrier of a single gene disorder and has one of the indication criteria for PGT-A, such as severe male factor infertility and/or advanced maternal age
ePGT *Extended preimplantation genetic testing*	Multifactorial and polygenic disorders are investigated ● The clinical application of NGS technologies and the genome-wide single nucleotide polymorphism sequence enable the investigation of non-Mendelian diseases ● Familial full penetration disorders ● The application area is not yet clear

(*Continued*)

Table 21.2 (Continued)

Types of preimplantation genetic testing	
niPGT *Non-invasive PGT*	• The blastocyst BF of blastocysts and the embryo culture medium used provide suitable DNA templates for genetic analysis • A potential PGD tool that is cheaper, requires fewer micromanipulation skills, and poses a lower risk to embryos • DNA isolation and amplification protocols should be optimized to minimize contamination and obtain a reproducibly accurate clinical diagnosis • Its clinical potential is unknown

Abbreviations: BF, blastocyst fluid; CCS, comprehensive chromosome screening; FISH, fluorescent in situ hybridization; HLA, Human Leucocyte Antigen; IVF, in vitro fertilization; NGS, next-generation sequencing; PGD, preimplantation genetic diagnosis; PGT, preimplantation genetic testing.

is used to increase live birth rates and implantation success by screening the embryo at risk of aneuploidy (Chen et al., 2018). However, the application of PGS is still controversial due to the existence of euploid babies born after the transfer of aneuploid embryos to the uterus (Gleicher et al., 2016; Orvieto & Gleicher, 2016; Orvieto, 2016). In some European countries, such as Germany, the PGD / PGS practices are more stringent and polar body examination is preferred as the method applied, as it does not damage embryo integrity despite only showing maternal contribution (Chen et al., 2018; Montag et al., 2009).

In terminology, the detection of numerical chromosome anomalies was called "PGS", while the detection of single-gene diseases was called "PGD". Recently, the term Pre-Implantation Genetic Test (PGT) has begun to be used, using the terminology PGT-A to screen for numerical chromosomal abnormalities, PGT-SR for structural rearrangements such as translocation or inversion, and PGT-M for single gene diseases (Parikh et al., 2018).

FISH-based PGS application has ceased to be the primary choice in practice due to the development of genetic technologies such as quantitative polymerase chain reaction (qPCR), comparative genomic hybridization (aCGH) and next-generation sequencing (NGS) (Ma et al., 2016). In comprehensive chromosomal screening, the qPCR method has been reported to be the practice with the best results (Treff et al., 2012).

There are various ethical concerns, such as the application of PGD to save sibling life and its use in advanced age-onset diseases (Chen et al., 2018).

Table 21.3 Comparison of biopsy methods used in PGD with advantages and disadvantages (Fesahat et al., 2020; Kane et al., 2016; Sullivan-Pyke & Dokras, 2018)

PGT approaches	Methods	Technical characteristics	Applications	Limitations
PGT-A	FISH	Uses fluorescent probes specific to each chromosome First Examination	Analysis of numerical chromosome abnormalities Good compatibility with large nucleated blastomere in the cleavage stage	Analyzing a limited number of chromosomes
	aCGH	DNA extraction, amplification, and fluorochrome labeling, respectively Hybridization of the embryo's DNA with a dissimilar color-labeled reference DNA Scanning of color ratios for chromosomal variations	Whole-chromosome aneuploidy Translocations	Expensive Time- consuming Unable to detect mosaicism False positives
	qPCR	q- PCR amplification of each chromosome curves compared with each other and reference	All numerical anomalies Applicable to both the blastomere and TE biopsy Work easily Inexpensive Combined PGT	Segmental aneuploidy, mosaicism, and translocations cannot be detected

(Continued)

Table 21.3 (Continued)

PGT approaches	Methods	Technical characteristics	Applications	Limitations
	NGS	DNA extracted is amplified, broken, labeled, and sequenced Searching in databases Determine numerical and structural abnormalities	Comprehensive analysis of numerical abnormalities Applicable to both the blastomere and TE biopsy High sensitivity to mosaicism and subtle abnormalities Ability to automate and progressively cheap combined PGT	Detection of balanced chromosomal translocations is limited
PGT-M	Linkage Analysis + mini-sequencing	Single-gene mutations are investigated using specific primers Mini-sequencing is used for genotyping of amplicons	Direct and indirect detection of monogenic disorders and de novo mutations Cheap and powerful diagnostic power.	Requires a special probe and primer design The setup condition is time consuming
	Karyomapping	The DNA extracted is amplified and fluorochrome-labeled Thousands of SNP variants hybridize on a microarray slide The rates of SNPs determine the haplotype.	Indirect detection of single gene mutation by haplotyping Fast, easy Specific to the case	Needs sufficient SNP markers. PGT-M set-up required Not suitable for detecting de novo mutations Expensive.
	NGS	Direct investigation of the mutation using targeted amplification of known sequence	Simultaneous analysis of genes	Data analysis requires experts Expensive

Abbreviations: aCGH, array comparative genomic hybridization; FISH, fluorescent in situ hybridization; NGS, next-generation sequencing; PGT, preimplantation genetic testing; PGT-A, PGT for aneuploidies; PGT-M, PGT for single gene / monogenic disorders; qPCR, quantitative real-time PCR; SNP, Single Nucleotide Polymorphism; TE, trophectoderm.

Table 21.4 The diagnostic capacity of PGT techniques (Kane et al., 2016)

Diagnostic capacity	aCGH	SNP array	qPCR	NGS
24 chromosomes	+	+	+	+
UPD	-	+	+	-
Balanced chromosome rearrangements	-	+	-	-
Haploidy/polyploidy	±	+	+	±
Segmental aneuploidies (threshold)	+ 5 – 6 Mb	+ 2.4 – 5 Mb	-	+ ~3 Mb
Advantages	Widespread	Ability to detect the widest chromosomal abnormality	Time- consuming	Increased resolution and throughput detection of mosaicism
Disadvantages	Limited detection of mosaicism	Expensive	Evaluation of only a few loci per chromosome	Expensive cost

Abbreviations: aCGH, array comparative genomic hybridization; NGS, next-generation sequencing; PGT, preimplantation genetic testing; qPCR, quantitative real-time PCR; SNP, Single Nucleotide Polymorphism; UPD, Uniparental disomy.

Conclusion

To allow fresh embryo transfer, it is important to obtain maximum genetic information as soon as possible from the biopsy sample taken for genetic analysis. Although recent advances in genetic testing technologies are promising in improving IVF outcomes, they await confirmation by sufficiently robust prospective randomized trials (Kane et al., 2016). Data on the sensitivity and specificity of molecular PGT tests will expand our experience with the efficiency and accuracy of these technologies.

References

Basille, C., Frydman, R., El Aly, A., & Achour-Frydman, N. (2009). Preimplantation genetic diagnosis: state of the art. *European journal of obstetrics, gynecology, and reproductive biology, 145*(1), 9–13. https://doi.org/10.1016/j.ejogrb.2009.04.004

Brezina, P. R., Anchan, R., & Kearns, W. G. (2016). Preimplantation genetic testing for aneuploidy: what technology should you use and what are the differences? *Journal of assisted reproduction and genetics, 33*(7), 823–832. https://doi.org/10.1007/s10815-016-0740-2

Chen, H. F., Chen, S. U., Ma, G. C., & Chen, M. (2018). Preimplantation genetic diagnosis and screening: Current status and future challenges. *Journal of the Formosan Medical Association = Taiwan yi zhi, 117*(2), 94–100. https://doi.org/10.1016/j.jfma.2017.08.006

Fesahat, F., Montazeri, F., & Hoseini, S. M. (2020). Preimplantation genetic testing in assisted reproduction technology. *Journal of gynecology obstetrics and human reproduction, 49*(5), 101723. https://doi.org/10.1016/j.jogoh.2020.101723

Gleicher, N., Vidali, A., Braverman, J., & International PGS Consortium Study Group (2016). Accuracy of preimplantation genetic screening (PGS) is compromised by degree of mosaicism of human embryos. *Reproductive biology and endocrinology: RB&E, 14*(1), 54. https://doi.org/10.1186/s12958-016-0193-6

Handyside, A. H., Kontogianni, E. H., Hardy, K., & Winston, R. M. (1990). Pregnancies from biopsied human preimplantation embryos sexed by Y-specific DNA amplification. *Nature, 344*(6268), 768–770. https://doi.org/10.1038/344768a0

Handyside, A. H., Pattinson, J. K., Penketh, R. J., & Tuddenham, E. G. (1989). Biopsy of human preimplantation embryos and sexing by DNA amplification. *Lancet (London, England), 1*(8634), 347–349. https://doi.org/10.1016/s0140-6736(89)91723-6

Ingerslev, H. J., Degn, B., Hnida, C., & Pedersen, I. S. (2018). Preimplantation genetic diagnosis. *Ugeskr Laeger, 180*(14), V09170692

Kane, S. C., Willats, E., Bezerra Maia E Holanda Moura, S., Hyett, J., & da Silva Costa, F. (2016). Pre-Implantation Genetic Screening Techniques: Implications for Clinical Prenatal Diagnosis. *Fetal diagnosis and therapy, 40*(4), 241–254. https://doi.org/10.1159/000449381

Ma, G.C., Chen, H.F., Yang, Y.S, Lin, W. H., Tsai, F. P., Lin, C. F., Chiu, C., & Chen, M. A. (2016). A pilot proof-of-principle study to compare fresh and vitrified cycle preimplantation genetic screening by chromosome microarray and next generation sequencing. *Mol Cytogenet*, *9*,25. https://doi.org/10.1186/s13039-016 -0238-8

Wapner, R., Jenkins, T., & Khalek, N. (2009). Prenatal Diagnosis of Congenital Disorders. In: Creasy, R., Resnik, R., & Lockwood, C. (Eds), *Creasy and Resnik's Maternal-Fetal Medicine: Principles and Practice E-Book*, *6th Edition* (pp. 259-261). Saunders press. ISBN 978-1-4160-4224-2.

Montag, M., van der Ven, K., Rösing, B., & van der Ven, H. (2009). Polar body biopsy: a viable alternative to preimplantation genetic diagnosis and screening. *Reproductive biomedicine online*, *18 Suppl 1*, 6–11. https://doi.org/10.1016/s1472-6483(10)60109-5

Orvieto R. (2016). Preimplantation genetic screening- the required RCT that has not yet been carried out. *Reproductive biology and endocrinology: RB&E*, *14*(1), 35. https://doi.org/10.1186/s12958-016-0171-z

Orvieto, R., & Gleicher, N. (2016). Should preimplantation genetic screening (PGS) be implemented to routine IVF practice? *Journal of assisted reproduction and genetics*, *33*(11), 1445–1448. https://doi.org/10.1007/s10815-016-0801-6

Parikh, F. R., Athalye, A. S., Naik, N. J., & Madon, P. F. (2018). Preimplantation Genetic Testing: Its Evolution, Where Are We Today? *Journal of human reproductive sciences*, *11*(4), 306–314. https://doi.org/10.4103/jhrs.JHRS_132_18

Strom, C. M., Verlinsky, Y., Milayeva, S., & Applebaum, M. (1990). Preconception genetic diagnosis of cystic fibrosis. *Lancet (London, England)*, *336*(8710), 306–307. https://doi.org/10.1016/0140-6736(90)91835-x

Sullivan-Pyke, C., & Dokras, A. (2018). Preimplantation Genetic Screening and Preimplantation Genetic Diagnosis. *Obstetrics and gynecology clinics of North America*, *45*(1), 113–125. https://doi.org/10.1016/j.ogc.2017.10.009

Treff, N. R., Tao, X., Ferry, K. M., & Scott, R. T., Jr (2012). Development and validation of an accurate quantitative real-time polymerase chain reaction-based assay for human blastocyst comprehensive chromosomal aneuploidy screening. *Fertility and sterility*, *97*(4), 819–824. https://doi.org/10.1016/j.fertnstert.2012.01.115

Verlinsky, Y., Ginsberg, N., Lifchez, A., & Strom, C. M. (1990). Analysis of the first polar body: preconception genetic diagnosis. *Human reproduction (Oxford, England)*, *5*(7), 826–829. https://doi.org/10.1093/oxfordjournals.humrep.a137192

Chapter 22

Embryo and Oocyte Cryopreservation

Ümmügülsüm Önal, MD*

Department of Histology & Embryology, Selcuk University School of Medicine, Konya, Turkiye

Abstract

Cryopreservation offers solutions to potential legal or probable ethical issues in routine infertility procedures and provides advantages for fertility preservation for both medical and social reasons.

After cell freezing procedures, the vitrification technique used in embryo-oocyte cryopreservation is also no longer considered experimental. It has strengthened the clinical advantages of delayed embryo transfer with successful survivals. One of its rapidly growing indications is that it gives individual reproductive autonomy by preserving elective fertility. Evidence for a higher risk at implantation or during the obstetric or prenatal stages is currently insufficient. However, given that it has been 40 years since the first live birth after cryopreservation and that live births obtained from freezing cycles cannot be adequately followed, it is still unknown what problems infants born through freezing-thaw in vitro fertilization (IVF) pregnancy may have at older ages. When a recent technology is implemented in a clinical embryology laboratory, it is important to consider which technique produces better clinical findings and what the reliability outcomes of these will be in long-term research. Another important part is how clinical results vary in different indications in vitrification of oocytes or embryos. Here, the age of the mother and therefore the age of the oocyte is the most important factor.

Key Words: Fertility preservation, Embryo and blastocyst cryopreservation, Oocyte vitrification, Oocyte survival, Reproductive autonomy, SWOT analysis

---

* Corresponding Author's Email: ug.onal.md@gmail.com

In: Holistic Approach to Assisted Reproductive Technology
Editor: Kenan Demir and Rümeysa Yılmaz Göç
ISBN: 979-8-89113-017-3
© 2023 Nova Science Publishers, Inc.

Introduction

Cryopreservation technology first gained prominence with fertility preservation (FP) in cancer patients. From a conceptual standpoint, "freeze storage" describes the extremely low temperature storage of cells in liquid nitrogen (-196 °C) after freezing. Although cooling is not a physiological condition for human cells, the uncontrolled conversion of water into ice crystals may result in cell loss, particularly given the high concentration of water in living things. The human oocyte is particularly vulnerable to this process due to its size and its highly vulnerable meiotic spindle to degeneration. In 1980 (Figure 22.1) since the first freezing of human embryos, a breakthrough has been achieved in the current procedure with vitrification (amorphous, glass construction) thus achieving successful results for the oocyte. Cryopreservation therefore presents a choice for fertility preservation in cancer patients who will receive gonadotoxic therapy, as well as in patients with gonadal insufficiency, and even in those who seek to freeze germ cells for future use (Sciorio, 2020; Niederberger et al., 2018).

This chapter will focus mainly on indications, approaches, social, and medical clinical outputs for fertility preservations, which are currently available, beyond the technical procedure of oocyte and embryo cryopreservations.

First, what function does cryopreservation serve in invasive fertilization on a broad scale? (Rienzi et al., 2017)

- Increases the cumulative live birth rate for each cycle of oocyte pick-up.
- Offers egg banking services for the accumulation of oocytes
- Allows elective systematic implementation of the single embryo transfer policy.

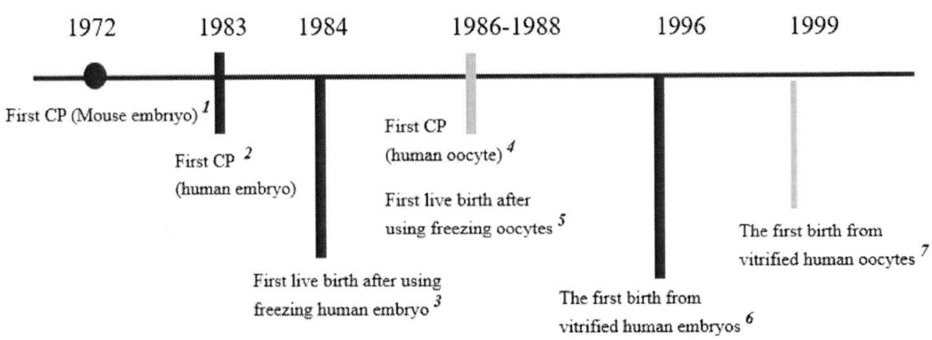

Figure 22.1 Cryopreservation timeline (approximate dates) (Whittingham, 1972; Testart et al., 1986; Ashwood-Smith, 1986; Friedler, 1988; Chen, 1986; Ohta, 1996; Kuleshova et al., 1999).

- Allows for preservation of fertility for medical and non-medical indications.
- Provides the possibility to perform cycle segmentation.

Who do we perform oocyte/embryo cryopreservation on to preserve fertility is another crucial issue. The first group includes cancer patients, as predicted, but there are other uses as well, including autoimmune diseases, people who need hematopoietic stem cell transplantation, and non-oncological medical conditions such as ovarian failure (POI) (Martinez, 2017). The aging of the oocyte is one of the substances that is especially emphasized and discussed. Therefore, to avoid this, the practice of freezing oocytes during times of high fertility and then using them to conceive children has undergone significant development, particularly in the last 10 years, and has sparked intense ethical discussion. Stoop changed the word "oocyte banking" to "age banking" in 2014, giving the literature a much more accurate language (Stoop et al., 2014).

When we examine the use of embryo cryopreservation specifically for fertility preservation, we can observe from the literature that earlier research used this technique mainly in cancer patients.

However, with the successful implementation of oocyte cryopreservation with the vitrification technique, a very important advantage was noted: it provides reproductive autonomy to the woman; at this point, we see that CP has advanced a lot. When we look at the data for the last 10 years, oocyte cryopreservation has almost entirely replaced embryo cryopreservation in fertility preservation because it continues to be performed with similar success.

Failure to freeze oocytes in previous years was the main factor in the widespread adoption of embryo cryopreservation. Slow freezing of the oocytes could not produce satisfactory results, but by the end of the 2000s, particularly in young patients with vitrification technique; Successful results were obtained, close to fresh, so it began to be used more widely in clinics. It began to be widely used for all indications, not just to preserve fertility. It also led to higher survival success rates. Therefore, oocyte cryopreservation emerges as a pioneer in fertility preservation compared to the embryo (Maheshwari et al., 2022)

Technically speaking, what process should we employ in the IVF lab to freeze oocytes or blastocysts? Now, cohort and final meta-analyses in the literature unequivocally show that vitrification is a more effective technique than slow freezing at every stage of development. Therefore, it is extremely valuable to have a competent vitrification program in the laboratory if freezing is to be performed for any indication. In addition to clinical effectiveness, the reliability of long-term technology will also be important. To date, studies show that there is no increased risk either at implantation or at the obstetric or prenatal stage due to vitrification of the oocyte or blastocyst-embryo. Therefore, the vitrification process is currently used in the IVF laboratory safely and effectively (Rienzi et al., 2017).

Again, if we look at what should be the criterion of being able to successfully perform a technique in an IVF laboratory; there are a number of performance indicators that should be used, and this should be monitored on a regular basis. For oocytes, data from The Alpha consensus meeting on cryopreservation can be consulted; in the clinical IVF laboratory, at least 70% viability should be targeted with the vitrification method. The target value is especially in young patients; we expect to achieve almost as much viability as a fresh oocyte by vitrification of the oocyte. When looking for embryo - blastocyst in your IVF laboratory, especially in the blastocyst stage; it can achieve a survival rate of 90% or even 100%. In other words, vitrification is a very successful technology in every stage of development (Alpha Scientists in Reproductive Medicine, 2012; ESHRE, 2020; ESHRE & Alpha Scientists in Reproductive Medicine, 2017).

In whom do we use vitrification of oocytes within the scope of fertile preservation? Oocyte vitrification has been widely used in cancer patients and especially in cases of endometriosis among other medical diseases, which has been increasing in recent years.

Other reason; the group with the most ethical discussions, especially on social indications; In the past this was called a social indication, but today the terminology is used as an elective fertility preservation. Because perhaps decreased ovarian reserve should not be considered a social reason, but rather a medical reason, and elective fertility preservation would be a more accurate *definition.*

What is the patient coverage of elective fertility preservation? In order to protect the reproductive autonomy of single women who do not want to use donor sperm; the majority of this group consists of women who want to freeze their oocytes at a younger age when their fertility is better and then preserve their chances of having children. In other words, with this technology, women are given a very valuable awareness. Community studies show that many women do not realize that their fertility will actually decrease until the age of 38, or rather that their oocytes will age. This shows us that the widespread use of fertility preservation for this purpose will increase the awareness of many women at an earlier stage. Therefore, we can say that it is a very valuable method in the elective group.

Clinical Results (Social and Medical)

In a multicenter study of Rienzi L. and his group published in 2012; A model for decision making for infertile patients based on birth rates after oocyte vitrification is presented; and still has a realistic predictive value that both clinicians and embryologists can use very effectively in patient consultation. The most important outcome of the study; The same success cannot be achieved with vitrification of the oocytes in every patient. First, the patient must be informed about this issue; In this study, it is clearly seen that the live birth rate almost doubles in patients with 6–8 or more oocytes. When we look at women with less than 8 oocytes and older age (over 38 years), this rate drops to 12%. When we evaluate patients with a good prognosis, that is, in patients with 8 or more Oocytes, if the 3rd day has a large number of good quality embryos and can be transferred to the blastocyst stage, success can increase up to 60% (Rienzi et al., 2012).

Again in a similar study; In patients who have undergone oocyte vitrification for elective and medical reasons: it shows how many mature oocytes need to be collected, frozen and used in women of that age group in order to have 1-3 children in different age groups. When each age group is looked at independently of each other, there is actually a similar trend; the more metaphase II oocytes you have, the more you increase the probability of having 1-3 children. There is one more thing to pay particular attention to; Considering the 30-34 age group and the 41-42 age group together, age is the most important factor in these 2 groups; The age of the oocyte stands out as the most important predictive factor in oocyte vitrification cycles. In a 41-42-year-old woman, the probability of having a child increases as the number of oocytes increases. But many more metaphase II Oocytes need to be frozen than a 30-34-year-old woman to have a similar probability of success (Doyle et al., 2016).

Clinicians may be in believing that; just like in blastocyst vitrification, every cell we freeze will survive 100% and this cell will be available for fertilization. Unfortunately, we cannot talk about such a situation in vitrification of oocytes. As a laboratory, we have to maintain a minimum of 70% viability, but other than that, different rates may be in question in different age groups and maybe even in different prognoses.

Another retrospective observational multicenter study pointed out that the viability rate can vary from 80% to 96%; emphasizes that it is a much more sensitive cell and that 100% viability should never be expected in every patient group (Cobo et al., 2016; Cobo et al., 2013).

The number of Metaphase II (M II) oocytes collected from patients under and over 35 years of age was compared with the cumulative birth rates in the same group study. In both groups, there are very serious differences between 5 oocytes collected and 15 oocytes collected in the same age group. The live birth rate can rise from 15% to 85% for those under the age of 35 years, and a rate that rises from 5% to 35% in the over-35 age group. In terms of age; if you can freeze 15 metaphase II in a young woman, the cumulative probability of live birth increases to 85%, so this study tells us that vitrification is a very effective method if you can do it at a young age. When we consider the older age group, the cumulative rate of living birth increases as the number of M II oocytes rises over the age of 35, but when we look at the situation where 10 oocytes can be collected on both sides, the older oocytes do not give us the same cumulative birth rate as a young oocyte, at least even when we use the same number of oocytes.

In the work of a pioneering group in 2017; It gives an estimated value for clinicians and patients by revealing how many metaphase II Oocytes need to be frozen for the probability of obtaining at least one live birth in different age groups. Figure 22.2 presented by Goldman and his team also has data similar to the literature: The number of mature oocytes that should be used to achieve the same live birth rate in a woman at 35 and a woman at 44 is very different from each other.

In another comprehensive study, the clinical results of vitrification performed in patients between the ages of 35 and older for various indications (poor response, elective FP). We observe significant differences between older women with a poor prognosis and younger women in both survival rate and cumulative live birth each cycle/patient (50% to 30% in the poor response group and 62% to 24% in the elective FP group). Put simply, the younger the

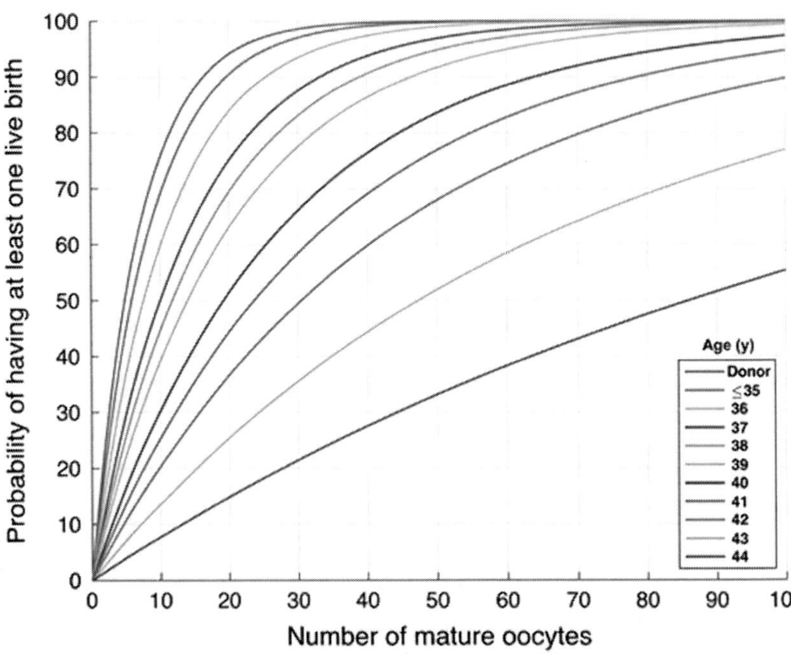

Figure 22.2 Live birth predictions by age and number of mature oocytes recovered (R.H. Goldman et al., 2017)

female age, the more metaphase 2 oocytes and the correspondingly higher cumulative live birth rates increase the rate of successful clinical output in both indications (even with a good or bad prognosis).

To reconsider cryopreservation in terms of its indications; In a study in 2018, which parameters were taken into account as a determinant in the success of IVF results in the elective and oncofertility groups. And interestingly, although clinical success (implantation rate) is lower in cancer patients, when the main variables are fixed (here the age of the woman and the controlled ovarian stimulation protocol used are known to be the most important variables); statistical difference disappears, that is, cancer disease alone is not related to poor clinical outcome (Cobo et al., 2018). Therefore, today, is the reason for the worsening of clinical outcomes in oncofertility patients the type of cancer in the patient? or instead, just like in other patients, is the age of the woman, the controlled-ovarian stimulation (COS) protocol applied, and the number of eggs collected the main related factor?

The literature has not yet explained this. Of course, we know very well that in the elective group, the age of the woman (hence the age of the egg) and the number of eggs are the main factors, but in the cancer patient group, perhaps the age at which the woman was diagnosed with cancer may also be a major factor. However, our current conclusion is the following. The age of the egg seems to be the most important factor in the oncofertility group, also ahead of the cancer type.

We can review this study from 2021 to see what the current clinical data indicate, and we see that the outcomes of the oncofertility group are actually rather good (Cobo et al., 2021). Perhaps making a distinction according to age and cancer type in the onko-fertility patient group, and looking at the success factors and predictive reasons here, may provide us with much clearer results. In the continuation of the study, when we look at patients under the age of 35 and over the age of 35, these are the elective group, the patients with endometriosis, and the patients with oncofertility preservation; there is a similar trend in each group regardless of age; the more eggs (M II oocyte), the better the cumulative live birth rate. But, of course, patients over the age of 36 need to use much more eggs. Again, in the continuation of the study, similar to the previous paragraph, when we look at the oncofertility group, there are no significant differences compared to other groups with similar egg numbers. Maybe the factor here is; Could it be the age at which the woman was diagnosed with cancer, adding this information will be useful in the future.

So what if we look at the SWOT analysis for the cases of elective FP oocyte vitrification (Gil-Arribas et al., 2022);

SWOT analysis identifies the strengths, weaknesses, opportunities and threats of the method and assesses the risks from various angles.

STRENGTHS. This is a very effective procedure for vitrification, particularly in the young age range, and it can currently be carried out very successfully, especially for vitrification of oocytes. Up to date, in studies, it has good perinatal reliability and an important advantage is that it provides the opportunity to make family planning during periods when the woman's fertility is good, as it provides awareness to the patient; This is one of the strengths of the method.

OPPORTUNITIES. However, when we look at the opportunities it provides; patients are concerned about the safety of the hormone therapy they will receive for the cycle, however; Studies of structures, at least to date, show that there is no increase in cases of gynecological cancer. In addition, when fertility education is increased at a global level, it provides a very serious opportunity to women; In terms of their chances of having children in the future. As is known, the most important age in terms of career is 30s and 40s. Similarly, when a woman freezes her eggs at the age of 30, she has the opportunity to continue her career in a more stress-free and motivated way. In fact, the risks of going to oocyte donation in the future are reduced.

WEAKNESSES. It is an expensive technology considering the number of cycles. In addition, there is currently no prognostic biomarker for ovarian reserve. Furthermore, freezing eggs does not always guarantee fertilization. Additionally, it is critical that women in this regard undergo thorough evaluation and be given a realistic plan of action. Its usage rate in the literature varies between 6% and 12.5%, which makes it another weakness that makes it a strategy that is not cost-effective. After all, the patient will receive medical treatment; this has minimal risks. The quality or maturity of the egg collected never guarantees the quality of the embryo or pregnancy.

THREATS. When we consider threats, we can see that they can result in late pregnancy difficulties or neonatal complications, and if there are legal limitations in the country, this drives women to look for alternatives elsewhere. Of course, not every laboratory will be able to reach the ideal outcomes described in the literature at the beginning of this chapter. Here, the experience and track record of the IVF laboratory with CP difficulties are crucial. Interestingly, research reveals that the majority of women who attempt egg freezing are women with higher economic and educational levels. Could this actually steer a woman who does not want children in this direction, forcing her to become a single mother because she is already in a superior socioeconomic group and is less likely to find a partner in the future? There have been such debates recently. Many single mothers in Spain, for example, have frozen and used their oocytes in this way. This appears to be one of the most controversial social issues.

Conclusion

Slow freezing is rapidly replacing by vitrification since it has a higher survival probability after thawing. New clinical indications, such as preservation of fertility, have begun to emerge as a result of the rapid spread of vitrification in both oocytes and embryos.

Elective reasons continue to spark debate not only about their cost-effectiveness but also about ethical and medical issues. In general, even if vitrification is a leading method of treating infertility, the benefits and drawbacks of elective freezing should be discussed. So, based on their age and the number of accessible oocytes, this group should receive guidance.

Women who choose fertility preservation should be informed that doing so would only increase their chances of conceiving a biological child with individual real success rates and cannot ensure that they will become mothers in the future.

Numerous research on the physiology of oocytes and embryos during cryopreservation has been published since it was first used, but larger studies and follow-up of vitrified IVF cycles are required, particularly to confirm the impact of new cryopreservation procedures at the cell level. Embryo obtained from IVF cycles using freezing gametes or cryopreserved embryos, especially later in life, after live birth; It should be followed systematically and in a large population in all developmental stages, including geriatric. We don't know much about these babies' long-term prognosis except their live birth rate.

Because of this, oocyte vitrification is a suggested technology for elective CP, currently defined as age banking, for women who are at risk of losing their ovarian function due to a medical condition, such as cancer patients, or women who are at risk of having a low genetic reserve, as well as women who want to put off having children by preventing age-related fertility drops.

Although the evidence is still less, studies currently available indicate successful results in all indications. However, several factors affect the outcomes:

The results in all populations are significantly influenced by the patient's age at the time of oocyte collection. It should be suggested to women in this demographic to decide on their reproductive preservation when they are still young (≤ 35 years old).

To achieve generally acceptable success rates (cumulative living rate based on the number of oocytes used per patient from 40% to 70%), it is preferable to obtain 10-15 oocytes in patients under 35 years of age. These many oocytes can be produced over a few cycles (Cobo et al., 2021). In the case of older women, the statistics must be individualized.

Furthermore, the prevalence of fertility preservations may have an impact on success rates because endometriosis and cancer patients have worse clinical outcomes (the implantation rate in cancer patients is significantly lower), although in cancer patients; the effect of cancer type on success rates and the role of cancer in clinical outcomes has not yet been established (Dolmans and Manavella, 2018).

Within the framework of assisted reproductive technology, a cryopreservation method that is optimal for each IVF laboratory must be developed.

According to recent literature, the optimal course of freezing for all stages of development is vitrification. Since embryo survival rates are almost 100%, it can be said that current vitrification technologies are quite effective.

The long-term follow-up results of children born with freezing oocyte fertilization are limited and, although this is not an alarming finding, this ambiguity should be clearly resolved with comprehensive studies (Noyes et al., 2009).

Women should be informed about the risk of losing reproductive autonomy and the possibility of preserving it, with accurate success rates.

Within the scope of further studies; making the freezing procedure standardized and traceable for each IVF laboratory will be an important advantage to both clearly demonstrate clinical results and improve the procedure.

References

Alpha Scientists in Reproductive Medicine. (2012). The Alpha consensus meeting on cryopreservation key performance indicators and benchmarks: proceedings of an expert meeting. *Reproductive BioMedicine Online*, *25*(2), 146-167. https://doi.org/10.1016/j.rbmo.2012.05.006.

Ashwood-Smith, M. J. (1986).The cryopreservation of human embryos. *Hum Reprod.*, *1*(5), 319-32. https://doi.org/10.1093/oxfordjournals.humrep.a136413

Chen, C. (1986). Pregnancy after human oocyte cryopreservation. *The Lancet*, *327*(8486), 884-886. https://doi.org/10.1016/s0140-6736(86)90989-x.

Cobo A, Castellò D, Vallejo B, Albert C, de los Santos JM, Remohí J. Cobo, A., Castellò, D., Vallejo, B., Albert, C., de los Santos, J. M., & Remohí, J. (2013). Outcome of cryotransfer of embryos developed from vitrified oocytes: double vitrification has no impact on delivery rates. *Fertility and sterility*, *99*(6), 1623-1630. https://doi.org/10.1016/j.fertnstert.2013.01.106.

Cobo, A., García-Velasco, J., Domingo, J., Pellicer, A., & Remohí, J. (2018). Elective and onco-fertility preservation: factors related to IVF outcomes. *Human Reproduction*, *33*(12), 2222-2231. https://doi.org/10.1093/humrep/dey321.

Cobo, A., García-Velasco, J. A., Coello, A., Domingo, J., Pellicer, A., & Remohí, J. (2016). Oocyte vitrification as an efficient option for elective fertility preservation. *Fertility and sterility*, *105*(3), 755-764. https://doi.org/10.1016/j.fertnstert.2015.11.027.

Cobo, A., García-Velasco, J. A., Remohí, J., & Pellicer, A. (2021). Oocyte vitrification for fertility preservation for both medical and nonmedical reasons. *Fertility and Sterility*, *115*(5), 1091-1101. https://doi.org/10.1016/j.fertnstert.2021.02.006.

Dolmans, M. M., & Manavella, D. D. (2019). Recent advances in fertility preservation. *Journal of Obstetrics and Gynaecology Research*, *45*(2), 266-279. https://doi .org/10.1111/jog.13818.

Doyle, J. O., Richter, K. S., Lim, J., Stillman, R. J., Graham, J. R., & Tucker, M. J. (2016). Successful elective and medically indicated oocyte vitrification and warming for autologous in vitro fertilization, with predicted birth probabilities for fertility preservation according to number of cryopreserved oocytes and age at retrieval. *Fertility and sterility*, *105*(2), 459-466. https://doi.org/10.1016/j .fertnstert.2015.10.026.

ESHRE (2020). ESHRE guideline: female fertility preservation. Human reproduction open, 2020(4), hoaa052. https://doi.org/10.1093/hropen/hoaa052.

ESHRE Special Interest Group of Embryology, & Alpha Scientists in Reproductive Medicine. (2017). The Vienna consensus: report of an expert meeting on the development of art laboratory performance indicators. *Human Reproduction Open*, *2017*(2), hox011. https://doi.org/10.1016/j.rbmo.2017.06.015.

Friedler, S., Giudice, L. C., & Lamb, E. J. (1988). Cryopreservation of embryos and ova. *Fertility and sterility*, *49*(5), 743-764. https://doi.org/10.1016/s0015 -0282(16)59879-3.

Gil-Arribas, E., Blockeel, C., Pennings, G., Nekkebroeck, J., Velasco, J. A. G., Serna, J., & De Vos, M. (2022). Oocyte vitrification for elective fertility preservation: a SWOT analysis. *Reproductive BioMedicine Online*, *44*(6), 1005-1014. https:// doi.org/10.1016/j.rbmo.2022.02.001.

Goldman, R. H., Racowsky, C., Farland, L. V., Munné, S., Ribustello, L., & Fox, J. H. (2017). Predicting the likelihood of live birth for elective oocyte cryopreservation: a counseling tool for physicians and patients. *Human reproduction*, *32*(4), 853-859. https://doi.org/10.1093/humrep/dex008

Kuleshova, L., Gianaroli, L., Magli, C., Ferraretti, A., & Trounson, A. (1999). Birth following vitrification of a small number of human oocytes: case report. *Human Reproduction*, *14*(12), 3077-3079. https://doi.org/10.1093/humrep/14.12.3077.

Maheshwari A, Bell JL, Bhide P, Brison D, Child T, Chong HY, Cheong Y, Cole C, Coomarasamy A, Cutting R, Hardy P, Hamoda H, Juszczak E, Khalaf Y, Kurinczuk JJ, Lavery S, Linsell L, Macklon N, Mathur R, Pundir J, Raine-Fenning N, Rajkohwa M, Scotland G, Stanbury K, Troup S, Bhattacharya S. (2022). Elective freezing of embryos versus fresh embryo transfer in IVF: a multicentre randomized controlled trial in the UK (E-Freeze). *Human Reproduction*, *37*(3), 476-487. https://doi.org/10.1093/humrep/deab279.

Martinez, F. (2017). Update on fertility preservation from the Barcelona International Society for Fertility Preservation–ESHRE–ASRM 2015 expert meeting: indications, results and future perspectives. *Fertility and sterility*, *108*(3), 407-415. https://doi.org/10.1093/humrep/dex218.

Niederberger, C, Pellicer A, Cohen J, Gardner DK, Palermo GD, O'Neill CL, Chow S, Rosenwaks Z, Cobo A, Swain JE, Schoolcraft WB, Frydman R, Bishop LA, Aharon D, Gordon C, New E, Decherney A, Tan SL, Paulson RJ, Goldfarb JM, Brännström M, Donnez J, Silber S, Dolmans MM, Simpson JL, Handyside AH,

Munné S, Eguizabal C, Montserrat N, Izpisua Belmonte JC, Trounson A, Simon C, Tulandi T, Giudice LC, Norman RJ, Hsueh AJ, Sun Y, Laufer N, Kochman R, Eldar-Geva T, Lunenfeld B, Ezcurra D, D'Hooghe T, Fauser BCJM, Tarlatzis BC, Meldrum DR, Casper RF, Fatemi HM, Devroey P, Galliano D, Wikland M, Sigman M, Schoor RA, Goldstein M, Lipshultz LI, Schlegel PN, Hussein A, Oates RD, Brannigan RE, Ross HE, Pennings G, Klock SC, Brown S, Van Steirteghem A, Rebar RW, LaBarbera AR. (2018). Forty years of IVF. *Fertil Steril., 110*(2):185-324.e5. https://doi.org/10.1016/j.fertnstert.2018.06.005.

Noyes, N., Porcu, E., & Borini, A. (2009). Over 900 oocyte cryopreservation babies born with no apparent increase in congenital anomalies. *Reproductive biomedicine online*, *18*(6), 769-776. https://doi.org/10.1016/s1472-6483(10)60025-9.

Ohta, N. (1996). Ultrarapid freezing of human embryos by vitrification method-a case of delivery. *Jpn J Fertil Steril*, *41*, 276-279.

Rienzi, L, Cobo, A, Paffoni, A, Scarduelli C, Capalbo A, Vajta G, Remohí J, Ragni G, Ubaldi FM. (2012). Consistent and predictable delivery rates after oocyte vitrification: an observational longitudinal cohort multicentric study. *Hum Reprod.*, *27*(6):1606-12. https://doi.org/10.1093/humrep/des088.

Rienzi, L, Gracia C, Maggiulli R, LaBarbera AR, Kaser DJ, Ubaldi FM, Vanderpoel S, Racowsky C. (2017). Oocyte, embryo and blastocyst cryopreservation in ART: systematic review and meta-analysis comparing slow-freezing versus vitrification to produce evidence for the development of global guidance. *Hum Reprod,* 23(2):139-155. https://doi.org/10.1093/humupd/dmw038.

Sciorio, R. (2020). Cryopreservation of human embryos and oocytes for fertility preservation in cancer and non cancer patients: a mini review. *Gynecol Endocrinol.,* 36(5):381-388. https://doi.org/10.1080/09513590.2020.1719402.

Stoop, D., Cobo, A., & Silber, S. (2014). Fertility preservation for age-related fertility decline. *The Lancet*, *384*(9950), 1311-1319. https://doi.org/10.1016/S0140-6736(14)61261-7

Testart, J., Lassalle, B., Belaisch-Allart, J., Hazout, A., Forman, R., Rainhorn, J. D., & Frydman, R. (1986). High pregnancy rate after early human embryo freezing. *Fertility and Sterility*, *46*(2), 268-272. https://doi.org/10.1016/s0015-0282(16)49524-5. PMID: 3732533.

Whittingham, D. G., Leibo, S. P., Mazur, P. (1972). Survival of mouse embryos frozen to -196 degrees and -269 degrees C. *Science.*, *178*(4059), 411-4.

Chapter 23

Cryopreservation of Human Spermatozoa

Berrin Yangın Doğru, MD*
IVF Center, Konya City Hospital, Konya, Turkiye

Abstract

Since about 1964, infertility has ceased to be a problem for many men with the successful application of human sperm cryopreservation. Nowadays, assisted reproductive technologies (ART) are used as an effective method to preserve the fertility of cancer patients after surgery, radiotherapy (RT), and chemotherapy (CT) procedures. Modern cancer treatments have improved survival rates. This has led to the desire to improve quality of life and preserve fertility. Sperm cells that are frozen and thawed have reduced motility, altered acrosome integrity, altered membrane structure, and increased DNA fragmentation. All these changes reduce the fertilization capacity of sperm. The success of pregnancy and live birth after intrauterine insemination (IUI) and conventional invitro fertilization (conventional IVF) procedures with these spermatozoa is low. Intracytoplasmic sperm injection (ICSI) is now routinely used. Even a single sperm cell is important in the ICSI procedure. This is because even a single sperm cell has the potential to fertilize the oocyte and cause pregnancy. ICSI using frozen thawed spermatozoa and ICSI using fresh spermatozoa have similar success in fertilization, pregnancy, and live birth. For all these reasons, sperm cryopreservation has become a successful method of routine use in IVF centers today.

Key Words: ART, IVF, Sperm cryopreservation, Cryoprotectant, Slow freezing, Vitrification, Thawing

---

* Corresponding Author's E-mail: berrinyangindogru@gmail.com

In: Holistic Approach to Assisted Reproductive Technology
Editor: Kenan Demir and Rümeysa Yılmaz Göç
ISBN: 979-8-89113-017-3
© 2023 Nova Science Publishers, Inc.

Introduction

Cryopreservation is a term made up of the words cold and preserve. Cryopreservation is a method that, unlike freezing, allows cells to be preserved at subzero temperatures, allowing them to be recycled and reused when necessary by thawing them without losing their viability. Thanks to this technique, male and female reproductive cells, embryos at various stages, and testicular and ovarian tissue can be preserved in tanks filled with liquid nitrogen at -196° C for years, preserving individual reproductive ability (Ferrari et al., 2016; Rienzi et al., 2017).

Male infertility can have primary or secondary causes. Causes of acquired infertility include autoimmune diseases that disrupt the blood-testicular barrier, such as diabetes mellitus, neurological diseases such as spinal injury of the medulla, testicular failure, ejaculatory dysfunction, severe malignancies such as testicular tumors, and surgical, radiotherapy (RT), chemotherapy (CT) procedures used to treat these diseases (Agarwal et al., 2014; Botchan et al., 2013; Ferrari et al., 2016; Pening et al., 2022).

Gonadal cells rapidly dividing are more adversely affected by chemotherapeutic agents and radiation therapy (Dohle, 2010; Ragheb & Sabanegh, 2010; Tournaye et al., 2014). In certain chromosomal diseases, azoospermia and infertility can occur later in life (Davila Garza & Patrizio, 2013). Spermatogenic serial cells obtained from such azoospermic patients by surgical methods such as testicular sperm extraction (TESE), percutaneous testicular sperm aspiration (PTSA), percutaneous epididymal sperm aspiration (PESA), and epididymal microsurgical sperm aspiration (MESA) can be cryopreserved. In this way, expensive and invasive procedures, such as biopsies, are avoided and patient fertility is preserved. Sperm obtained from obstructive and non-obstructive azoospermic patients by surgical methods is preserved by freezing (Di Santo et al., 2012; Donnelly et al., 2001). Lazaro Spallanzani first succeeded in preserving semen by freezing it in snow about two hundred years ago (Menezo et al., 1999). Sperm were then successfully frozen using glycerol to protect them from the harmful effects of ice crystals produced by conventional freezing by Polge et al. (1949). The use of thawed sperm after semen cryopreservation resulted in the first live birth, reported in a cow in 1951. The first live birth in humans was reported in 1953 (Stewart, 1951).

Successful sperm cryopreservation was achieved long before cryopreservation of oocytes and embryos (Hezavehei et al., 2018). With the use of liquid nitrogen in the following years, this technique developed rapidly and took its place in routine ART applications (Bunge & Sherman, 1953). Freeze-thawed sperm have been used in procedures such as intrauterine insemination (IUI), classical in vitro fertilization (IVF), and intracytoplasmic sperm injection (ICSI) (Dohle, 2010).

ICSI is preferred as the ART method because sperm quality is adversely affected to some extent after freeze-thaw protocols. There are no significant differences between pregnancy and live birth rates after ICSI with frozen sperm and fresh sperm (Verza & Esteves, 2004).

Indications for sperm freezing; In countries where it is legal, donor sperm can be frozen and stored in sperm banks. In addition, sperm samples can be frozen before treatments that are likely to affect fertility, and possible infertility of the patient can be tried to prevent. In ART procedures, frozen sperm can be used in patients who cannot obtain fresh sperm. Also, in patients who cannot give a sample on the day of the procedure due to psychological, etc. For these reasons, a sample can be taken and frozen before the procedure. Sperm can be frozen to minimize the risk of transmission of infections such as HIV and can be used to achieve pregnancy with ART methods (Sharma et al., 2015). Sperm can be frozen so that genetic diagnostic tests can be performed on sperm cells. Sperm that are difficult to obtain using surgical procedures such as TESE can be frozen. This avoids invasive procedure for the patient that can lead to frequent repetition of testicular fibrosis. Furthermore, each TESE procedure requires a team of specialists (operating room conditions, urologists and anesthesiologists, operating room nurses, embryologists, etc.) and is costly (Di Santo et al., 2012; Sharma et al., 2015; Sherman, 1973).

Cryoprotectants

Cryoprotectants are highly permeable substances with a low molecular weight. The working principle of cryoprotectants is to prevent the formation of glacial crystals by lowering the freezing point of the substance (Royere et al., 1996). Cryoprotectants are divided into permeable and nonpermeable. Permeable cryoprotectants are glycerol, propylene glycol, and dimethylsulfoxide. Non-permeable cryoprotectants, for that matter, are sucrose, raffinose, and glycine (Sieme et al., 2016). Permeable cryoprotectants stabilize the plasma membrane, while impermeable cryoprotectants minimize intracellular ice formation. They often enhance each other's effectiveness by being used together (Henry et al., 1993). Glycerol was the first cryoprotectant used (Polge et al., 1949). However, in human sperm cells, glycol is the cryoprotectant with the best results (Crabbe et al., 1999; Curry, 2000).

The motility, functionality, acrosome integrity, and viability of thawed spermatozoa after cryopreservation are significantly reduced. The biochemical mechanisms of cryopreservation and reduced sperm fertilization ability after thawing are still not fully understood (Hezavehei et al., 2018; Nijs et al., 2009; Ozkavukcu et al., 2008).

However, sperm cryopreservation is still the most effective and only method to preserve male fertility for many patients (Nijs et al., 2009; Ozkavukcu et al., 2008).

Due to the decrease in sperm vitality and motility after thawing, some substances had to be added. Different and more complex solutions containing many substances have been developed for this purpose. The most commonly used in humans; Glycerol egg yolk citrate (GEYC), human sperm preserving medium (HSPM) containing albumin and HEPES, N-tris methyl 2-amino ethane sulfonic acid (TES), tris hydroxymethyl amino methane (TRIS), the solution containing sodium citrate, glycerol, egg yolk (TESTCY), etc. (Fabozzi et al., 2016). Studies have shown that even after three repeated series of freeze-thaw protocols, viable, motile sperm counts sufficient for fertilization are still maintained (Bandularatne & Bongso, 2002).

Cryopreservation

There are currently two main ways of freezing male reproductive cells. Traditional slow freezing and vitrification, which is a fast method. Vitrification of sperm with liquid nitrogen is a fast, easy, and economical method. This method avoids the formation of intracellular ice crystals that cause damage (Tao et al., 2020). In many IVF Laboratories, sperm samples are frozen using fast- or slow-freezing techniques, while testicular tissue is frozen using a slow-freezing protocol (Agarwal & Tvrda, 2017).

Between 2012 and 2015, Reed et al. analyzed all frozen embryo transfers performed in their clinic. Vitrification has been found to show higher vitality and equal rates of implantation to pregnancy compared to traditional slow freezing (Reed et al., 2015). The slow freezing and vitrification of spermatozoa were compared by Ali Mohamed, and vitrification was shown to be less toxic, easier and economical (Ali Mohamed, 2015). Similarly, studies comparing vitrification with traditional slow freezing have shown that vitrification results in higher sperm vitality and motility after thawing (Vutyavanich et al., 2010; Zhou et al., 2021; Nawroth et al., 2002; Szczygiel et al., 2002; Centola et al., 1992; Cross & Hanks, 1991; Esteves et al., 1996; Moskovtsev et al., 2012; Pabon et al., 2019). In a meta-analysis of 2428 articles using vitrification and conventional slow freezing, sperm thawed after vitrification were analyzed for total motility, progressive motility, morphology and DNA fragmentation. It was concluded that rapid vitrification freezing was more successful in terms of motility than the traditional slow freezing method. There was no difference in DNA fragmentation. Similarly, testicular and epididymal sperm have been shown to have higher sperm vitality and motility (Li et al., 2019). Although the success of vitrification depends on the vitrification protocol, the choice of agents used, the sensitivity of the cell to freezing, the technical skill of the practitioner, the sperm count, motility, and quality of the sample, it is better than traditional slow freezing (Botchan et al., 2013; Ferrari et al., 2016; Li et al., 2019; Pening et al., 2022; Dupesh et al., 2018).

Spermatozoa vitrification is not as successful as embryo and oocyte vitrification. This is because the male gonadal cell has higher osmotic fragility (Gilmore et al., 1997). In contrast to oocyte and embryo vitrification, permeable cryoprotectants are not preferred for sperm vitrification. Because the hypertonic environment during the cryopreservation process may cause osmotic shock in the sperm and prevent tail movements by tail curling (O'Connell et al., 2002; Oldenhof et al., 2013; Schuster et al., 2003). Vitrification with nonpermeable cryoprotectant showed better sperm motility, less DNA fragmentation, and better mitochondrial membrane potential compared to conventional slow freezing (Aizpurua et al., 2017; Reed et al., 2015; Riva et al., 2018). Substances such as egg yolk and glycerol are added to cryoprotective solutions to reduce sperm osmotic stress (Anger et al., 2003; Tao et al., 2020). Some studies suggest that DNA fragmentation is slightly increased in frozen thawed sperm compared to fresh sperm and that embryo quality is slightly reduced as a result (Gosalvez et al., 2011). Frozen sperm samples can now be stored using a variety of apparatuses such as cryoloop, VitriSafe, cryopette, cryoLogic, cryostraws, and cryovials (Stein et al., 2015; Cohen et al., 1997; Herrler et al., 2006). There is a low risk of cross-contamination due to direct contact of the sperm with liquid nitrogen if the freezing apparatus used is an open system. The storage of sperm samples in liquid nitrogen vapor for approximately 3 months can be considered as an alternative method, as it prevents the risk of contamination (Sharma et al., 2015; Tao et al., 2020). To eliminate the risk of cross-contamination, high-security pipettes (HSV) can be used (Desai et al., 2012).

There are many different thawing protocols. To find the optimal thawing temperature, many researchers have conducted studies at different temperatures. All of these studies obtained similar results at different temperatures (room temperature, 37° C, 38° C, 40° C, 42° C, 44° C). This shows us that at an ideal temperature, the thawing procedure is flexible (Ali Mohamed, 2015; Le et al., 2019; Mansilla et al., 2016; Martinez-Soto et al., 2011; Sanchez et al., 2013). Once the sample has been rapidly vitrified, it must be rapidly heated again to thaw it without ice crystals forming inside. This prevents the formation of ice crystals (Li et al., 2019). When comparing vitrification with conventional 0.25 ml-0.5 ml and small-size micropipettes (50-100 μl), it was observed that sperm frozen using micropipettes had better motility after thawing. This has been attributed to faster vitrification due to the small volume (Liu et al., 2017).

On the contrary, some studies show that the cooling rate does not need to be very fast (Isachenko et al., 2004). In a study comparing a method in which the sample was kept at room temperature for 10 minutes and then heated at 37° C for 10 minutes with a method in which the sample was melted at 37° C for 20 minutes, it was observed that the number of fast linear motile sperm and sperm vitality were higher and DNA fragmentation rates were lower due to better glycerol dilution in the second method (Martinez-Soto et al., 2011).

In another study, liquid nitrogen was removed from the tank and the sample was kept at room temperature for about 5 minutes and then placed in 37° C water for 20 minutes for successful thawing (Verza & Esteves, 2004).

After thawing, spermatozoa are evaluated according to Kruger criteria and WHO procedural guidelines (Kruger et al., 1986; Labs et al., 2016; WHO, 1999).

There is still no clear view of the temperature and speed at which mammalian spermatozoa should be thawed (Malo et al., 2019; Verza & Esteves, 2004).

Cryopreservation Methods

There are two basic methods. Slow freezing and vitrification.

Conventional slow freezing can be done using manual or programmable freezers. With manual slow freezing, a 1:1 ratio of cryoprotectant is slowly added to the semen sample at room temperature after it has liquefied. The sample is then loaded into the freezing apparatus. It is first cooled from room temperature to 5° C at a rate of 0.5-1 ° C / min, then gradually cooled to -80° C at a rate of 1-10° C / min. Then the mixture was immersed in liquid nitrogen at -196° C. This can also be done using programmable freezers and takes about 2-4 hours in total (Di Santo et al., 2012; Said et al., 2010; Sharma et al., 2015). Rapid freezing was first introduced by Sherman in 1990 (Keel & Webster, 1990). The amount of sample to be frozen is determined prior to the procedure, and a sufficient freezing apparatus is prepared. The patient is informed about the freezing procedure. Written informed consent is obtained. The necessary forms are filled out. Information about the patient (name, surname, date of birth, T.R. identification number, file number, etc.), the name of the sample, the method of collection, the time of collection, the amount, sperm count, progression, vitality, the procedures performed (washing, gradient, etc.), the cryoprotectant used, the method to be applied and who performed the freezing process are written on these forms. After 3 days of sexual abstinence, the patient's identity information is checked and he or she is taken to the sperm donation room. The sample is collected by masturbation in a sterile container labeled with the patient's name according to the criteria of the World Health Organization (WHO). The quantity is measured (WHO, 1999).

A semen sample is allowed to liquefy at 37° C for 30 minutes. Viscous samples with slow liquefaction can be mechanically pipetted in and out. In this way, liquefaction is achieved. The cryoprotectant is heated in a laminar chamber at room temperature or 37° C for approximately 30 minutes. The liquefied semen sample can optionally be frozen raw or processed after sperm selection procedures such as washing, flotation, and density gradient. The sample and cryoprotectant are mixed very slowly dropwise in a 1:1 ratio (Depending on the cryoprotectant medium used, this ratio may vary as recommended by the manufacturer). Gently in and out with the pipette, taking care not to create air bubbles. It could take approximately 2 min. The mixture is allowed to rest for a while to stabilize. The sample is then loaded into various freezing apparatuses (cryostraw, cryovial, etc.) and sealed so that it does not come into contact with air. Care is taken to work under aseptic conditions and not to completely fill containers (Verza & Esteves, 2004). Information such as the patient's name and surname, date of birth, date the sample was frozen, and patient file number is written on the freezing apparatus or labels with an indelible pen. In the freezer, the sperm sample is first treated with liquid nitrogen vapor for approximately 15 minutes. It is then suspended about 15-20 cm from liquid nitrogen in the tank at -80° C and then quickly immersed in liquid nitrogen at -196° C (Figure 23.1). If a cryostraw is used as a loading device, it should be preferred to place it horizontally on a floating foam pallet in a foam box filled with liquid nitrogen instead of hanging it in the tank so that the liquid nitrogen vapor reaches every point equally (Figure 23.2). The cryostraw or cryovial loaded sample is carefully placed in its prelocalized location in the preservation tank using metal clamps and protective gloves; maximum care and diligence must be taken to avoid confusion in all these transactions due to legal liability (Di Santo et al., 2012; Schuster et al., 2003; Sharma et al., 2015; Irvine Scientific, n.d.).

Vitrification is also possible without the use of cryoprotectants. The sample is washed and prepared using the swim-up method after the sample is liquefied. It is loaded into a freezing apparatus and quickly immersed in liquid nitrogen at -196° C. In this way, the cytotoxic effect of cryoprotectants on sperm is avoided (Di Santo et al., 2012; Nawroth et al., 2002; Sharma et al., 2015). To maximize the efficiency of cryopreservation, studies suggest the use of techniques such as density gradient and flotation before freezing or after thawing (Chan et al., 2006). However, some studies recommend freezing the semen sample without any treatment, such as washing, swimming, and

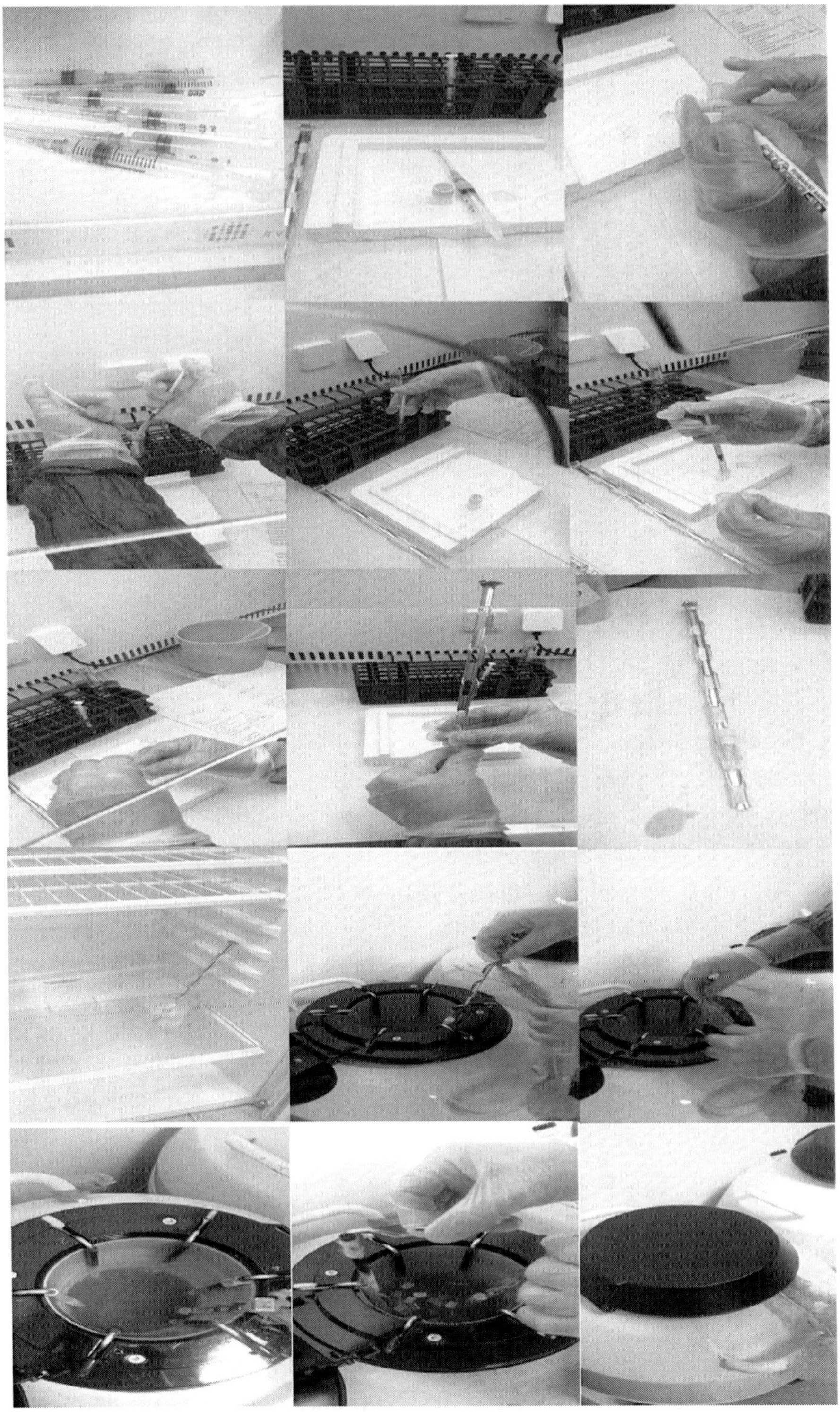

Figure 23.1 Sample freezing with Cryovial. (Pictures are taken from our own laboratory archive.)

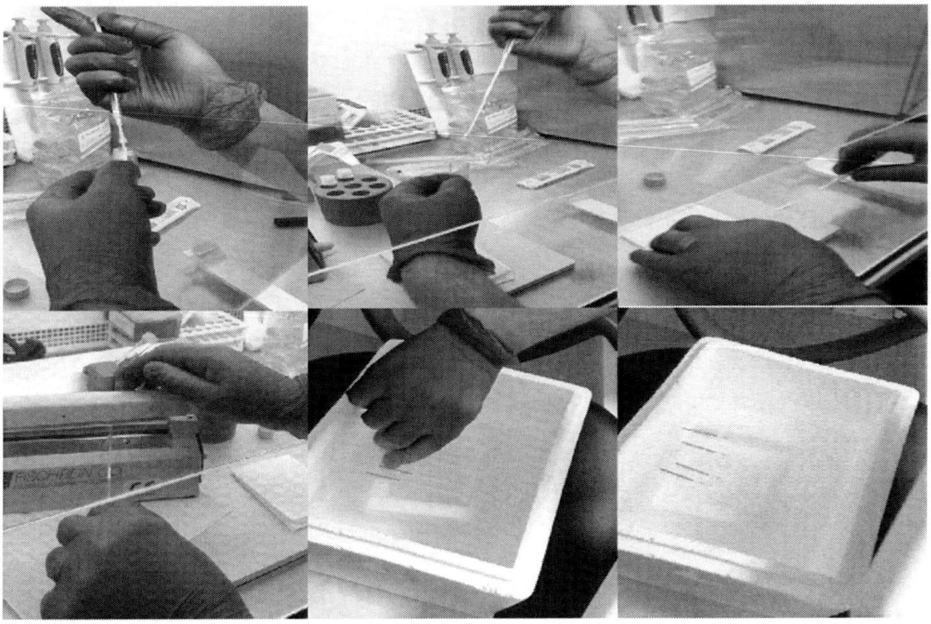

Figure 23.2 Sample freezing with Cryostraw. (Pictures are taken from our own laboratory archive.)

density gradient. In these studies, direct freezing and thawing of untreated semen resulted in less exposure of sperm to cryosurgery and less DNA fragmentation. The presence of antioxidants in semen has been attributed to this situation (Brotherton, 1990; Jang et al., 2017).

Thawing protocol

While there is no established protocol, the method preferred by many laboratories is as follows.

The patient is informed about the thawing of the sample and informed written consent is obtained. The forms are filled in. The frozen sample is removed from the storage tank filled with liquid nitrogen after the records are checked. The cryovial or cryostraw is kept at room temperature for about 15 minutes. Meanwhile, 2x15 ml of conical bottom sterile tubes with the patient's name and information written on them are prepared in a laminar cabinet. If the sample was frozen without the use of sperm selection techniques (flotation, density gradient, etc.), a gradient is used after thawing. Different concentrations of gradient solution (1.5-2mL) preheated at 37° C are carefully poured into a conical bottom tube. This should be done very slowly and in a way that creates a level. The freezer loader apparatus is dried and opened in the laminar cabinet. Using a sterile pipette, 1 ml of the sample is carefully added to the conical tube. It is centrifuged (300 xg) for about 15 min. Centrifugation speed and duration may vary according to the quality of the sperm. Working aseptically with a clean pipette, the upper portion is discarded and the lower 0.5 ml pellet is resuspended with sperm wash solution and collected (Figure 23.3). This washing process is repeated twice.

If the sample has been frozen using sperm selection techniques (such as density gradient), the sample is thawed and poured into a 15 ml conical bottom tube. It is slowly and carefully mixed with the sperm wash solution that was previously warmed at room temperature. It is centrifuged (300 xg) for 10 min. The top side is discarded with a sterile pipette. The 0.5ml pellet is resuspended

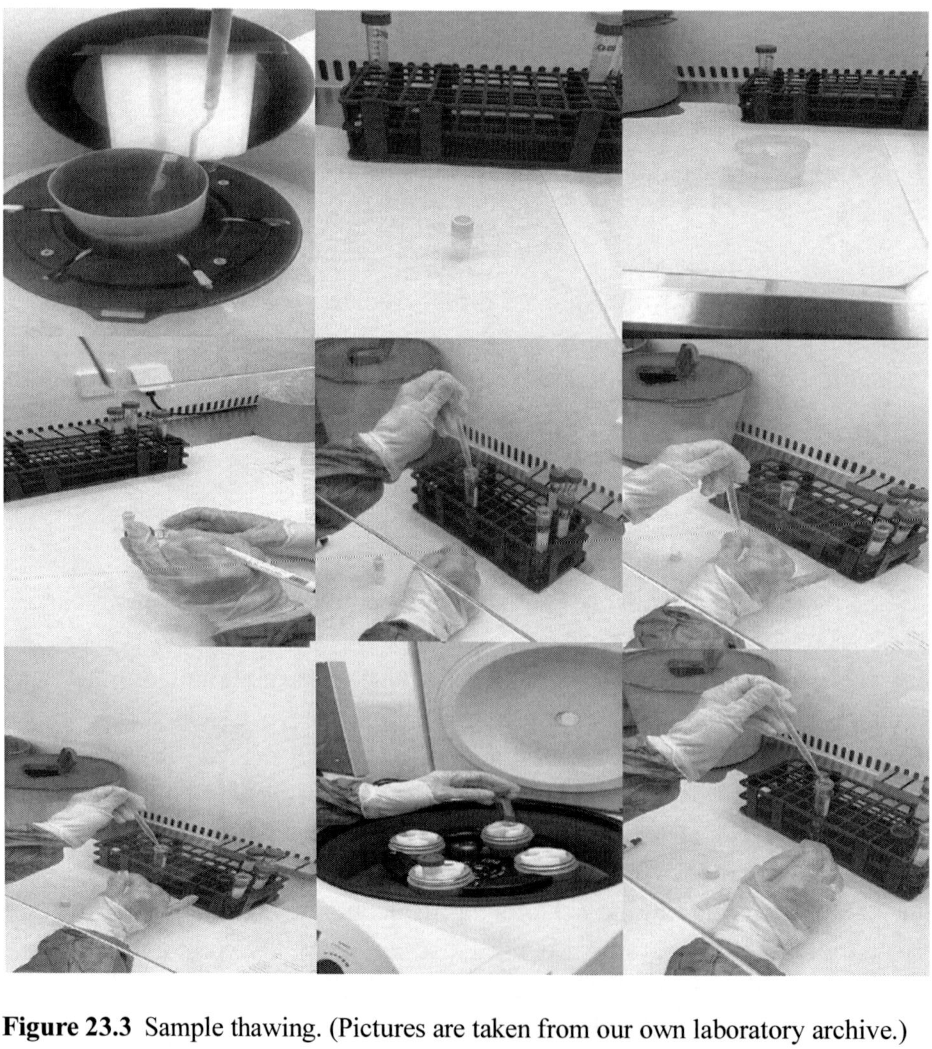

Figure 23.3 Sample thawing. (Pictures are taken from our own laboratory archive.)

with sperm wash solution, collected, and used in the desired ART technique (Irvine Scientific, n.d.).

Freezing a very small number of spermatozoa that are difficult to obtain:

The routine use of ICSI in IVF centers has increased the importance and usability of the small number of sperm obtained from patients with oligozoospermia, since pregnancy can be achieved even with a single sperm (Liu et al., 2020; Ohashi et al., 2001; Shibahara et al., 1999). TESE is invasive and expensive. The patient's tissue samples should be separated from erythrocytes and similar cells that do not belong to the spermatogenic series and free oxygen radicals. For this purpose, the sample was treated with a buffered culture solution such as HEPES in a laminar cabinet. The seminiferous tubules are dissected using an insulin syringe with the needle at a 90-degree angle on the stereomicroscope, and the spermatogenic series cells are separated from the tissue. If necessary, enzymes such as trypsin/DNase and type 1 collagenase can be added to the solution to lyse the tissue. The tissue and cells released are collected with a pipette and mixed by vortexing for approximately 30 seconds. It is incubated in an incubator with 5% CO_2 for about 60 min. After incubation, the sample was centrifuged in conical bottom tubes, washed, and examined in detail under an inverted microscope. Live sperm found are used in fresh cycles or frozen and stored for later use (Javed et al., 2019; van Wely et al., 2015; Yu et al., 2018). The sample obtained after TESE can be frozen with the sperm freezing protocol by washing and gradient study. It is not an easy process to find, freeze, and thaw these few, precious sperm, and then find them again. In recent years, numerous methods have been tried to ensure that these few spermatozoa can be safely frozen and easily found and used after thawing. For this, the researchers used the zona pellucida left behind after the oocyte was evacuated with a microinjection needle. Insertion of a small number of spermatozoa in the zona pellucida and freezing with the oocyte freezing protocol. Therefore, it is easier to find sperm after thawing. Since these spermatozoa are not in direct contact with the cryoprotectant solution, their motility is not reduced and DNA fragmentation is not observed. (Cohen et al., 1997; Walmsley et al., 1998; Ye et al., 2009). However, this procedure was not preferred due to its technical difficulty and the need for zona pellucida, a biological material, and alternative methods were sought. A small number of sperm cells are stored in microdroplets and frozen. Cryopreserved using agarase capsules or microdrops of arginic acid (Craft & Tsirigotis, 1995; Gil-Salom et al., 2000; Hatakeyama et al., 2017; Herrler et al., 2006). There are also studies in which a small number of sperm collected with an ICSI pipette were filled into volvox globator spheres, which were frozen with a classical sperm freezing protocol (Just et al., 2004). An alternative method is to freeze a small number of sperm using cryotop or cryoloop. But there is a risk of contamination as these sperm come into direct contact with liquid nitrogen (Chen et al., 2015; Endo et al., 2012; F. Nawroth et al., 2002; Schuster et al., 2003).

Conclusion

Today, sperm cryopreservation procedures are successfully applied. It has entered routine use in donor sperm banks, IVF centers, and ART Techniques. The surgically obtained spermatozoa can be safely stored thanks to cryopreservation. In this way, repeated expensive and invasive procedures can be avoided. Furthermore, for many patients at risk for infertility due to various autoimmune diseases, and malignancies and their treatment (oncosurgery, RT, CT, varicocele, etc.), sperm is an effective fertility preservation method. To date, many different freeze-thaw protocols have been used for sperm cryopreservation. Each laboratory has its own practices based on its own familiarity, experience, and practice. In addition, in most laboratories, slow freezing is replaced by rapid vitrification. Freezing, thawing, and easy availability of very small numbers of sperm after thawing are difficult and require separate technical equipment. Many methods have been tried for this in recent years. Although the quality of sperm can be adversely affected to some extent after freezing and thawing protocols, this can be ignored when ICSI is preferred over IUI and classical IVF as ART methods. Similar pregnancy and live birth rates were obtained after ICSI with frozen and thawed sperm and fresh sperm. The effects of cryopreservation on sperm DNA are still not fully understood. But for many patients, sperm cryopreservation remains the only way to preserve fertility. Studies continue to be conducted to find the most appropriate, practical, and successful protocol (cryoprotectant, freezing loading device, freezing thaw temperature, and time) for sperm cryopreservation.

References

Agarwal, A., Durairajanayagam, D., & du Plessis, S. S. (2014). Utility of antioxidants during assisted reproductive techniques: an evidence based review. *Reproductive Biology and Endocrinology, 12*. https://doi.org/Artn/11210.1186/1477-7827-12-112

Agarwal, A., & Tvrda, E. (2017). Chapter 5 Slow Freezing of Human Sperm. *Methods Mol Biol, 1568*, 67-78. https://doi.org/10.1007/978-1-4939-6828-2_5

Aizpurua, J., Medrano, L., Enciso, M., Sarasa, J., Romero, A., Fernandez, M. A., & Gomez-Torres, M. J. (2017). New permeable cryoprotectant-free vitrification method for native human sperm. *Human Reproduction*, *32*(10), 2007-2015. https://doi.org/10.1093/humrep/dex281

Ali Mohamed, M. S. (2015). Slow cryopreservation is not superior to vitrification in human spermatozoa; an experimental controlled study. *Iran J Reprod Med*, *13*(10), 633-644. https://www.ncbi.nlm.nih.gov/pubmed/26644792

Anger, J. T., Gilbert, B. R., & Goldstein, M. (2003). Cryopreservation of sperm: indications, methods and results. *J Urol*, *170*(4 Pt 1), 1079-1084. https://doi.org/10.1097/01.ju.0000084820.98430.b8

Bandularatne, E., & Bongso, A. (2002). Evaluation of human sperm function after repeated freezing and thawing. *J Androl*, *23*(2), 242-249. https://www.ncbi.nlm.nih.gov/pubmed/11868818

Botchan, A., Karpol, S., Lehavi, O., Paz, G., Kleiman, S. E., Yogev, L., Yavetz, H., & Hauser, R. (2013). Preservation of sperm of cancer patients: extent of use and pregnancy outcome in a tertiary infertility center. *Asian J Androl*, *15*(3), 382-386. https://doi.org/10.1038/aja.2013.3

Brotherton, J. (1990). Cryopreservation of human semen. *Arch Androl*, *25*(2), 181-195. https://doi.org/10.3109/01485019008987609

Bunge, R. G., & Sherman, J. K. (1953). Fertilizing capacity of frozen human spermatozoa. *Nature*, *172*(4382), 767-768. https://doi.org/10.1038/172767b0

Centola, G. M., Raubertas, R. F., & Mattox, J. H. (1992). Cryopreservation of human semen. Comparison of cryopreservatives, sources of variability, and prediction of post-thaw survival. *J Androl*, *13*(3), 283-288. https://www.ncbi.nlm.nih.gov/pubmed/1601749

Chan, P. J., Jacobson, J. D., Corselli, J. U., & Patton, W. C. (2006). A simple zeta method for sperm selection based on membrane charge. *Fertil Steril*, *85*(2), 481-486. https://doi.org/10.1016/j.fertnstert.2005.07.1302

Chen, Y., Li, L., Qian, Y., Xu, C., Zhu, Y., Huang, H., Jin, F., & Ye, Y. (2015). Small-volume vitrification for human spermatozoa in the absence of cryoprotectants by using Cryotop. *Andrologia*, *47*(6), 694-699. https://doi.org/10.1111/and.12320

Cohen, J., Garrisi, G. J., Congedo-Ferrara, T. A., Kieck, K. A., Schimmel, T. W., & Scott, R. T. (1997). Cryopreservation of single human spermatozoa. *Human Reproduction*, *12*(5), 994-1001. https://doi.org/10.1093/humrep/12.5.994

Crabbe, E., Verheyen, G., Tournaye, H., & Van Steirteghem, A. (1999). Freezing of testicular tissue as a minced suspension preserves sperm quality better than whole-biopsy freezing when glycerol is used as cryoprotectant. *Int J Androl*, *22*(1), 43-48. https://doi.org/10.1046/j.1365-2605.1999.00149.x

Craft, I., & Tsirigotis, M. (1995). Simplified recovery, preparation and cryopreservation of testicular spermatozoa. *Human Reproduction*, *10*(7), 1623-1626. https://doi.org/10.1093/oxfordjournals.humrep.a136142

Cross, N. L., & Hanks, S. E. (1991). Effects of cryopreservation on human sperm acrosomes. *Human Reproduction*, *6*(9), 1279-1283. https://doi.org/10.1093/oxfordjournals.humrep.a137526

Curry, M. R. (2000). Cryopreservation of semen from domestic livestock. *Rev Reprod*, *5*(1), 46-52. https://doi.org/10.1530/ror.0.0050046

Davila Garza, S. A., & Patrizio, P. (2013). Reproductive outcomes in patients with male infertility because of Klinefelter's syndrome, Kartagener's syndrome, round-head sperm, dysplasia fibrous sheath, and 'stump' tail sperm: an updated literature review. *Curr Opin Obstet Gynecol*, *25*(3), 229-246. https://doi.org/10.1097/GCO.0b013e32835faae5

Desai, N., Goldberg, J., Austin, C., Sabanegh, E., & Falcone, T. (2012). Cryopreservation of individually selected sperm: methodology and case report of a clinical pregnancy. *J Assist Reprod Genet*, *29*(5), 375-379. https://doi.org/10.1007/s10815-012-9733-y

Di Santo, M., Tarozzi, N., Nadalini, M., & Borini, A. (2012). Human Sperm Cryopreservation: Update on Techniques, Effect on DNA Integrity, and Implications for ART. *Adv Urol*, *2012*, 854837. https://doi.org/10.1155/2012/854837

Dohle, G. R. (2010). Male infertility in cancer patients: Review of the literature. *Int J Urol*, *17*(4), 327-331. https://doi.org/10.1111/j.1442-2042.2010.02484.x

Donnelly, E. T., McClure, N., & Lewis, S. E. (2001). Cryopreservation of human semen and prepared sperm: effects on motility parameters and DNA integrity. *Fertil Steril*, *76*(5), 892-900. https://doi.org/10.1016/s0015-0282(01)02834-5

Dupesh, S., Rasappan, P., Shila, S., & Gunasekaran, K. (2018). Human Sperm Freezing: Mini Update. *Advances in Reproductive Sciences*, *6*(3), 59-69.

Endo, Y., Fujii, Y., Kurotsuchi, S., Motoyama, H., & Funahashi, H. (2012). Successful delivery derived from vitrified-warmed spermatozoa from a patient with nonobstructive azoospermia. *Fertil Steril*, *98*(6), 1423-1427. https://doi.org/10.1016/j.fertnstert.2012.07.1128

Esteves, S. C., Sharma, R. K., Thomas, A. J., Jr., & Agarwal, A. (1996). Suitability of the hypo-osmotic swelling test for assessing the viability of cryopreserved sperm. *Fertil Steril*, *66*(5), 798-804. https://www.ncbi.nlm.nih.gov/pubmed/8893688

Fabozzi, G., Starita, M. F., Rega, E., Alteri, A., Colicchia, A., Piscitelli, C., & Giannini, P. (2016). Evaluation of the Efficiency of Two Different Freezing Media and Two Different Protocols to Preserve Human Spermatozoa from Cryoinjury. *Int J Reprod Med*, *2016*, 6059757. https://doi.org/10.1155/2016/6059757

Ferrari, S., Paffoni, A., Filippi, F., Busnelli, A., Vegetti, W., & Somigliana, E. (2016). Sperm cryopreservation and reproductive outcome in male cancer patients: a systematic review. *Reprod Biomed Online*, *33*(1), 29-38. https://doi.org/10.1016/j.rbmo.2016.04.002

Gil-Salom, M., Romero, J., Rubio, C., Ruiz, A., Remohi, J., & Pellicer, A. (2000). Intracytoplasmic sperm injection with cryopreserved testicular spermatozoa. *Mol Cell Endocrinol*, *169*(1-2), 15-19. https://doi.org/10.1016/s0303-7207(00)00345-2

Gilmore, J. A., Liu, J., Gao, D. Y., & Critser, J. K. (1997). Determination of optimal cryoprotectants and procedures for their addition and removal from human spermatozoa. *Human Reproduction*, *12*(1), 112-118. https://doi.org/10.1093/humrep/12.1.112

Gosalvez, J., Nunez, R., Fernandez, J. L., Lopez-Fernandez, C., & Caballero, P. (2011). Dynamics of sperm DNA damage in fresh versus frozen-thawed and gradient processed ejaculates in human donors. *Andrologia*, *43*(6), 373-377. https://doi.org/10.1111/j.1439-0272.2010.01022.x

Hatakeyama, S., Tokuoka, S., Abe, H., Araki, Y., & Araki, Y. (2017). Cryopreservation of very low numbers of spermatozoa from male patients undergoing infertility treatment using agarose capsules. *Hum Cell*, *30*(3), 201-208. https://doi.org/10.1007/s13577-017-0166-x

Henry, M. A., Noiles, E. E., Gao, D., Mazur, P., & Critser, J. K. (1993). Cryopreservation of human spermatozoa. IV. The effects of cooling rate and warming rate on the maintenance of motility, plasma membrane integrity, and mitochondrial function. *Fertil Steril*, *60*(5), 911-918. https://www.ncbi.nlm.nih.gov/pubmed/8224279

Herrler, A., Eisner, S., Bach, V., Weissenborn, U., & Beier, H. M. (2006). Cryopreservation of spermatozoa in alginic acid capsules. *Fertil Steril*, *85*(1), 208-213. https://doi.org/10.1016/j.fertnstert.2005.06.049

Hezavehei, M., Sharafi, M., Kouchesfahani, H. M., Henkel, R., Agarwal, A., Esmaeili, V., & Shahverdi, A. (2018). Sperm cryopreservation: A review on current molecular cryobiology and advanced approaches. *Reprod Biomed Online*, *37*(3), 327-339. https://doi.org/10.1016/j.rbmo.2018.05.012

Irvine Scientific (n.d.). *Semen and Sperm Freezing Protocol*. Retrieved from. https://irvinescientific-art-eu.fujifilm.com/images/download/fujifilm-irvine-scientific/protocols/002126_Sperm_Freezing_Protocol.pdf

Isachenko, V., Isachenko, E., Katkov, II, Montag, M., Dessole, S., Nawroth, F., & Van Der Ven, H. (2004). Cryoprotectant-free cryopreservation of human spermatozoa by vitrification and freezing in vapor: effect on motility, DNA integrity, and fertilization ability. *Biol Reprod*, *71*(4), 1167-1173. https://doi.org/10.1095/biolreprod.104.028811

Jang, T. H., Park, S. C., Yang, J. H., Kim, J. Y., Seok, J. H., Park, U. S., Choi, C. W., Lee, S. R., & Han, J. (2017). Cryopreservation and its clinical applications. *Integr Med Res*, *6*(1), 12-18. https://doi.org/10.1016/j.imr.2016.12.001

Javed, A., Ramaiah, M. K., & Talkad, M. S. (2019). ICSI using fresh and frozen PESA-TESA spermatozoa to examine assisted reproductive outcome retrospectively. *Obstet Gynecol Sci*, *62*(6), 429-437. https://doi.org/10.5468/ogs.2019.62.6.429

Just, A., Gruber, I., Wober, M., Lahodny, J., Obruca, A., & Strohmer, H. (2004). Novel method for the cryopreservation of testicular sperm and ejaculated spermatozoa from patients with severe oligospermia: a pilot study. *Fertil Steril*, *82*(2), 445-447. https://doi.org/10.1016/j.fertnstert.2003.12.050

Keel, B. A., & Webster, B. W. (1990). CRC handbook of the laboratory diagnosis and treatment of infertility.

Kruger, T. F., Menkveld, R., Stander, F. S., Lombard, C. J., Van der Merwe, J. P., van Zyl, J. A., & Smith, K. (1986). Sperm morphologic features as a prognostic factor in in vitro fertilization. *Fertil Steril*, *46*(6), 1118-1123. https://doi.org/10.1016/s0015-0282(16)49891-2

Labs, E. G. G. o. G. P. i. I., De los Santos, M. J., Apter, S., Coticchio, G., Debrock, S., Lundin, K., Plancha, C. E., Prados, F., Rienzi, L., Verheyen, G., Woodward, B., & Vermeulen, N. (2016). Revised guidelines for good practice in IVF laboratories (2015). *Human Reproduction*, *31*(4), 685-686. https://doi.org/10.1093/humrep/dew016

Le, M. T., Nguyen, T. T. T., Nguyen, T. T., Nguyen, V. T., Nguyen, T. T. A., Nguyen, V. Q. H., & Cao, N. T. (2019). Cryopreservation of human spermatozoa by vitrification versus conventional rapid freezing: Effects on motility, viability, morphology and cellular defects. *Eur J Obstet Gynecol Reprod Biol*, *234*, 14-20. https://doi.org/10.1016/j.ejogrb.2019.01.001

Li, Y. X., Zhou, L., Lv, M. Q., Ge, P., Liu, Y. C., & Zhou, D. X. (2019). Vitrification and conventional freezing methods in sperm cryopreservation: A systematic review and meta-analysis. *Eur J Obstet Gynecol Reprod Biol*, *233*, 84-92. https://doi.org/10.1016/j.ejogrb.2018.11.028

Liu, F., Zou, S. S., Zhu, Y., Sun, C., Liu, Y. F., Wang, S. S., Shi, W. B., Zhu, J. J., Huang, Y. H., & Li, Z. (2017). A novel micro-straw for cryopreservation of small number of human spermatozoon. *Asian J Androl*, *19*(3), 326-329. https://doi.org/10.4103/1008-682X.173452

Liu, H., Xie, Y., Gao, L., Sun, X., Liang, X., Deng, C., Gao, Y., & Liu, G. (2020). Impact on using cryopreservation of testicular or epididymal sperm upon intracytoplasmic sperm injection outcome in men with obstructive azoospermia: a systematic review and meta-analysis. *J Assist Reprod Genet*, *37*(11), 2643-2651. https://doi.org/10.1007/s10815-020-01940-1

Malo, C., Elwing, B., Soederstroem, L., Lundeheim, N., Morrell, J. M., & Skidmore, J. A. (2019). Effect of different freezing rates and thawing temperatures on cryosurvival of dromedary camel spermatozoa. *Theriogenology*, *125*, 43-48. https://doi.org/10.1016/j.theriogenology.2018.07.037

Mansilla, M. A., Merino, O., Risopatron, J., Isachenko, V., Isachenko, E., & Sanchez, R. (2016). High temperature is essential for preserved human sperm function during the devitrification process. *Andrologia*, *48*(1), 111-113. https://doi.org/10.1111/and.12406

Martinez-Soto, J. C., Garcia-Vazquez, F. A., Gumbao, D., Landeras, J., & Gadea, J. (2011). Assessment of two thawing processes of cryopreserved human sperm in pellets. *Cryobiology*, *63*(3), 131-136. https://doi.org/10.1016/j.cryobiol.2011.08.001

Menezo, Y. J., Chouteau, J., Torello, J., Girard, A., & Veiga, A. (1999). Birth weight and sex ratio after transfer at the blastocyst stage in humans. *Fertil Steril*, *72*(2), 221-224. https://doi.org/10.1016/s0015-0282(99)00256-3

Moskovtsev, S., Lulat, A. G.-M. I., & Librach, C. L. (2012). Cryopreservation of Human Spermatozoa by Vitrification vs. Slow Freezing: Canadian Experience.

Nawroth, F., Isachenko, V., Dessole, S., Rahimi, G., Farina, M., Vargiu, N., Mallmann, P., Dattena, M., Capobianco, G., & Peters, D. (2002). Vitrification of human spermatozoa without cryoprotectants. *CryoLetters*, *23*(2), 93-102.

Nijs, M., Creemers, E., Cox, A., Janssen, M., Vanheusden, E., Castro-Sanchez, Y., Thijs, H., & Ombelet, W. (2009). Influence of freeze-thawing on hyaluronic acid binding of human spermatozoa. *Reprod Biomed Online*, *19*(2), 202-206. https://doi.org/10.1016/s1472-6483(10)60073-9

O'Connell, M., McClure, N., & Lewis, S. E. (2002). The effects of cryopreservation on sperm morphology, motility and mitochondrial function. *Human Reproduction*, *17*(3), 704-709. https://doi.org/10.1093/humrep/17.3.704

Ohashi, Y., Miharu, N., Honda, H., Samura, O., & Ohama, K. (2001). High frequency of XY disomy in spermatozoa of severe oligozoospermic men. *Human Reproduction*, *16*(4), 703-708. https://doi.org/10.1093/humrep/16.4.703

Oldenhof, H., Gojowsky, M., Wang, S., Henke, S., Yu, C., Rohn, K., Wolkers, W. F., & Sieme, H. (2013). Osmotic stress and membrane phase changes during freezing of stallion sperm: mode of action of cryoprotective agents. *Biol Reprod*, *88*(3), 68. https://doi.org/10.1095/biolreprod.112.104661

Ozkavukcu, S., Erdemli, E., Isik, A., Oztuna, D., & Karahuseyinoglu, S. (2008). Effects of cryopreservation on sperm parameters and ultrastructural morphology of human spermatozoa. *J Assist Reprod Genet*, *25*(8), 403-411. https://doi.org/10.1007/s10815-008-9232-3

Pabon, D., Meseguer, M., Sevillano, G., Cobo, A., Romero, J. L., Remohi, J., & de Los Santos, M. J. (2019). A new system of sperm cryopreservation: evaluation of survival, motility, DNA oxidation, and mitochondrial activity. *Andrology*, *7*(3), 293-301. https://doi.org/10.1111/andr.12607

Pening, D., Constant, M., Bruynbroeck, M., Delbaere, A., & Demeestere, I. (2022). Impact of cancer on cryopreserved sperm quality and fertility: A cohort study. *Health Sci Rep*, *5*(4), e726. https://doi.org/10.1002/hsr2.726

Polge, C., Smith, A. U., & Parkes, A. S. (1949). Revival of spermatozoa after vitrification and dehydration at low temperatures. *Nature*, *164*(4172), 666. https://doi.org/10.1038/164666a0

Ragheb, A. M., & Sabanegh, E. S., Jr. (2010). Male fertility-implications of anticancer treatment and strategies to mitigate gonadotoxicity. *Anticancer Agents Med Chem*, *10*(1), 92-102. https://doi.org/10.2174/1871520611009010092

Reed, M. L., Said, A. H., Thompson, D. J., & Caperton, C. L. (2015). Large-volume vitrification of human biopsied and non-biopsied blastocysts: a simple, robust technique for cryopreservation. *J Assist Reprod Genet*, *32*(2), 207-214. https://doi.org/10.1007/s10815-014-0395-9

Rienzi, L., Gracia, C., Maggiulli, R., LaBarbera, A. R., Kaser, D. J., Ubaldi, F. M., Vanderpoel, S., & Racowsky, C. (2017). Oocyte, embryo and blastocyst cryopreservation in ART: systematic review and meta-analysis comparing slow-freezing versus vitrification to produce evidence for the development of global guidance. *Hum Reprod Update*, *23*(2), 139-155. https://doi.org/10.1093/humupd/dmw038

Riva, N. S., Ruhlmann, C., Iaizzo, R. S., Marcial Lopez, C. A., & Martinez, A. G. (2018). Comparative analysis between slow freezing and ultra-rapid freezing for human sperm cryopreservation. *JBRA Assist Reprod*, *22*(4), 331-337. https://doi.org/10.5935/1518-0557.20180060

Royere, D., Barthelemy, C., Hamamah, S., & Lansac, J. (1996). Cryopreservation of spermatozoa: a 1996 review. *Hum Reprod Update*, *2*(6), 553-559. https://doi.org/10.1093/humupd/2.6.553

Said, T. M., Gaglani, A., & Agarwal, A. (2010). Implication of apoptosis in sperm cryoinjury. *Reprod Biomed Online*, *21*(4), 456-462. https://doi.org/10.1016/j.rbmo.2010.05.011

Sanchez, R., Fontecilla, J., Isachenko, E., Mora, B., Isachenko, V., & Cabrillana, M. E. (2013). Temperatures in the Devitrification Process Is Essential for Preserved Morphological Membrane Integrity and Sperm Function in Human Spermatozoon. *Fertility and Sterility*, *100*(3), S183-S183. https://doi.org/DOI 10.1016/j.fertnstert.2013.07.1433

Schuster, T. G., Keller, L. M., Dunn, R. L., Ohl, D. A., & Smith, G. D. (2003). Ultra-rapid freezing of very low numbers of sperm using cryoloops. *Human Reproduction*, *18*(4), 788-795. https://doi.org/10.1093/humrep/deg162

Sharma, R., Kattoor, A. J., Ghulmiyyah, J., & Agarwal, A. (2015). Effect of sperm storage and selection techniques on sperm parameters. *Syst Biol Reprod Med*, *61*(1), 1-12. https://doi.org/10.3109/19396368.2014.976720

Sherman, J. K. (1973). Synopsis of the use of frozen human semen since 1964: state of the art of human semen banking. *Fertil Steril*, *24*(5), 397-412. https://doi.org/10.1016/s0015-0282(16)39678-9

Shibahara, H., Hamada, Y., Hasegawa, A., Toji, H., Shigeta, M., Yoshimoto, T., Shima, H., & Koyama, K. (1999). Correlation between the motility of frozen-thawed epididymal spermatozoa and the outcome of intracytoplasmic sperm injection. *Int J Androl*, *22*(5), 324-328. https://doi.org/10.1046/j.1365-2605.1999.00187.x

Sieme, H., Oldenhof, H., & Wolkers, W. F. (2016). Mode of action of cryoprotectants for sperm preservation. *Anim Reprod Sci*, *169*, 2-5. https://doi.org/10.1016/j.anireprosci.2016.02.004

Stein, A., Shufaro, Y., Hadar, S., Fisch, B., & Pinkas, H. (2015). Successful use of the Cryolock device for cryopreservation of scarce human ejaculate and testicular spermatozoa. *Andrology*, *3*(2), 220-224. https://doi.org/10.1111/andr.12007

Stewart, D. (1951). Storage of bull spermatozoa at low temperature. *Vet Rec*, *63*, 65-66.

Szczygiel, M. A., Kusakabe, H., Yanagimachi, R., & Whittingham, D. G. (2002). Intracytoplasmic sperm injection is more efficient than in vitro fertilization for generating mouse embryos from cryopreserved spermatozoa. *Biol Reprod*, *67*(4), 1278-1284. https://doi.org/10.1095/biolreprod67.4.1278

Tao, Y., Sanger, E., Saewu, A., & Leveille, M. C. (2020). Human sperm vitrification: the state of the art. *Reprod Biol Endocrinol*, *18*(1), 17. https://doi.org/10.1186/s12958-020-00580-5

Tournaye, H., Dohle, G. R., & Barratt, C. L. (2014). Fertility preservation in men with cancer. *Lancet*, *384*(9950), 1295-1301. https://doi.org/10.1016/S0140-6736(14)60495-5

van Wely, M., Barbey, N., Meissner, A., Repping, S., & Silber, S. J. (2015). Live birth rates after MESA or TESE in men with obstructive azoospermia: is there a difference? *Human Reproduction*, *30*(4), 761-766. https://doi.org/10.1093/humrep/dev032

Verza, S., Jr., & Esteves, S. C. (2004). Feasibility of refreezing human spermatozoa through the technique of liquid nitrogen vapor. *Int Braz J Urol*, *30*(6), 487-493. https://doi.org/10.1590/s1677-55382004000600006

Vutyavanich, T., Piromlertamorn, W., & Nunta, S. (2010). Rapid freezing versus slow programmable freezing of human spermatozoa. *Fertil Steril*, *93*(6), 1921-1928. https://doi.org/10.1016/j.fertnstert.2008.04.076

Walmsley, R., Cohen, J., Ferrara-Congedo, T., Reing, A., & Garrisi, J. (1998). The first births and ongoing pregnancies associated with sperm cryopreservation within evacuated egg zonae. *Human Reproduction*, *13 Suppl 4*, 61-70. https://doi.org/10.1093/humrep/13.suppl_4.61

WHO (1999). *WHO laboratory manual for the examination of human semen and sperm-cervical mucus interaction*. Cambridge university press.

Ye, Y., Xu, C., Qian, Y., Jin, F., & Huang, H. (2009). Evaluation of human sperm function after being cryopreserved within the zona pellucida. *Fertil Steril*, *92*(3), 1002-1008. https://doi.org/10.1016/j.fertnstert.2008.07.1737

Yu, G., Liu, Y., Zhang, H., & Wu, K. (2018). Application of testicular spermatozoa cryopreservation in assisted reproduction. *Int J Gynaecol Obstet*, *142*(3), 354-358. https://doi.org/10.1002/ijgo.12537

Zhou, D., Wang, X. M., Li, R. X., Wang, Y. Z., Chao, Y. C., Liu, Z. Z., Huang, Z. H., Nie, H. C., Zhu, W. B., Tan, Y. Q., & Fan, L. Q. (2021). Improving native human sperm freezing protection by using a modified vitrification method. *Asian J Androl*, *23*(1), 91-96. https://doi.org/10.4103/aja.aja_29_20

Chapter 24

Embryo Transfer

Aysın Pınar Türkmen, MD*
Department of Histology and Embryology, Faculty of Medicine, Ondokuz Mayıs University, Samsun, Turkiye

Abstract

Studies conducted since 1972 have focused on the quality of transferred embryos. The quality, number, and morphological stage of embryos, single good-quality blastocyst transfers, and frozen embryo transfers came to the fore. It is possible to reveal the superiority of the embryo's variables over each other with the standardized transfer process. Practitioners should be familiar with preparation before transfer, catheter loading technique, posttransfer control, and recording phase. The highest pregnancy success may be achieved by being aware of the factors that will affect the success of the transfer and its consequences.

Key Words: ART, IVF, Technique of embryo transfer, Good practice

Introduction

Patrick Steptoe and Robert Edwards have broken new ground in infertility treatment using human reproductive cells. The two scientists, who started to work together in the field of in vitro fertilization in 1968, performed the first human embryo transfer (ET) in 1972. Six years later, they achieved their first live birth success with their consistent work in the field of in vitro fertilization. In this process, 102 embryo transfers by Steptoe and Edwards failed and

---

* Corresponding Author's Email: turkmenaysin@gmail.com

In: Holistic Approach to Assisted Reproductive Technology
Editor: Kenan Demir and Rümeysa Yılmaz Göç
ISBN: 979-8-89113-017-3
© 2023 Nova Science Publishers, Inc.

an ectopic pregnancy developed in one of their cases (Brinsden, 2009; King, 1978). With this satisfactory result, studies in the field of in vitro fertilization have gained momentum. As in vitro fertilization has become widespread worldwide, experiences have been collected and evaluated, and guidelines have been published to increase success criteria.

With the intensification of research in the field of reproductive medicine, scientific societies have been established to increase the safety and quality of laboratory procedures. Universal developments in the clinical and laboratory field and sharing of experiences have resulted in the development of advanced techniques in reproductive health. According to the report of the International Committee for Monitoring Assisted Reproductive Technologies (ICMART) obtained from 75 countries, 344,317 babies were born out of 1,160,474 embryo transfers performed in 2013 (Banker et al., 2021). Over the years, better results have been obtained with in vitro fertilization in the treatment of infertility. In the report of the European IVF Monitoring Consortium (EIM) of the European Society for Human Reproduction and Embryology in 2018, which includes data from 39 countries, the pregnancy rate per transfer was reported to be 34.1% (Wyns et al., 2022). The increasing number of children born with medically assisted reproduction (MAR) since 1978 has led to the support of treatment worldwide and its development with new suggestions and technologies.

In light of scientific experience, selective approaches have been developed on the number, quality, and stage of development of embryos to be transferred, considering risky pregnancies caused by MAR, fetal development problems, and birth rates. Although fresh blastocyst stage ET is known to contribute more to the clinical pregnancy rate than cleavage stage ET, more research is needed to strengthen the evidence in this area (Glujovsky et al., 2016; Glujovsky et al., 2022; Li et al., 2021).

Intrauterine placement of two or more embryos in ET has led to the problem of high multiple pregnancy rates (MPR) over the years. Due to the risks of multiple pregnancies that threaten maternal and newborn health, single embryo transfers (sET) have come to the fore. Various algorithms for ET have been proposed to prevent multiple pregnancies without reducing birth rates. Some countries changed their legal regulations and aimed to reduce perinatal mortality and morbidity by supporting sET transfer (Cutting et al., 2008; Harbottle et al., 2015; McLernon et al., 2010). Babies born from pregnancies developed as a result of embryo transfer have a higher rate of preterm birth and low birth weight than those born as a result of spontaneous pregnancies. When sET and double embryo transfer were compared, the rate of preterm birth and low birth weight infants was found to be lower after sET (Grady et al., 2012).

The aim of transfer, which is the last step for success in MAR, should be to make ET as perfect as possible in light of clinical experience. This is closely related to the quality and number of the embryo and an appropriate transfer procedure. The experience gained in embryo transfer indicates that the cotransfer of good quality embryo (GQE) and poor quality embryo (PQE) does not make any difference in clinical pregnancy or live birth rates compared to single GQE transfer. On the other hand, the transfer of pairs of GQE and PQE embryos increases multiple pregnancies. Especially in women under 40 years of age, a single good GQE transfer may be preferred. More studies are still needed for those over 40 (Ma et al., 2022; Xiao et al., 2022).

Accessing the technology to store oocytes and embryos by freezing has made it necessary to compare the results of frozen embryo transfer with fresh transfers. A review of eight studies concluded that single fresh blastocyst transfer had higher live birth rates than single cryopreserved thawed embryo transfer (Zeng & Li, 2019). Clinical pregnancy and live birth rates are higher in fifth day blastocyst transfers (Bourdon et al., 2019). When transfers and pregnancy outcomes were compared, low birth weight and small babies were found to be risky after fresh ET, while large baby risk was found after frozen ET (Elias et al., 2020).

However, some studies support the view that low ovarian hyperstimulation syndrome and high live birth rates are achieved, although the implantation rate is not different as a result of frozen ET (FET) (Zhang et al., 2018).

Taking into account the stage reached in ET from the past to the present, many studies have revealed the importance of the quality, number, and developmental stage of the embryo in the success of the transfer. The efforts to create a pregnancy in 1972 have been replaced today by the goal of achieving a healthy live birth. The goal of achieving a healthy live birth may be crowned with a standardized embryo transfer technique in experienced hands. This section has been prepared for the practical needs of histology and embryology specialists. We aim to create resources for the current approach to ET techniques. The subject is grouped under two main headings that are compatible with daily practice. In order to develop pregnancy as a result of ET, based on technical approaches during the procedure, the preparation and transfer phases before and after ET are presented.

Practical Approach

Pre-Transfer Preparation and Placement of the Embryo

Embryo transfer is defined as the selection of an embryo that has been fertilized in vitro and whose developmental stage has been followed, loaded into the carrier catheter with standard techniques, and placed in the uterine cavity. Transcervical embryo placement is the most preferred method (Giulia Mariani, 2017).

After the transfer day is decided, the patient is informed of the scheduled day and time one day earlier. Preliminary information is provided on the general condition of embryos (Gameiro et al., 2015). Approximately 3 ml of transfer medium (5% O_2, 6% CO_2) is placed in the incubator the day before the procedure (Halvaei et al., 2013). On the day of transfer, the patient identification information and the patient file are reviewed. The patient is interviewed about the final stage of development of the embryos and the embryo to be transferred.

The transfer Petri dish is placed on the heated laminar cabinet surface for heating. Commonly used single central well Petri dishes may be selected for transfer. In the preference of the Petri dish, its use in the field of in vitro fertilization (IVF) must be approved and the possibility of toxic effects on the embryo must be tested. The preparation materials are completed by adding an ET catheter, sterile surgical gloves, and 1 ml of syringe. The catheter preference for ET may be soft or rigid. Rigid catheters are especially preferred for challenging transfers. It is recommended that routine ET be performed with a soft transfer catheter (McDonald & Norman, 2002; Mizrachi & McQueen, 2022; Penzias et al., 2017; van Weering et al., 2002). The preference for the syringe may be Hamilton or tuberculin. Due to possible toxic effects, products that do not contain plastic seals and have undergone embryo toxicity tests should be used. Sterile powder-free surgical gloves are still preferred. Although its adverse effects have not been proven, it is predicted that the powder may contaminate the embryo (Hannoun et al., 2009). The type of glove is not recommended, as no adverse effects have been observed according to the ASRM embryo transfer guideline in 2017 (Practice Committee of the American Society for Reproductive Medicine. Electronic address & Practice Committee of the American Society for Reproductive, 2017). The assisted hatching process is applied when necessary. Embryo(s) are prepared just prior to transfer. After the patient is taken to the operating room and prepared for ET, the information of the embryo file and the patient's ID are matched for the last time (WHO, 2008). Embryo loading into the catheter can be done from a sub-oil culture drop or via a transfer Petri dish. Catheter loading methods have similar pregnancy rates (D'Angelo et al., 2022; Halvaei et al., 2013). Drop 1 ml of preprepared transfer medium in a single well (Centre Well Dish) transfer Petri dish, into the central well and into the ring-shaped groove around it. Embryo(s) selected for transfer are transferred from the culture Petri dish to the transfer Petri dish (Figure 24.1). The embryo is moved to the first groove. After it is washed, it is placed in the center of the central chamber. Embryos that have developed, except those that are to be transferred, are quickly returned to the incubator.

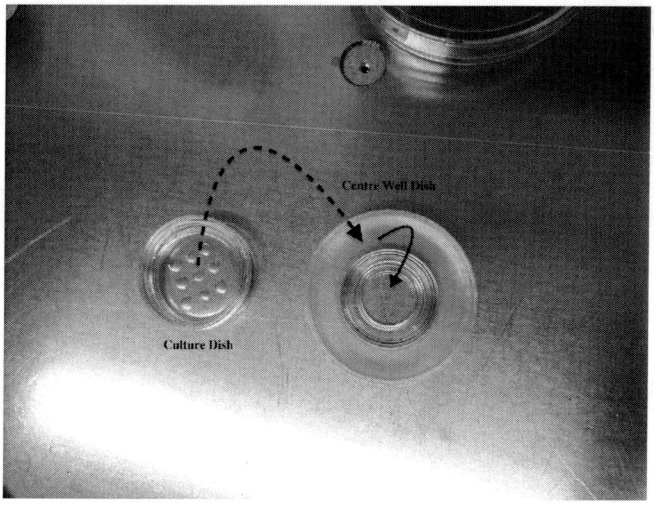

Figure 24.1 Transfer of embryo from culture petri dish to transfer petri dish (author's own archive).

After patient preparation, the embryo(s) taken into the transfer Petri dish are immediately loaded into the catheter. It is recommended that the processing time should be less than 120 seconds. Increased duration is associated with a decrease in pregnancy rate. Studies suggesting that the highest pregnancy rate is achieved in cases where the loading and release process time is <44 seconds support the need for embryo transfer in a short time. (D'Angelo et al., 2022; Matorras et al., 2004).

The loading can be performed with the air-liquid-embryo or with the technique that contains only liquid-embryo (Figure 24.2). The inside of the catheter is washed with the transfer medium drawn into the syringe. Depending on the technique, loading can be done as air bubble-medium and embryo(s)-air bubble-medium or medium and embryo(s).

It is recommended to transfer the embryo with a loading volume of 10–30 µl. In low volume (<10 µl) transfers, implantation and pregnancy rates are low. In large-volume (>60 µl) transfers, the embryo may not be stable where it was transferred. This may pose a risk of an ectopic pregnancy. It is recommended to leave the embryo at a distance of 1.5-2 cm from the fundus endometrium. A high pregnancy rate was achieved when the fundus and air bubble distance was <10 mm. It is recommended to push the syringe plunger at constant pressure. An automated syringe system can be used for this process (Bayram et al., 2021; Cenksoy et al., 2014; D'Angelo et al., 2022; Ebner et al., 2001; Penzias et al., 2017).

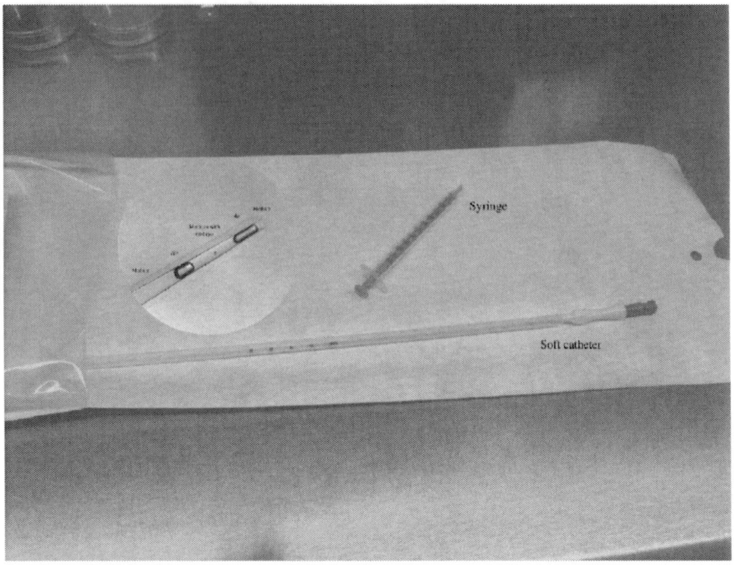

Figure 24.2 Catheter loading methods (author's own archive).

Today, ultrasonography-guided embryo transfer (USG) allows for instant evaluation of where the embryo will be placed. The pregnancy rate is higher than the traditional transfer (clinical touch). Due to the air bubbles, an idea about the placement of the embryo can be obtained immediately after transfer. Myometrial contractions, an undesirable side effect of the transfer approach, may cause the embryo to migrate from the transfer site. The view that myometrial contractions cause negative effects on pregnancy is supported. With instant observation (USG) transfer, endometrial damage and transfer to the lower parts of the uterus may be minimized (Brown et al., 2016; Practice Committee of the American Society for Reproductive Medicine. Electronic address & Practice Committee of the American Society for Reproductive, 2017; Saravelos & Li, 2019; Teixeira et al., 2015).

Post-Transfer Approaches

After intrauterine placement of the embryo(s), the catheter and outer sheath are slowly removed from the cervical canal. The catheter is pulled at a constant speed while holding the syringe plunger. Catheter tip control is performed. The embryologist examines the catheter under the stereo microscope for embryo retention. When the embryo is seen during examination, the transfer is repeated. Since implantation and clinical pregnancy outcomes are similar, retransfer is supported by recent studies (Kadour-Peero et al., 2022; Practice

Committee of the American Society for Reproductive Medicine. Electronic address & Practice Committee of the American Society for Reproductive, 2017; Saravelos & Li, 2019). After the procedure, the transferred embryo number, developmental stage, transfer catheter type, blood on the catheter, mucus, application time, and practitioners should be recorded.

Conclusion

Studies show that practitioners who transfer the embryo have similar pregnancy outcomes. On the other hand, the success of embryo transfer is affected by many factors, such as the experience of the clinician and embryologist, synchronized studies, difficulty in catheterization, embryo loading technique, prolonged transfer time, properties of the culture medium, injection pressure, and speed. Obstetricians and embryologists who will work in the field of reproductive medicine should have experience with standard procedures, and even experienced embryologists should be monitored according to key performance indicators.

References

Banker, M., Dyer, S., Chambers, G. M., Ishihara, O., Kupka, M., de Mouzon, J., Zegers-Hochschild, F., & Adamson, G. D. (2021). International Committee for Monitoring Assisted Reproductive Technologies (ICMART): world report on assisted reproductive technologies, 2013. *Fertil Steril*, *116*(3), 741-756. https://doi.org/10.1016/j.fertnstert.2021.03.039

Bayram, A., De Munck, N., Elkhatib, I., Arnanz, A., El-Damen, A., Abdala, A., Coughlan, C., Garrido, N., Vidales, L. M., Lawrenz, B., & Fatemi, H. M. (2021). The position of the euploid blastocyst in the uterine cavity influences implantation. *Reprod Biomed Online*, *43*(5), 880-889. https://doi.org/10.1016/j.rbmo.2021.02.008

Bourdon, M., Pocate-Cheriet, K., Finet de Bantel, A., Grzegorczyk-Martin, V., Amar Hoffet, A., Arbo, E., Poulain, M., & Santulli, P. (2019). Day 5 versus Day 6 blastocyst transfers: a systematic review and meta-analysis of clinical outcomes. *Human Reproduction*, *34*(10), 1948-1964. https://doi.org/10.1093/humrep/dez163

Brinsden, P. R. (2009). Thirty years of IVF: The legacy of Patrick Steptoe and Robert Edwards. *Human Fertility*, *12*(3), 137-143. https://doi.org/10.1080/14647270903176773

Brown, J., Buckingham, K., Buckett, W., & Abou-Setta, A. M. (2016). Ultrasound versus 'clinical touch' for catheter guidance during embryo transfer in women. *Cochrane Database Syst Rev*, *3*, CD006107. https://doi.org/10.1002/14651858.CD006107.pub4

Cenksoy, P. O., Ficicioglu, C., Yesiladali, M., Akcin, O. A., & Kaspar, C. (2014). The importance of the length of uterine cavity, the position of the tip of the inner catheter and the distance between the fundal endometrial surface and the air bubbles as determinants of the pregnancy rate in IVF cycles. *Eur J Obstet Gynecol Reprod Biol*, *172*, 46-50. https://doi.org/10.1016/j.ejogrb.2013.09.023

Cutting, R., Morroll, D., Roberts, S. A., Pickering, S., Rutherford, A., Bfs, & Ace. (2008). Elective single embryo transfer: guidelines for practice British Fertility Society and Association of Clinical Embryologists. *Hum Fertil (Camb)*, *11*(3), 131-146. https://doi.org/10.1080/14647270802302629

D'Angelo, A., Panayotidis, C., Alteri, A., Mcheik, S., & Veleva, Z. (2022). Evidence and consensus on technical aspects of embryo transfer. *Human Reproduction Open*, *2022*(4). https://doi.org/ARTN hoac03810.1093/hropen/hoac038

Ebner, T., Yaman, C., Moser, M., Sommergruber, M., Polz, W., & Tews, G. (2001). The ineffective loading process of the embryo transfer catheter alters implantation and pregnancy rates. *Fertil Steril*, *76*(3), 630-632. https://doi.org/10.1016/s0015-0282(01)01980-x

Elias, F. T. S., Weber-Adrian, D., Pudwell, J., Carter, J., Walker, M., Gaudet, L., Smith, G., & Velez, M. P. (2020). Neonatal outcomes in singleton pregnancies conceived by fresh or frozen embryo transfer compared to spontaneous conceptions: a systematic review and meta-analysis. *Arch Gynecol Obstet*, *302*(1), 31-45. https://doi.org/10.1007/s00404-020-05593-4

Gameiro, S., Boivin, J., Dancet, E., de Klerk, C., Emery, M., Lewis-Jones, C., Thorn, P., Van den Broeck, U., Venetis, C., Verhaak, C. M., Wischmann, T., & Vermeulen, N. (2015). ESHRE guideline: routine psychosocial care in infertility and medically assisted reproduction-a guide for fertility staff. *Human Reproduction*, *30*(11), 2476-2485. https://doi.org/10.1093/humrep/dev177

Giulia Mariani, J. B. (2017). Embryo Transfer. In C. S. David K. Gardner (Ed.), *Handbook of In Vitro Fertilization* (Vol. 4). CRC Press. https://doi.org/10.1201/9781315157269

Glujovsky, D., Farquhar, C., Quinteiro Retamar, A. M., Alvarez Sedo, C. R., & Blake, D. (2016). Cleavage stage versus blastocyst stage embryo transfer in assisted reproductive technology. *Cochrane Database Syst Rev*(6), CD002118. https://doi.org/10.1002/14651858.CD002118.pub5

Glujovsky, D., Quinteiro Retamar, A. M., Alvarez Sedo, C. R., Ciapponi, A., Cornelisse, S., & Blake, D. (2022). Cleavage-stage versus blastocyst-stage embryo transfer in assisted reproductive technology. *Cochrane Database Syst Rev*, *5*(5), CD002118. https://doi.org/10.1002/14651858.CD002118.pub6

Grady, R., Alavi, N., Vale, R., Khandwala, M., & McDonald, S. D. (2012). Elective single embryo transfer and perinatal outcomes: a systematic review and meta-analysis. *Fertil Steril*, *97*(2), 324-331. https://doi.org/10.1016/j.fertnstert.2011.11.033

Halvaei, I., Khalili, M. A., Razi, M. H., Agha-Rahimi, A., & Nottola, S. A. (2013). Impact of different embryo loading techniques on pregnancy rates in in vitro fertlization/embryo transfer cycles. *J Hum Reprod Sci*, *6*(1), 65-69. https://doi.org/10.4103/0974-1208.112385

Hannoun, A., Zreik, T. G., Ghaziri, G., Abu Musa, A., & Awwad, J. (2009). Effect of powdered gloves, worn at the time of embryo transfer, on the pregnancy outcome of IVF cycles. *Journal of Assisted Reproduction and Genetics*, *26*(1), 25-27. https://doi.org/10.1007/s10815-008-9285-3

Harbottle, S., Hughes, C., Cutting, R., Roberts, S., Brison, D., Association Of Clinical, E., & The British Fertility, S. (2015). Elective Single Embryo Transfer: an update to UK Best Practice Guidelines. *Hum Fertil (Camb)*, *18*(3), 165-183. https://doi.org/10.3109/14647273.2015.1083144

Kadour-Peero, E., Tulandi, T., Feferkorn, I., Hiszkiahu, R., & Buckett, W. (2022). Effects of embryo retention during embryo transfer on IVF outcomes. *J Assist Reprod Genet*, *39*(5), 1065-1068. https://doi.org/10.1007/s10815-022-02450-y

King, K. (1978). Life after Birth - Imagery in Beckett,Samuel Trilogy - Solomon,Ph. *Southern Humanities Review*, *12*(1), 84-84. <Go to ISI>://WOS:A1978FZ01200035

Li, Y., Liu, S., & Lv, Q. (2021). Single blastocyst stage versus single cleavage stage embryo transfer following fresh transfer: A systematic review and meta-analysis. *Eur J Obstet Gynecol Reprod Biol*, *267*, 11-17. https://doi.org/10.1016/j.ejogrb.2021.10.004

Ma, S., Peng, Y., Hu, L., Wang, X., Xiong, Y., Tang, Y., Tan, J., & Gong, F. (2022). Comparisons of benefits and risks of single embryo transfer versus double embryo transfer: a systematic review and meta-analysis. *Reprod Biol Endocrinol*, *20*(1), 20. https://doi.org/10.1186/s12958-022-00899-1

Matorras, R., Mendoza, R., Exposito, A., & Rodriguez-Escudero, F. J. (2004). Influence of the time interval between embryo catheter loading and discharging on the success of IVF. *Human Reproduction*, *19*(9), 2027-2030. https://doi.org/10.1093/humrep/deh366

McDonald, J. A., & Norman, R. J. (2002). A randomized controlled trial of a soft double lumen embryo transfer catheter versus a firm single lumen catheter: significant improvements in pregnancy rates. *Human Reproduction*, *17*(6), 1502-1506. https://doi.org/DOI 10.1093/humrep/17.6.1502

McLernon, D. J., Harrild, K., Bergh, C., Davies, M. J., de Neubourg, D., Dumoulin, J. C., Gerris, J., Kremer, J. A., Martikainen, H., Mol, B. W., Norman, R. J., Thurin-Kjellberg, A., Tiitinen, A., van Montfoort, A. P., van Peperstraten, A. M., Van Royen, E., & Bhattacharya, S. (2010). Clinical effectiveness of elective single versus double embryo transfer: meta-analysis of individual patient data from randomised trials. *BMJ*, *341*, c6945. https://doi.org/10.1136/bmj.c6945

Mizrachi, Y., & McQueen, D. B. (2022). Embryo transfer success: It is in our hands. *Fertility and Sterility*, *118*(5), 815-819. https://doi.org/10.1016/j.fertnstert.2022.08.858

Penzias, A., Bendikson, K., Butts, S., Coutifaris, C., Falcone, T., Fossum, G., Gitlin, S., Gracia, C., Hansen, K., La Barbera, A., Mersereau, J., Odem, R., Paulson, R., Pfeifer, S., Pisarska, M., Rebar, R., Reindollar, R., Rosen, M., Sandlow, J., Vernon, M., & Practice Committee of the American Society for Reproductive Medicine (2017). Performing the embryo transfer: a guideline. *Fertility and Sterility*, *107*(4). https://doi.org/10.1016/j.fertnstert.2017.01.025

Practice Committee of the American Society for Reproductive Medicine & Practice Committee of the American Society for Reproductive, M. (2017). Performing the embryo transfer: a guideline. *Fertil Steril*, *107*(4), 882-896. https://doi.org/10.1016/j.fertnstert.2017.01.025

Saravelos, S. H., & Li, T. C. (2019). Embryo transfer techniques. *Best Pract Res Clin Obstet Gynaecol*, *59*, 77-88. https://doi.org/10.1016/j.bpobgyn.2019.01.004

Teixeira, D. M., Dassuncao, L. A., Vieira, C. V. R., Barbosa, M. A. P., Neto, M. A. C., Nastri, C. O., & Martins, W. P. (2015). Ultrasound guidance during embryo transfer: a systematic review and meta-analysis of randomized controlled trials. *Ultrasound in Obstetrics & Gynecology*, *45*(2), 139-148. https://doi.org/10.1002/uog.14639

van Weering, H. G., Schats, R., McDonnell, J., Vink, J. M., Vermeiden, J. P., & Hompes, P. G. (2002). The impact of the embryo transfer catheter on the pregnancy rate in IVF. *Human Reproduction*, *17*(3), 666-670. https://doi.org/10.1093/humrep/17.3.666

WHO. (2008). *World alliance for patient safety: forward programme 2008-2009.* https://apps.who.int/iris/handle/10665/70460 Access Date: 31 Jan 2023

Wyns, C., De Geyter, C., Calhaz-Jorge, C., Kupka, M. S., Motrenko, T., Smeenk, J., Bergh, C., Tandler-Schneider, A., Rugescu, I. A., Goossens, V., Consorti, E. I. M., & ESHRE. (2022). ART in Europe, 2018: results generated from European registries by ESHRE dagger. *Human Reproduction Open*, *2022*(3). https://doi.org/ARTN hoac02210.1093/hropen/hoac022

Xiao, Y., Wang, X., Gui, T., Tao, T., & Xiong, W. (2022). Transfer of a poor-quality along with a good-quality embryo on in vitro fertilization/intracytoplasmic sperm injection-embryo transfer clinical outcomes: a systematic review and meta-analysis. *Fertil Steril*, *118*(6), 1066-1079. https://doi.org/10.1016/j.fertnstert.2022.08.848

Zeng, M., & Li, L. (2019). Single fresh blastocyst transfer or single cryopreserved-thawed blastocyst transfer: which is preferable for infertile patients in IVF/ICSI cycles? A meta-analysis. *Gynecol Endocrinol*, *35*(1), 17-22. https://doi.org/10.1080/09513590.2018.1490408

Zhang, W., Xiao, X., Zhang, J., Wang, W., Wu, J., Peng, L., & Wang, X. (2018). Clinical outcomes of frozen embryo versus fresh embryo transfer following in vitro fertilization: a meta-analysis of randomized controlled trials. *Arch Gynecol Obstet*, *298*(2), 259-272. https://doi.org/10.1007/s00404-018-4786-5

Chapter 25

Quality Control and Quality Assurance in the IVF Laboratory

Alper Şişmanoğlu, MD*
Department of Obstetrics and Gynecology, Faculty of Medicine, Altınbaş University, Istanbul, Turkiye.

Abstract

The most critical outcome factors of an in vitro fertilization (IVF) laboratory are pregnancy results and live birth rates. For these successful outcomes, the performance of the IVF laboratory is of compulsory necessity. Gametes and embryos are very sensitive to environmental effects, and small fluctuations of external conditions may compromise their viability. So, it is essential to establish optimal conditions for the human eggs, sperm cells, and the resulting embryos. In order to maintain these very specific conditions, quality control (QC) routines need to be established with quality specifications for each quality parameter. After establishing the parameters, we should asses them regularly, and at the end if necessary, we can adjust them to bring back the optimal laboratory environment. This evaluation and fine-tuning should be repeated daily, weekly, monthly, and annually to provide perfect conditions. Quality control aims to give the same results with different elements at different times in a laboratory. For this, performance indicators (PIs) (Performance Indicators) should be defined and used, and at the same time, PI indicators should be measurable. PIs are studied in three main areas: Structural PIs, Process PIs and Conclusion PIs. To achieve and maintain particular conditions in the IVF laboratory, quality specifications and quality control routines must be established for each quality parameter. These parameters are evaluated daily, weekly, monthly, or yearly to determine if they meet certain specifications, and then they should be fine-tuned to bring the levels to

* Corresponding Author's Email: Alper.sismanoglu@altinbas.edu.tr

In: Holistic Approach to Assisted Reproductive Technology
Editor: Kenan Demir and Rümeysa Yılmaz Göç
ISBN: 979-8-89113-017-3
© 2023 Nova Science Publishers, Inc.

acceptable limits of measurement uncertainty. These quality parameters are temperature, pH, CO2 & other gas mixtures, air quality, and infection control of the IVF laboratory. All of these should be included in the periodic quality control and quality assurance process in IVF laboratories.

Key Words: IVF laboratory, Performance indicators, IVF success, Laboratory parameters

Introduction

The IVF laboratory has special importance in ART treatments. There should be standardization in all procedures performed in the IVF laboratory and the processes should be kept under control. The quality control program is planned to evaluate the laboratory as a whole. In this way, the aim is not only to detect and correct the problems and errors in the laboratory but also to increase the efficiency of the laboratory and, at the same time, its performance.

Examination of Performance in Art Center

Quality management includes quality assurance and quality control and improvement. Quality assurance is the review of everything related to quality in the laboratory and clinic, and it includes not only transactions, but also results and user satisfaction. It also includes comparing and criticizing other laboratories by performing the same procedures with the same samples. On the other hand, quality control aims to give the same results with different elements at different times in a laboratory. Therefore, performance indicators (PIs) should be defined and used, while PI indicators should be measurable. In addition, an accurate process evaluation is necessary to provide the given service efficiently (De Los Santos et al., 2016; Fabozzi et al., 2020).

PIs are studied in three main areas.

1. Structural
2. Process
3. Conclusion

Structural PI s

It measures environmental quality in general. It needs to be examined separately as facilities, equipment, and staff. The working area of the facility and the laboratory environment should be reliable and the risk of accidents should be minimized. The laboratory should be suitable for the working system and compatible with the number of personnel. The equipment, the materials used, and the number of tools must be appropriate for the workload. The incubators, working cabinets, and consumables should be maintained and calibrated on time. The staff requires reliable teamwork for successful IVF treatment, and trained and qualified staff updated with continuing education are essential. Having sufficient team members alleviates the workload and creates a more productive working environment (Practice Committee of the American Society for Reproductive Medicine, & Practice Committee of the Society for Assisted Reproductive Technology, 2008, Català et al. 2015).

Process PI

All laboratory operations must be performed on time within the framework of specific procedures and protocols. The temperature, PH, and osmolarity values of the culture media used for embryo development are critical (Wale & Gardner, 2016). The rapid and timely completion of procedures such as ICSI (Intracytoplasmic sperm injection) and PGD (Preimplantation genetic diagnosis) by the experienced embryology team prevents fluctuations in these values. Process measurements are direct measurements of the quality and are the most sensitive to differences in the quality of care (Mant, 2001).

Protective measures, especially ensuring that contamination does not occur in communicable diseases and taking precautions, ensure the safety of personnel and patients. All procedures involving gametes and embryos should be performed in controlled media in protective cabinets. VOCs (volatile organic compounds) measurements should be made and HEPA filters should be changed regularly. Appropriate clothing and gloves, regular hand washing, and sterile and disposable materials should be used. Proper waste disposal and surface cleaning are essential.

Identification and Traceability

Identifying patients and the traceability of gametes, embryos, products, and materials are critical in ART treatments. Labeling, small chips, and electronic alarm systems are used today. Such a system increases safety and patient satisfaction and minimizes mismatch risk (Rienzi et al., 2017).

Conclusion PI

The results indicators can be evaluated using quality control (QC). In monitoring the performance of the ART laboratory, the results of fertilization rate, embryo quality, pregnancy rate, multiple pregnancy rate, implantation rate, and the development of a laboratory's QC can be monitored based on the "correct procedure practice rules" of the ESHRE guideline. The control chart is one of the most common tools used for this purpose.

Adherence to PI values enables early detection of problems and the adoption of corrective action plans. As a result, monitoring the PI values nswers the question, "Is everything OK in the lab?". Each laboratory should develop its control mechanism. The KPIs should be monitored constantly in every ART laboratory; control charts are the most commonly used (Fabozzi et al., 2020). Shewhart and Levey Jennings's quality control charts are widespread charts to be used in such a manner. (Fig. 25.1)

Achieving a healthy live birth on an ART results from a multidisciplinary clinical effort. Numerous factors contribute to this goal from the very beginning. Initial interview with the patient and ending embryo transfer from the selection of stimulation to protocols and laboratory procedures. Unfortunately, although there are many studies on the appropriate laboratory criteria, there is limited consensus on the clinical side of the appropriate laboratory, and this is a severe limitation because the clinical and laboratory perspectives are closely linked in IVF. Any technological advance implemented in the laboratory includes the potential for clinicians to change the direction of treatment and adopt innovations (Franco Jr. et al., 2017). For example, standardization and a more significant application of blastocyst culture, cryopreservation by vitrification, and/or trophectoderm biopsy in IVF laboratories have allowed clinicians to modify ovarian stimulation protocols aimed at maximizing ovarian

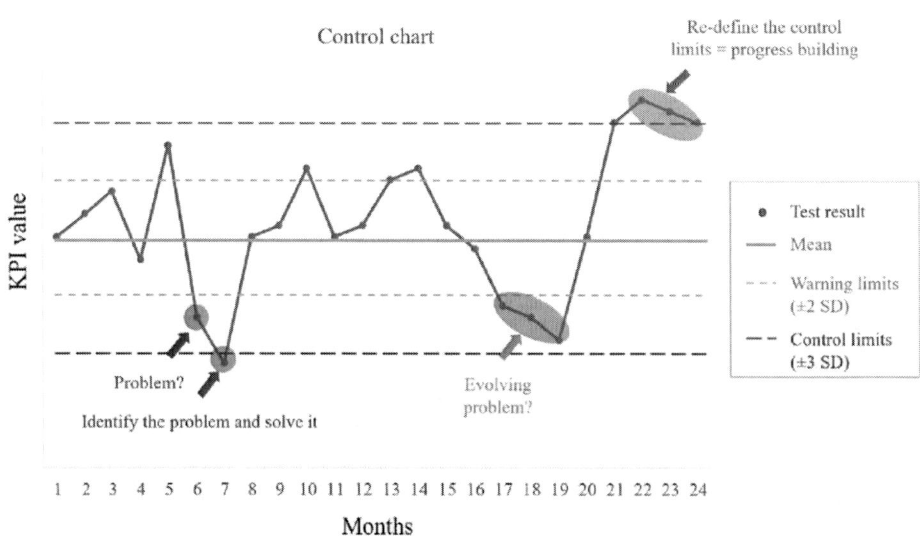

Figure 25.1 Representative scheme of a control chart (Fabozzi et al., 2020).

response; To minimize the risk of overstimulated ovaries, an ovulation-inducing agonist was adopted while elective single embryo transfer was accepted for use to maximize implantation.

In some cases, the time taken to achieve this success has been shortened by increasing pregnancy success rates and taking a healthy baby home through comprehensive chromosome test-based preimplantation genetic testing, thanks to advanced freezing and thawing protocols in IVF laboratories. Therefore, clinical KPIs (Key performance indicators) and shared KPIs between clinicians and embryologists are essential for improving quality. The laboratory KPIs of all future IVF treatments mainly cover care's safety, effectiveness, efficiency, and timeliness dimensions. By including clinical KPIs, an IVF center can also encompass equity and patient-centeredness, thus considering all six dimensions of care.

Evaluation of the Performance of the Embryology Laboratory

Embryology laboratory performance is essential for successfully completing an in vitro fertilization (IVF) cycle. Small fluctuations in their media can compromise the development and viability of gametes and embryos; therefore, creating optimal culture conditions in which gametes and embryos are obtained and preserved is crucial. To achieve and maintain these particular conditions, quality specifications and quality control (QC) routines must be established for each quality parameter. These parameters are evaluated daily, weekly, monthly, or yearly to determine if they meet certain specifications and then fine-tuned to bring the levels to acceptable limits of measurement uncertainty (Montag & Morbeck, 2017).

Temperature

The temperature of the culture medium must be consistent during manipulations and use in the culture outside and inside the incubators. Manipulation and use outside the incubator include microscope-heated stages, laminar flow-heated surfaces, and heating blocks. The set temperature of these devices must first be determined by a series of measurements of the temperature in a particular dish or tube, along with the corresponding surface temperature. The aim is to determine the set surface temperature (as shown on the equipment display) required to maintain 37.0° C in the medium vessel/tube. The final settings will vary depending on the type of culture dish used, the conductivity, the oil layer, etc. If more than one plate type is used on the heated surface, this set-point verification must be repeated for each plate type, and the risk of overheating one plate over the other should be considered. Usually, the set-point of results for the heated stage or block is higher than 37.0°C. Once the set-point has been determined, the corresponding surface temperature (measured using a surface probe) can be used for temperature mapping. Once the set point for the heater has been determined, there can be significant differences between the different heated areas. Therefore, temperature mapping is required for each heated stage and surface to indicate temperature changes. Temperature mapping is done every three months; temperature is measured at different locations to reveal which locations support the desired temperature; these locations are marked as 'safe to use' and the rest as 'not suitable for use'. After verification, daily routine QC measurements can be made in "safe-to-use" areas using a standard surface probe. Maintaining a constant temperature inside the incubator is crucial for a successful embryo culture. Types of incubator include standard large box incubators, which can have a single interior door or multiple interior doors, and smaller benchtop incubators that recover more quickly after opening and closing the door. Risk assessment is required to determine the number of plates the incubator can support without temperature loss.

Regardless of the model, all incubators require temperature mapping over 24 hours to identify possible temperature inconsistencies under different conditions over time. Similarly to heated surfaces, temperature mapping is done when a new incubator is installed, and containers or tubes are placed in different parts of the room every three months after that. Therefore, consistent and accurate readings are essential for the daily monitoring of incubator temperature. Unfortunately, the type K microprobe used for temperature mapping is susceptible to electromagnetic fields and is therefore susceptible to errors and lacks the sensitivity to detect differences of ±0.1° C at 37° C. For this purpose, PT100 probes with more sensitive platinum sensors are used in all incubators. These probes can be connected daily to a thermocouple for manual daily readings (noted in the logbook) or to a continuous monitoring system where temperature data are acquired and transmitted via a wireless link to a base station. Data are checked daily according to the device display and weekly to verify no fluctuations over time.

Additionally, external control is provided by activating alarm options that include remote alarms such as Short Message Service (SMS) and alarm relay when temperatures fall outside the acceptable range. Daily temperature measurements (or continuous) should also include laboratory ambient room temperature (RT; normally 23 ± 2° C; Not F) and refrigerator and freezer temperatures (adjusted according to the recommendations of the media manufacturers).

Logbook records should include current, minimum, and maximum temperatures and personnel signatures.

pH

An acceptable narrow pH range is crucial for a complete QC program to optimize the culture system. Weekly pH verification is essential for the culture medium used and for all incubators. The pH should be checked each time a premixed gas cylinder is replaced or before a new lot of culture media is used. Media are equilibrated in plates or loose-capped tubes overnight prior to testing, excluding media handling. The processing media are heated to 37° C in a capped tube placed in a heating block. Monitoring pH using a blood gas analyzer provides highly accurate measurements. After initial calibration (according to the manufacturer's instructions), the preequilibrated culture medium is loaded into the blood gas analyzer, and a pH value is usually obtained along with other blood gas parameters (Note G). The traditional method of using a benchtop pH meter to measure pH may not be fully accurate if it is not used quickly and efficiently, and the negative impact of elevated ambient protein levels on the pH probe needs to be considered. Alternatively, custom pH meters can measure continuous pH inside the incubator under the same volumes and conditions the embryos are exposed to, but these pH meters are less accurate.

Calibration and pH Measurements Using a pH Meter

1. Calibrate the pH meter according to the manufacturer's instructions. Set the pH meter to 37° C or place the automatic temperature compensation probe in a tube containing water in a heating block.
2. Place new split calibration standards in capped tubes.
3. Let the standards reach 37° C.
4. Place the pH electrode at standard pH 4. When the pH is stabilized and calibrated, rinse the electrode with deionized H_2O and gently dry. Repeat the procedure by placing the electrode first at standard pH 7 and then at standard pH 10.
5. After calibration, return the electrode to standard pH 7 and verify the reading (~6,98 ± 0,02). If the reading is not within the range, repeat the calibration.
6. Remove the test tube containing the media from the incubator and quickly seal the tube. Place the tube on a 37° C heating block and place the electrodes in the medium. Save when the reading is fixed.

7. Repeat for the other tube of the same medium and average the two readings.
8. Repeat the process for all different media and all incubators used.
9. Cover the electrodes with 3 M KCL solution when all measurements are complete. Calibration records are kept along with maintenance records for probe and probe performance. If the measured values differ significantly from the target values, the electrodes should be replaced. Cleaning the electrodes with detergents can cause damage and the electrodes are not always efficient; therefore, the electrodes should be replaced after 12 months of use.

CO_2 and Gas Mixtures

Daily monitoring of incubator CO_2 concentration (and O_2 if appropriate) is required. The CO_2 set point can vary between incubators and is determined based on weekly pH verification (adjusted if necessary). No further action is required if all pH measurements are within the acceptable range. If the pH is out of range for a given incubator, the CO_2 level is adjusted to raise or lower the pH. The pH can also be affected by gas quality and possible leaks. Therefore, certificates must be submitted from the gas company, including gas purity and specifications in accordance with international standards, and leak checks should be done annually. A blood gas analyzer that passes two levels of external liquid QC (provided by the manufacturer) can be used for accurate readings of CO_2 and O_2 levels in the culture medium and pH readings. Before testing, two sets of tubes containing culture medium are equilibrated for 24 hours in each incubator. Several CO_2 meters are available. If daily QC is performed using this device, it must be calibrated against a standard certified gas before and after each series of readings (Note K). Thermal conductivity sensors are calibrated in an H_2O-saturated atmosphere, and incubator covers should not be opened for at least 15 minutes before taking a reading. Infrared sensors can also detect CO_2 and O_2 levels with the advantage of not requiring high humidity levels to operate.

Portable devices are available simultaneously, taking CO_2, O_2, relative humidity, and temperature readings (Note L). Some of the newer tech incubators come with built-in gas and temperature sensors and readings that can be reviewed and downloaded. Alternatively, each incubator's external CO2 and humidity sensors can be used with multi-input data loggers (such as an automatic monitoring and alarm system for temperature). No matter which instrument is used, CO_2 and O_2 measurements are made daily and records are kept for all incubators. The values obtained should correspond to both the set-point and the incubator display. For benchtop incubators using premixed gas, accurate control of the gas mixture is sometimes not possible because of the possibility of the tube being clogged by condensation. In this case, pH measurement is crucial to confirm the premixed gas. Additionally, the purge rate of the gas incoming for this type of incubator must be monitored (set at approximately 15–25 ml/min).

Air Quality

In the IVF laboratory, clean ultrapure air is required, and this is achieved by an air handling unit that automatically changes the air along with the heating, ventilation, and air conditioning (HVAC) system. A positive air pressure in the laboratory 10 to 15 Pa more than in adjacent rooms is required to prevent air from entering the laboratory from adjacent rooms. The temperature should not fluctuate significantly (±1° C) between seasons and the HVAC system should be adjusted when necessary. The HVAC system helps cool the air and removes moisture. Relative humidity levels in the laboratory should be between 40% and 60% to minimize fungal growth. The number and size of particles in a cubic meter of air can define how clean the air is. High-efficiency particulate air (HEPA) filters are installed on the laboratory ceiling to remove airborne contaminants. Laminar flow hoods also include HEPA filtration; all filters are regularly checked and replaced. The European Union Cell and Tissue Directive 16 determines the norm of particle and microorganism contamination, which suggests that particle counts and microbial colony counts should be equivalent to grade A with a grade B background. Prefilters, along with activated carbon filters and potassium permanganate filters, are also required to maintain the air quality inside the laboratory by absorbing VOCs (Note N). Independent filtration units can also be used for this purpose.

Contamination and Infection Control

Despite the use of antibiotics in the culture medium and strict aseptic techniques by embryologists, there is still a risk of contamination if the medium is not controlled. Therefore, the laboratory is cleaned and decontaminated daily; All surfaces are rinsed with sterile water to remove toxic residues from laboratory disinfectants (preferably commercially available embryo-tested spray or 70% ethanol). In addition, all incubators are cleaned and autoclaved every three to six months.

Other Parameters

The scope of routine QC can be unlimited, and although this section aims to cover the basics, others apply to specific laboratories and conditions. For example, if a laboratory is weighing a sperm sample to determine volume, the QC should include routine weighing of standard weights. It must be recognized that monitoring staff performance is a significant part of quality assurance, but their processes are particular to each laboratory. Therefore, it is essential to evaluate each process and ask what parameters might affect the outcome of this process. These parameters will need to be included in the routine QC process.

Monitoring Standard Operating Procedure

All parameters need to be monitored (frequency in parentheses). The monitoring logbook should contain the measurement value, the acceptable range, and the action taken when a measurement falls outside the given range. Each entry requires a signature of the staff.

1. Temperature measurements of "safe to use" heated areas of all heated appliances (daily)
2. Temperature measurements of all incubators (continuous or daily)
3. Control of temperature data loggers (daily and weekly for continuous systems)
4. Ambient room temperature (daily)
5. Temperatures in the refrigerator and freezer (daily)
6. Temperature mapping for heated appliances and incubators (every three months and for all new equipment before it goes into use)
7. pH measurements (weekly or for a new medium LOT and a new premixed gas bottle)
8. CO2 concentration for all incubators (daily or continuous)
9. O2 concentration for all incubators (daily or continuous when low oxygen culture is applied)
10. Positive pressure (daily)
11. Laboratory humidity (daily)
12. Particle count (twice a day at rest and work)
13. VOCs (daily)
14. Contact plates or swabs of all work surfaces (three times a month)
15. Active air samplers and layout plates

All commercial embryo culture media have a recommended pH ranging from 7.1 to 7.45. Some manufacturers recommend the same range for all media, while others have different ranges for different media. An alternative option is to use the IVF chamber, an isolated system with integrated temperature and gas control and air filtration without interaction with the outside environment. Suppose that temperature mapping reveals that the locations most commonly used by embryologists fall outside the desired temperature range. In that case, an alternative option is to change the set temperature of the heated surface accordingly and remap the temperatures until the desired areas correspond to the desired temperature range. Temperature matching is also required for tube holders used during oocyte collection. If transport incubators are also used, temperature mapping is required for all tube insertion points under the conditions under which gametes/embryos are transferred. The laboratory room temperature (RT) is debatable. Some say higher temperatures reduce the risk of cooling when samples are kept outside incubators. However, it should be considered that higher RT also increases the risk of bacterial/fungal contamination. Blood gas analyzers can be expensive, but most IVF labs in larger hospitals can use hospital analyzers located in the central lab or emergency/birth ward. Using media instead of blood does not alter the accuracy of the measurement or damage the equipment. A tight seal between the electrode and the walls of the test tube is required for accurate measurements. A rubber gasket can be placed around the electrode to create a seal and stabilize pH readings.

In its classic use, quality control in the IVF laboratory is simple documentation showing that equipment and instruments are working and doing so within a predetermined range of standards. This evidence is archived physically in folders or electronically on a server unless received for accreditation purposes. The timely discovery of defective equipment/instruments, followed by prompt corrective action through effective quality management practices, is the gold standard of quality control (Gardner & Pool, 2019).

Conclusion

Success in IVF laboratories requires dedicated quality control and assurance, implemented at the appropriate level (Mortimer & Mortimer, 2015). In recent years, increasing demand on laboratory staff to ensure optimal environment and better IVF results, such as pregnancy and live birth, increased the complexity of IVF laboratories which faced embryologists with increasing responsibility and risks of uncorrectable errors (Alikani et al., 2014). Systemic PI monitoring is crucial for early detection of the problems, and this can give a chance for early corrective actions before the clinical impacts are seen (Liperis & Sjöblom, 2017). Laboratory with internal control programs and external assurance routines are able to maintain the optimal laboratory environment and are giving the human fertility treatment to benefit from these QC measurements by giving the chance to have the best IVF results (Matson, 1998). In given periods of time, ASRM reviews and publishes updated guidelines in the form of minimum standards for IVF laboratories intended to enhance the already high standards practiced by ART programs (The American Society for Reproductive Medicine, 1998). Clearly, the achievement of a healthy live birth in an ART clinic is the result of multidisciplinary effort. A multitude of factors contribute to this goal, starting from the very first consultation, passing through the choice of the stimulation protocols, and ending in the laboratory procedures down to embryo transfer.

References

Alikani, M., Go, K. J., McCaffrey, C., & McCulloh, D. H. (2014). Comprehensive evaluation of contemporary assisted reproduction technology laboratory operations to determine staffing levels that promote patient safety and quality care. *Fertility and Sterility*, *102*(5), 1350-1356. https://doi.org/10.1016/j.fertnstert.2014.07.1246

Català, V., Calafell, J. M., Santaló, J., Badenas, J., Munné, S., Estop, A., & Egozcue, J. (2015). The Alpha Consensus Meeting on the professional status of the clinical embryologist: proceedings of an expert meeting. *Reproductive BioMedicine Online*, *30*, 431-451.

De los Santos, M. J., Apter, S., Coticchio, G., Debrock, S., Lundin, K., Plancha CE, Prados F, Rienzi L, Verheyen G, Woodward B, & Vermeulen, N. (2016). Revised guidelines for good practice in IVF laboratories (2015). *Human Reproduction*, *31*(4), 685-686. https://doi.org/10.1093/humrep/dew016.

Fabozzi, G., Cimadomo, D., Maggiulli, R., Vaiarelli, A., Ubaldi, F. M., & Rienzi, L. (2020). Which key performance indicators are most effective in evaluating and managing an in vitro fertilization laboratory? *Fertility and Sterility*, *114*(1), 9-15. https://doi.org/10.1016/j.fertnstert.2020.04.054

Franco Jr, J. G., Petersen, C. G., Mauri, A. L., Vagnini, L. D., Renzi, A., Petersen, B., Mattila MC, Comar VA, Ricci J, Dieamant F, Oliveira JBA, & Baruffi, R. L. (2017). Key performance indicators score (KPIs-score) based on clinical and laboratorial parameters can establish benchmarks for internal quality control in an ART program. *JBRA Assisted Reproduction*, *21*(2), 61. https://doi.org/10.5935/1518-0557.20170016.

Gardner, D. K., & Pool, T. B. (2019). Contemporary quality control in the IVF laboratory: heading to the cloud? *Reproductive Biomedicine Online*, *39*(1), 1-2. https://doi.org/10.1016/j.rbmo.2019.05.002

Liperis, G., & Sjöblom, C. (2017). Quality control in the IVF laboratory. In Montag, M. H., & Morbeck, D. E. (Eds.), *Principles of IVF laboratory practice: Optimizing performance and outcomes*. Cambridge University Press.

Mant, J. (2001). Process versus outcome indicators in the assessment of quality of health care. *International journal for quality in health care*, *13*(6), 475-480.

Matson, P. L. (1998). Internal quality control and external quality assurance in the IVF laboratory. *Human Reproduction*, *13*(suppl_4), 156-165. https://doi.org/10.1093/humrep/13.suppl_4.156

Montag, M. H., & Morbeck, D. E. (Eds.). (2017). *Principles of IVF laboratory practice: Optimizing performance and outcomes*. Cambridge University Press.

Mortimer, S. T., & Mortimer, D. (2015). *Quality and risk management in the IVF laboratory* (2nd Ed.). Cambridge University Press.

Practice Committee of the American Society for Reproductive Medicine, & Practice Committee of the Society for Assisted Reproductive Technology. (2008). Revised guidelines for human embryology and andrology laboratories. *Fertility and sterility*, *90*(5), S45-S59. https://doi.org/10.1016/j.fertnstert.2008.08.099

Rienzi, L., Bariani, F., Dalla Zorza, M., Albani, E., Benini, F., Chamayou, S., Chamayou S, Minasi MG, Parmegiani L, Restelli L, Vizziello G, & Costa AN; Italian Society of Embryology, Reproduction and Research (SIERR) (2017). Comprehensive protocol of traceability during IVF: the result of a multicentre failure mode and effect analysis. *Human Reproduction*, *32*(8), 1612-1620. https://doi.org/10.1093/humrep/dex144

The American Society for Reproductive Medicine. (1998). Revised minimum standards for in vitro fertilization, gamete intrafallopian transfer, and related procedures. *Fertility and Sterility*, *70*(4), 1-5. https://doi.org/10.1016/s0015-0282(98)00299-4

Wale, P. L., & Gardner, D. K. (2016). The effects of chemical and physical factors on mammalian embryo culture and their importance for the practice of assisted human reproduction. *Human reproduction update*, *22*(1), 2-22. https://doi.org/10.1093/humupd/dmv034

Index

F

G

H

M

N

O

P

Q

R

S

T